DIAGNOSIS AND TREATMENT OF GENITOURINARY MALIGNANCIES

Diagnosis and Treatment of Genitourinary Malignancies

edited by

KENNETH J. PIENTA
Department of Internal Medicine
Division of Hematology/Oncology
University of Michigan
Ann Arbor, MI 48109-0680

Contents

DIAGNOSIS AND TREATMENT OF GENITOURINARY MALIGNANCIES

1. Epidemiology of prostate cancer and bladder cancer: an overview

Ronald K. Ross

The category of genitourinary cancer potentially includes a large number of cancers with diverse epidemiology and etiology. We limit discussion in this chapter to an update of recent activity in the areas of prostate cancer and bladder cancer epidemiology, since these are far and away the most common genitourinary malignancies. Since each of these topics is extensive in its own right and both have been recently reviewed in some detail [1,2], we only briefly summarize historical risk factor data for each of these cancers and then provide an overview of current and, from our perspective, likely future foci of research into the epidemiology of these malignancies.

Prostate cancer

Prostate cancer is now the most commonly diagnosed cancer in the United States. An estimated 200,000 men were diagnosed in 1994, and an estimated 38,000 men died of prostate cancer, making it the second leading cause of cancer deaths in men (exceeded only by lung cancer) [3]. Prostate cancer rates exploded in the U.S. beginning in the late 1980s. In most segments of the U.S. population, prostate cancer incidence rates approximately doubled between 1988 and 1992 [1]. This rapid increase in incidence was not accompanied by a change in mortality and is likely due almost entirely to increased utilization of serologic assays for prostate-specific antigen to detect subclinical disease in otherwise healthy men.

The two most important known risk factors for prostate cancer are demographic — age and race–ethnicity (or international variation) [4]. Prostate cancer is the most age-related of all epithelial cancers — rare prior to age 40 and increasing at the 8th–9th power of age thereafter. African-American men have long been known to have the highest prostate cancer rates in the world. Japanese and Chinese men native to those countries and probably other Asian ethnicities such as Koreans have the lowest. The difference in risk between these high- and low-risk extremes has been reported to be as much as 50-fold, although a substantial part of this difference may be due to differences in detection strategies among populations [5].

Pienta, K.J., (ed.), DIAGNOSIS AND TREATMENT OF GENITOURINARY MALIGNANCIES.

There has been interest in the role of dietary factors in prostate cancer etiology for at least two decades. Dietary fat has been the most studied of many dietary components evaluated over these years. Both case–control and cohort studies, which have attempted either to estimate individual fat consumption or have simply looked at foods rich in fat, have rather consistently shown that men who develop prostate cancer consume more fat than men who do not. These studies have been conducted in target populations varying widely in age, underlying risk of prostate cancer, and socioeconomic status [1]. Nonetheless, this relationship cannot be considered totally established as a causal one, since these studies have varied considerably in quality; some have suffered from incompleteness in their dietary histories or from questionable reliability and/or validity of their dietary instruments; the case–control studies (which constitute the majority of these studies) suffer from the very real possibility that men who have been diagnosed with prostate cancer may change their diets or, more importantly, may report their dietary histories differently (i.e., provide invalid results due to 'recall bias'). Finally, many of these studies, even the better-designed ones, while finding an overall relationship between dietary fat and prostate cancer risk, nevertheless find inconsistencies in dose–response relationships or in subgroup analyses. These inconsistencies raise doubts regarding the causal nature of these associations. The recently reported Health Professionals Follow-Up prospective study of dietary fat and prostate cancer illustrates the latter problem [6]. This ongoing study involves 47,855 men aged 40–75 years who completed a comprehensive 131-item food-frequency questionnaire at baseline (i.e., at study entry). After four years of follow-up, 300 men had developed prostate cancer. After excluding stage A (largely occult) lesions, there was a modest association between prostate cancer risk and increasing quintile of fat consumption (RRs of 1.0 (low), 1.2, 1.1, 1.1, and 1.4 (high)) — a relationship that, however, did not achieve statistical significance. When the analysis was limited to more advanced disease (stages C and D), the association strengthened (RRs of 1.0 (low), 1.2, 1.3, 1.3, and 1.6), and approached statistical significance ($p = .08$).

The other major focus of dietary research on prostate cancer over the past decade has been the possible protective role of vitamin A or its precursor molecule, beta-carotene. The former compound is of interest principally due to its role in inducing differentiation of epithelial cells, whereas the latter serves as a potent antioxidant, binding free radicals that can damage DNA. The large series of observational studies that have tested this hypothesis have, as a group, offered no strong evidence that these compounds play any important role in modifying prostate cancer risk [1].

Two relatively recent dietary hypotheses concerning prostate cancer deserve mention. The active form of vitamin D, 1,25-dihydroxyvitamin D, can induce differentiation and reduce proliferation of both healthy and malignant prostatic epithelium [7]. A recent prospective serologic study suggested that men with high circulating levels of this compound have a much reduced risk of prostate cancer [8]. Phytoestrogens, such as isoflavonoids found in soy products, are weak estrogens that have been hypothesized to compete with androgens at receptor sites or at a more central level, and thereby mildly reduce androgen activity in the prostate [9]. There have been no epidemiologic studies directly testing whether these compounds reduce prostate cancer risk.

Growth of both normal and, at least in the early stages of malignancy, malignant prostatic epithelium is dependent on androgens. This finding has resulted in longstanding interest in the possible role of androgens in the pathogenesis of prostate cancer. This concept is supported by experimental evidence; although it has proven difficult to produce adenocarcinomas of the prostate in animal models by any means, all the currently established, reproducible experimental models have an androgen requirement for tumor development [10]. The main circulating human androgen, testosterone, diffuses freely into prostate cells, where it is rapidly and irreversibly converted to its metabolically active reduced form, dihydrotestosterone, through the activity of the enzyme 5-alpha reductase. Dihydrotestosterone binds to the androgen receptor, and this complex activates androgen-responsive genes involved in the growth and proliferation of prostate epithelium.

There have been many attempts to compare circulating androgen levels in men with and without prostate cancer, with little consistency in results [1]. Such studies are problematic given the strong possibility that either the presence of the disease itself or the treatment for it can alter androgen secretion or metabolism. More informative have been studies comparing androgen profiles in healthy men at varying risk of prostate cancer, especially with regard to racial–ethnic and international variation in risk. Such studies have demonstrated that high-risk African-American men have higher circulating testosterone levels than lower-risk Asian or U.S. white men [11,12] and that low-risk Asian men have altered intraprostatic metabolism of testosterone compared to U.S. whites and blacks [13,14]. These differences in androgenic profiles among racial–ethnic groups appear sufficiently large when extended over a lifetime to fully explain the underlying differences in prostate cancer incidence among these populations [11]. Asian men native to China or Japan do not have low levels of testosterone, as might be predicted from this hypothesis, but do have substantially reduced levels of two 5-alpha androgens, androstanediol and androsterone, that are thought to indicate reduced 5-alpha reductase expression in the prostate. Thus, the racial–ethnic variation in prostate cancer incidence might be explicable, in part, by differences in testosterone secretion on the one hand and intraprostatic metabolism of testosterone on the other.

The reasons for these underlying hormonal differences among populations at varying risk of prostate cancer are unknown, but are likely due to a combination of environmental (e.g., diet) and genetic differences among these populations. A number of genes are involved in the production and metabolism of testosterone. Table 1-1 lists and describes the function of several of these. Although some preliminary data suggest, directly or indirectly, that at least some of these genes might affect prostate cancer risk, none have to date undergone serious epidemiologic investigation.

Table 1-1. 'Candidate' genes for prostate cancer: genes involved in testosterone metabolism

Candidate gene	Prostate function
Androgen receptor	Translates androgen effects
5-alpha reductase type II	Converts testosterone to dihydrotestosterone
CYP17	Catalyzes rate limiting steps in testosterone biosynthesis
HSD3B2	Deactivates dihydrotestosterone

The 5-alpha reductase type 2 gene, for example, like all four of the genes listed, has been shown to be polymorphic, providing opportunities to compare sequence variations in the gene among populations at varying risk of prostate cancer and among individuals with and without prostate cancer. The polymorphism that has been described is a dinucleotide (TA) microsatellite in the 3' UTR of the gene [15]. Although most individuals possess a single allelotype, being TA_0 homozygotes, between 15% and 25% of the population, depending on race–ethnicity, carry a variant allele. African-American men, in fact, possess a series of alleles (TA_{18}–TA_{22}) that appear to be unique to this population and, based on preliminary data, appear to convey an excess risk of prostate cancer [15]. Asian populations have a low frequency of variant alleles, based on this polymorphism. If these results are confirmed through more definitive epidemiologic studies, an important additional issue will be to determine the functional significance of this polymorphism; polymorphic microsatellites in the UTRs of other genes have been shown themselves to have functional significance.

The androgen receptor gene encodes the androgen receptor, which serves multiple functions related to androgen activity in the prostate. It binds dihydrotestosterone in the cytosol of prostatic epithelium, translocates dihydrotestosterone to the nucleus for DNA binding, and participates in the transactivation of androgen-responsive genes [16]. The androgen receptor gene is located on the X-chromosome, so men carry only a single copy. There have been two polymorphic trinucleotide repeat microsatellites described in the gene, both located in exon 1, the transcription modulatory domain. In healthy men, one of these microsatellites, a CAG repeat sequence, is approximately normally distributed with a range of some 8 to 31 repeats. Several observations have suggested that the length of this microsatellite correlates with androgen function. A rare adult-onset motor-neuron, X-chromosome-linked disorder, namely, Kennedy's disease, is caused by an expansion of this microsatellite, so men with this disease have a minimum of 40 repeats and a reduced ability to transactivate androgen-responsive genes [17]. Experimental results utilizing transfection assays suggest that, within the normal range of repeats, there are also differences in activation of reporter genes: the greater the number of repeats, the less activation [18]. This finding has led to the hypotheses that a low number of repeats results in a more 'supercharged' androgen receptor than does a high number of repeats, and as a result, carries with it a higher risk of prostate cancer [19]. Based on their respective incidence rates of prostate cancer, this hypothesis further suggests that African-American men would, on average, have a relatively short CAG microsatellite, whereas Asian men would, on average, have a relatively long CAG microsatellite, compared to whites. This phenomenon has been repeatedly observed [20,21]. There are no published data yet relating the length of this microsatellite to prostate cancer risk in any population.

The other two genes listed in table 1-1 are even less studied epidemiologically but are of interest for future studies. The steady-state circulating level of testosterone is determined to a large extent by the rates of steroid biosynthesis in the testes and adrenals, which, in turn, are determined in large part by the activity of the rate limiting enzyme 17α-hydroxylase; 17/20 lyase (CYP17) [22]. The gene for CYP17 on chromosome 10 contains a newly described C to T transition polymorphism in its 5' region [23]. The two alleles are designated A_1 and A_2; the A_2 allele creates an additional SP1-type *cis* promoter site that has been hypothesized to result in increased expression. No studies have yet been conducted on the distribution of genotypes across populations or in relation to prostate cancer risk.

The HSD3B2 gene encodes the type II 3B hydroxysteroid dehydrogenase that initiates the inactivation of dihydrotestosterone in the prostate [24,25]. A complex dinucleotide repeat microsatellite polymorphism has been reported in the third intron of the HSD3B2 gene. The initial description, based on a study of 52 Caucasians, described nine alleles of a $(TG)_n$, $(TA)_n$, $(CA)_n$ microsatellite, with frequencies ranging from a high of 48% for the most common allele down to 1% for the least common [25]. There are currently no published data on the distribution of alleles across racial–ethnic groups at varying risk of prostate cancer nor among prostate cancer patients and controls. Like most of the other genes of interest, no work has yet been done to determine if these alleles have functional significance.

Prostate cancer is a familial disease. The most detailed epidemiologic studies of this phenomenon have been reported by Steinberg and colleagues [27] and by Monroe et al. [28]. Steinberg et al. reported that for an individual with only one first-degree relative with prostate cancer, risk is elevated 2.2-fold, increasing to roughly 5-fold if two first-degree relatives are affected, and to more than 10-fold if more than two are affected, all in comparison to men with no family history of prostate cancer [27]. This type of observation has led to the postulate that there exist one or several 'susceptibility' genes for prostate cancer that, in their mutated form, carry a very high risk of developing the disease. Carter et al. have determined, for example, that one specific form of hereditary prostate cancer is consistent with an autosomal-dominant mode of inheritance and that the putative unknown locus might account for as much as 9% of all prostate cancer [29].

Monroe and colleagues confirmed and expanded previous results by Hayes et al. [30] and Narod et al. [31] of the complexity of the familial risk pattern using data from a large multi-ethnic cohort study. They demonstrated that the risk of prostate cancer is about twice as high if a brother is affected with the disease than if a father is affected in each of four racial–ethnic groups studied. These results suggest the possible involvement of an X-linked genetic component or a rare recessive trait in the familial risk of prostate cancer.

Bladder cancer

The two major causes of bladder cancer — cigarette smoking and occupational exposure to arylamines — have been known for almost half a century [2]. Over this time period, we have learned much about the details of these associations, but no other major risk factors have been identified, despite intense interest in such factors as coffee drinking and use of artificial sweeteners. Recently, epidemiologists' attention has been turning increasingly to understanding the mechanism for the smoking–bladder cancer relationship and to understanding factors that might modify individual and population susceptibility to bladder cancer among cigarette smokers.

Interest in the latter problem has been stimulated in part by unexplained discrepancies between the descriptive epidemiology of bladder cancer, on the one hand, and the descriptive epidemiology of lung cancer and, for that matter, of cigarette smoking itself, on the other. Epidemiologic studies, either case–control or cohort in design, beginning with a study by Lillienfeld and colleagues in 1956 [32], have very consistently demonstrated that cigarette smokers have an approximately two- to threefold elevation in bladder cancer risk overall compared to nonsmokers, and that risk tends to increase with increasing duration of use and increased number of cigarettes smoked daily. These associations have been demonstrated in both men and women, among multiple racial–ethnic groups, and in countries with highly variant underlying bladder cancer risk [2]. Nonetheless, during the past several decades, when lung cancer rates were increasing rapidly in response to the increasing smoking prevalence in the U.S. through the 1960s, bladder cancer mortality rates were stable in men and actually declined somewhat in women [33]. There exist many populations around the world characterized by high smoking rates and, correspondingly, high lung cancer rates but low rates of bladder cancer. For example, we have demonstrated that in Los Angeles, African-American, Chinese, Japanese, and non-Latino white men have comparable smoking rates but an approximately threefold difference in bladder cancer incidence. Non-Latino white men have by far the highest incidence rate, followed by African-American men with roughly half the rate of whites and then Japanese and Chinese men with even lower rates — roughly one-third that of white men [34].

Although occupational exposure to arylamines, such as that which historically occurred in the textile synthetic dye industry and the rubber tire industry, caused substantial increases in bladder cancer risk [35,36], the proportion of men sustaining such exposures was always exceedingly low, so these exposures never contributed substantially to the overall population occurrence of bladder cancer. Moreover, these exposures were largely eliminated from occupational settings in the U.S. several decades ago.

The precise mechanism for the association between cigarette smoking and bladder cancer has not yet been fully elucidated, but this relationship is presumptively due to the presence in cigarette smoke of small amounts of the same carcinogenic arylamines known to cause bladder cancer in occupational settings [37]. A model of bladder cancer pathogenesis based on exposure to carcinogenic arylamines is shown in figure 1-1. All the arylamines that are

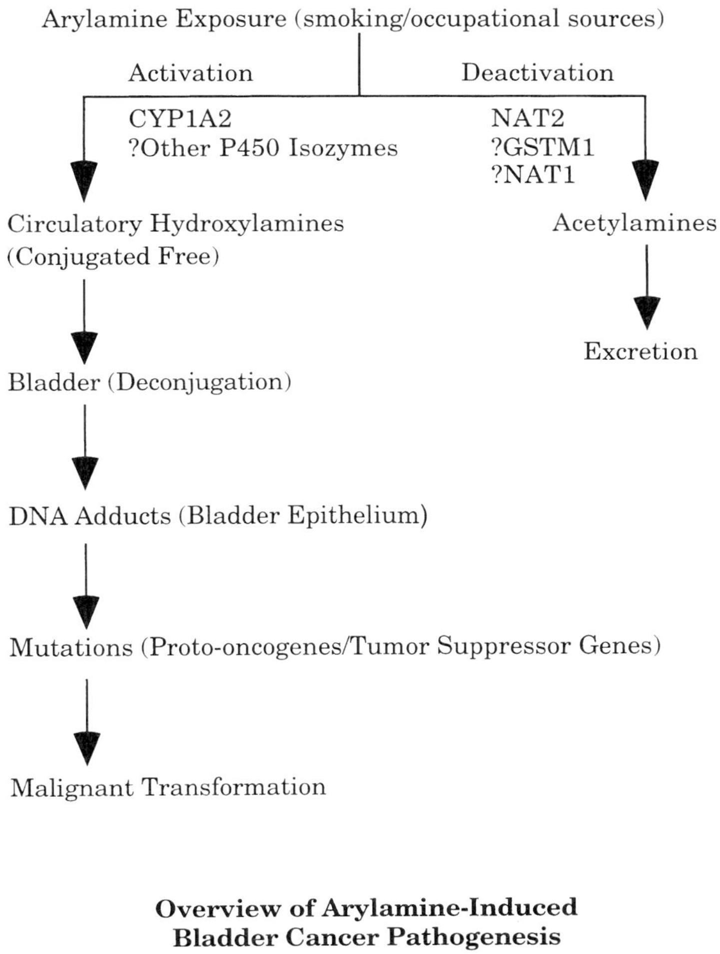

From: Ross RK, Jones PA, Yu MC. Bladder cancer epidemiology and pathogenesis. Semin Oncol (in press).

Figure 1.1. ••

established human bladder carcinogens must undergo metabolic activation to their fully carcinogenic forms. Metabolic activation is controlled, at least in part, through N-oxidation by the cytochrome P4501A2 isoenzyme (CYP1A2) [38]. This inducible enzyme system shows tremendous individual and population variability in activity. As described below, other p450 enzymes might also be involved in the metabolic activation of these arylamines. The metabolically active form of these arylamines, the hydroxylarylamines, can form adducts with hemoglobin or circulate either freely or as glucuronide conjugates and, subsequently, be excreted through the kidney [39]. These compounds can then be further modified in the acidic environment of the bladder, allowing adduct formation with bladder mucosal DNA. Misrepair of these adducts is hypothesized to be an important step in malignant transformation [40].

Alternatively, arylamines can be detoxified. A number of enzymes are likely to be involved in this process. Two of these, glutathione S-transferase mu and N-acetyltransferase, both of which are genetically regulated, have already undergone some epidemiologic investigation regarding their role in bladder cancer development following arylamine exposure.

There is no direct epidemiologic evidence linking the CYP1A2 phenotype to bladder cancer risk, although Kaderlik and Kadlubar have shown that levels of the hemoglobin adduct to 4-aminobiphenyl, a potent carcinogenic arylamine, are higher among individuals with a rapid CYP1A2 phenotype (assessed using a urine-based assay with caffeine as a test substance) [40]. The other p450 enzymatic phenotypes, CYP2D6 (using debrisoquine as a probe) and CYP3A4 (using dapsone as a probe), have been preliminarily explored in the context of bladder cancer risk, with somewhat complex results. One study found an overall positive relationship between high CYP2D6 activity and bladder cancer [41]; a second study found that extensive metabolizers were at high risk only for advanced bladder cancer [42]; and a third study found no relationship whatsoever [43]. Two studies have found significant, negative associations between high CYP3A4 enzyme activity and high-, but not low-, stage bladder cancer [44,45].

The relationship between N-acetyltransferase type II phenotype and/or genotype has been explored in 12 bladder cancer case–control studies, ranging considerably in size and quality. Hein combined data from all these studies in a variation of a meta-analysis and found a statistically significant 50% excess in slow versus rapid acetylators [46]; this is the predicted relationship, since rapid acetylators would be expected to more quickly detoxify and excrete these compounds. When the analyses were limited to persons with established arylamine exposure (typically through occupational sources), the risk for slow versus rapid acetylators was 2.2. It remains to be determined whether the differences in bladder cancer incidence among populations with similar smoking patterns can be explained in part by differences in acetylation capacity among these populations. However, indirect evidence suggests this is likely to be the case. Whites have a much higher population prevalence of slow acetylators (54%), compared to blacks (34%) or Asians (14%). Moreover, as expected, slow acetylators have higher levels of arylamine adducts to hemoglobin at every smoking level in each racial–ethnic group [47].

It has not been definitively determined whether glutathione S-transferase mu is actively involved in arylamine metabolism, but it clearly catalyzes the detoxification of other carcinogens present in cigarette smoke, especially the polycyclic aromatic hydrocarbons [48]. The GSTM1 gene is polymorphic, with about half the U.S. white population possessing the 'null' genotype; i.e., they lack both copies of the gene and exhibit no enzyme activity. Several studies have found that bladder cancer patients are more likely to possess the GSTM1 null genotype than are healthy controls, with the larger studies suggesting that persons with this genotype carry a 50% to 70% excess in bladder cancer risk [49,50]. One study among healthy men of various racial–ethnic groups found evidence that the GSTM1 genotype contributes to aminobiphenyl adduct levels. After adjusting for race, detailed smoking status, and N-acetyltransferase 2 phenotype, levels of aminobiphenyl-hemoglobin adduct levels were still significantly higher among individuals with the null genotype. Whites were considerably more likely to possess a 'high-risk' profile (slow N-acetyltransferase 2 phenotype, null GSTM1 genotype) than Asians (27% vs. 2.7%) and nearly twice as likely as African-Americans (27% vs. 15%) [51].

References

1. Ross RK, Coetzee GA (in press). The epidemiology and etiology of prostate cancer. In Diagnostic Imaging and Radiation Oncology Carcinoma of the Prostate, Petrovich Z, Baert L, Brady ZW (eds). Springer-Verlag: Berlin.
2. Ross RK, Jones PA, Yu MC (in press). Bladder cancer epidemiology and pathogenesis. Semin Oncol.
3. American Cancer Society. Cancer Facts and Figures, 1994.
4. Ross RK, Schottenfeld D (in press). Prostate cancer. In Cancer Epidemiology and Prevention, and ed., Schottenfeld D, Fraumeni JF (eds). WB Saunders: Philadelphia.
5. Shimizu H, Ross RK, Bernstein L (1991). Possible underestimation of incidence rate of prostate cancer in Japan. Jpn J Cancer Res 82:483–485.
6. Giovannucci E, Rimm EB, Colditz GA, et al. (1993). A prospective study of dietary fat and risk of prostate cancer. J Natl Cancer Inst 85:1571–1579.
7. Skowronski RJ, Peehl DM, Feldman D (1993). Vitamin D and prostate cancer: 1,25-dihydroxyvitamin D3 receptors and action in human prostate cancer cell lines. Endocrinology 132:1952–1960.
8. Corder EH, Guess HA, Hulka BS, et al. (1993). Vitamin D and prostate cancer: a prediagnostic study with stored sera. Cancer Epidemiol Biomarkers Prev 2:467–472.
9. Adlercreutz H, Markkanen H, Watanabe S (1993). Plasma concentrations of phytoestrogens in Japanese men. Lancet i:1209–1210.
10. Noble RL (1977). The development of prostatic adenocarcinoma in Nb rats following prolonged sex hormone administration. Cancer Res 37:1929–1933.
11. Ross RK, Bernstein L, Judd H, et al. (1986). Serum testosterone levels in young black and white men. J Natl Cancer Inst 76:45–48.
12. Ellis L, Nyburg H (1992). Racial/ethnic variations in male testosterone levels: a probable contributor to group differences in health. Steroids 57:72–75.
13. Ross RK, Bernstein L, Lobo RA, et al. (1992). 5-alpha-reductase activity and risk of prostate cancer among Japanese and U.S. white and black males. Lancet 339:887–890.

14. Lookingbill DP, Demers LM, Wang C, et al. (1991). Clinical and biological parameters of androgen action in normal healthy Caucasian versus Chinese subjects. J Clin Endocrinol Metab 72:1242–1248.
15. Reichardt JKV, Makridakis N, Henderson BE, et al. (1995). Genetic variability of the human SRD5A2 gene: implications for prostate cancer risk. Cancer Res 55:3973–3975.
16. Jenster G, Van der Korput HALM, Van Vroonhoven C, et al. (1992). Domains of the human androgen receptor involved in steroid binding, transcriptional activation, and subcellular localization. Mol Endocrinol 5:1396–1404.
17. Mhatre AN, Trifiro MA, Kaufman M, et al. (1993). Reduced transcriptional regulatory competence of the androgen receptor in X-linked spinal and bulbar muscular atrophy. Nature Genet 5:184–188.
18. Chamberlain NC, Driver ED, Miesfeld RL (1994). The length and location of CAG trinucleotide repeats in the androgen receptor N-terminal domain affect transactivation function. Nucleic Acids Res 22:3181–3186.
19. Coetzee GA, Ross RK (1994). Prostate cancer and the androgen receptor. J Natl Cancer Inst 86:872–873.
20. Edwards A, Hammond HA, Jin L, et al. (1992). Genetic variation at five trimeric and tetrameric tandem repeat loci in four human population groups. Genomics 12:241–253.
21. Irvine RA, Yu MC, Ross RK, Coetzee GA (1995). The CAG and GGC microsatellites of the androgen receptor gene are in linkage disequilibrium in men with prostate cancer. Cancer Res 55:1937–1940.
22. Picado-Leonard J, Miller WL (1987). Cloning and sequence of the human gene for P450c17 (steroid 17α-hydroxylase/17,20 lyase): similarity with the gene for P450c21. DNA 6:439–448.
23. Carey AH, Waterworth D, Patel Y, et al. (1994). Polycystic ovaries and premature male pattern baldness are associated with one allele of the steroid metabolism gene. Hum Mol Genet 3:1873–1876.
24. Berube D, Luu-The V, Lachance Y, et al. (1989). Assignment of the human 3B hydroxysteroid dehydrogenase gene to the p13 band of chromosome 1. Cytogenet Cell Genet 52: 199–200.
25. Labrie F, Simard J, Luu-The V, et al. (1992). Structure, function and tissue specific expression of 3B-hydroxysteroid dehydrogenase/5 ene-4-ene isomerase enzymes in classical and peripheral intracine steroidogenic tissue. J Steroid Biochem Mol Biol 43:805–826.
26. Rheaume E, Sanchez R, Mebarki F, et al. (1995). Identification and characterization of the G15D mutation found in a male with 3B-hydroxysteroid dehydrogenase (3B-HSD) deficiency: alteration of the putative NAD-binding domain of the type II3B-HSD. Biochemistry 34:2893–2900.
27. Steinberg GD, Carter BS, Beaty TH, et al. (1990). Family history and the risk of prostate cancer. Prostate 17:337–347.
28. Monroe KR, Yu MC, Kolonel LN, et al. (in press). Evidence of X-linked genetic component to prostate cancer risk. Nature Med.
29. Carter BS, Beaty TH, Steinberg GD, et al. (1992). Mendelian inheritance of familial prostate cancer. Proc Natl Acad Sci 89:3367–3371.
30. Hayes RB, Liff JM, Pottern LM, et al. (1995). Prostate cancer risk in US Blacks and Whites with a family history of prostate cancer. Int J Cancer 60:361–364.
31. Narod SA, Dupont A, Cusan L, et al. (1995). The impact of family history on early detection of prostate cancer. Nature Med 1:99–101.
32. Lillienfeld AM, Levin ML, Moore GE (1956). The association of smoking with cancer of the urinary bladder in humans. Arch Intern Med 98:129–135.
33. Devesa SS, Blot WJ, Stone BJ, et al. (1995). Recent cancer trends in the United States. J Natl Cancer Inst 87:175–182.
34. Bernstein L, Ross RK (1991). Cancer in Los Angeles County: A Portrait of Incidence and Mortality 1972–1987. Los Angeles: University of Southern California Press.
35. Case RAM, Hosker ME, McDonald DM, et al. (1954). Tumors of urinary bladder in workmen engaged in manufacture and use of certain dye-stuff intermediates in British chemical indus-

try: role of amiline, benzidine, alpha-naphthylamine, and beta-naphthylamine. Br J Industr Med 11:75–104.
36. Case RAM, Hosker ME (1954). Tumour of the urinary bladder as an occupational disease in the rubber industry in England and Wales. Br J Prev Soc Med 8:39–50.
37. Patrianakos C, Hoffman D (1979). On the analysis of aromatic amines in cigarette smoke. J Anal Toxicol 3:150–154.
38. Butler MA, Iwasaki M, Guengerich FP (1989). Human cytochrome $P450_{PA}$ (P-450IA2), the phenacetin O-deethylase, is primarily responsible for the hepatic 3-demethylation of caffeine and N-oxidation of carcinogenic arylamines. Proc Natl Acad Sci USA 86:7696–7700.
39. Bryant MS, Vineis P, Skipper PL, et al. (1988). Hemoglobin adducts of aromatic amines: associations with smoking status and type of tobacco. Proc Natl Acad Sci USA 85:9788–9791.
40. Kaderlik KR, Kadlubar FF (1995). Metabolic polymorphisms and carcinogen-DNA adduct formation in human populations. Pharmacogenetics 5:S108–S117.
41. Gough AC, Miles JS, Spurr NK, et al. (1990). Identification of the primary gene defect at the cytochrome P450 CYP2D locus. Nature 347:773–776.
42. Kaisary A, Smith P, Jaczq E, et al. (1987). Genetic predisposition to bladder cancer: ability to hydroxylate debrisoquine and mephenytoin as risk factors. Cancer Res 47:5488–5493.
43. Cartwright RA, Philip PA, Rogers HJ, et al. (1984). Genetically determined debrisoquine oxidation capacity in bladder cancer. Carcinogenesis 5:1191–1192.
44. Branch RA, Chern HD, Adedoyin A, et al. (1995). The procarcinogen hypothesis for bladder cancer: activities of individual drug metabolizing enzymes as risk factors. Pharmacogenetics 5:S97–S102.
45. Fleming CM, Persad R, Kaisary A, et al. (1994). Low activity of dapsone N-hydroxylation as a susceptibility risk factor in aggressive bladder cancer. Pharmacogenetics 4:199–207.
46. Hein DW (1988). Acetylator genotype and arylamine-induced carcinogenesis. Biochim Biophys Acta 948:37–66.
47. Yu MC, Skipper PL, Taghizadeh K (1994). Acetylator phenotype, aminobiphenyl-hemoglobin adduct levels, and bladder cancer risk in white, black, and Asian men in Los Angeles, California. J Natl Cancer Inst 86:712–716.
48. Board P, Coggan M, Johnston P, et al. (1990). Genetic heterogeneity of the human glutathione transferases: a complex of gene families. Pharmacol Ther 48:357–369.
49. Bell DA, Taylor JA, Paulson DF, et al. (1993). Genetic risk and carcinogen exposure: a common inherited defect of the carcinogen-metabolism gene glutathione S-transferase M1 (GSTM1) that increases susceptibility to bladder cancer. J Natl Cancer Inst 85:1159–1164.
50. Brockmoller J, Kerb R, Drakoulis N, et al. (1994). Glutathione S-transferase M1 and its variants A and B as host factors of bladder cancer susceptibility: a case–control study. Cancer Res 54:4103–4111.
51. Yu MC, Ross RK, Chan KK, et al. (in press). Glutathione S-transferase M1 genotype affects aminobiphenyl-hemoglobin adduct levels in white, black, and Asian smokers and non-smokers. Cancer Epidemiol Biomarkers Prev.

2. Von Hippel–Lindau syndrome: hereditary cancer arising from inherited mutations of the VHL tumor suppressor gene

Jeffrey S. Humphrey, Richard D. Klausner, and W. Marston Linehan

Von Hippel–Lindau syndrome (VHL) is an autosomal-dominant, multiple-tumor syndrome in which affected individuals are predisposed, over the course of their lifetime, to the formation of tumors or cysts in specific target organs such as the kidney, central nervous system (CNS), retina, adrenal gland, and pancreas. VHL is the most common syndrome of hereditary kidney cancer [1,2]. Metastatic clear cell kidney cancer and the neurologic sequelae of tumor growth in the CNS are the most common causes of morbidity and mortality of VHL patients. The VHL disease gene functions as a tumor suppressor gene (see below) [3] and places the VHL syndrome into a select group with diseases such as Li-Fraumeni syndrome, retinoblastomatosis, and familial breast–ovarian cancer, which are caused by mutations of the tumor suppressor genes p53, Rb, and BRCA1, respectively. An advance in the understanding of VHL and of sporadic clear cell kidney cancer occurred in 1993 when the gene responsible for the VHL syndrome was cloned [4].

VHL patients inherit a mutation of the VHL gene [4]. Tumors from VHL patients showed selective loss of the VHL allele inherited from the unaffected parent [5], as expected for a tumor suppressor protein (see below). Furthermore, an initial study of sporadic (i.e., nonfamilial) clear cell carcinoma identified VHL mutations in 57% of tumors, with loss of heterozygosity in 98% of those samples [6]. Further studies revealed VHL gene inactivation by hypermethylation in an additional 19% of sporadic clear cell tumors of the kidney [7]. Therefore, the VHL gene, like the Rb and p53 genes, appears to play a role in an uncommon familial cancer syndrome as well as in a common sporadic cancer. Because metastatic clear cell carcinoma of the kidney is so deadly and is currently refractory to chemotherapy and hormonal therapy [8], fresh approaches are need. It is hoped that an understanding of the function of the VHL gene product at a molecular and cell biology level will provide new insights into the genesis and clinical behavior of clear cell kidney cancer and stimulate the rational development of effective treatments of metastatic disease.

Pienta, K.J., (ed.), DIAGNOSIS AND TREATMENT OF GENITOURINARY MALIGNANCIES.

Overview of the VHL syndrome

History

The VHL syndrome is named after Eugene von Hippel, who recognized that distinctive retinal tumors, angiomas, were hereditary [9], and Arvid Lindau, who recognized that these tumors were part of a larger 'angiomatous lesion of the central nervous system' [10]. Over the first several decades of this century, families were described in which affected members had not only hemangioblastomas of the retina and CNS but also cysts and tumors of visceral organs, including the kidney, adrenal gland, pancreas, and epididymis. These tumors specifically include clear cell carcinoma of the kidney, pheochromocytoma, pancreatic cystadenoma, pancreatic islet cell tumors, and epididymal cystadenomas. Melmon and Rosen coined the eponym 'von Hippel–Lindau' in 1964 and proposed the widely accepted criteria for diagnosis: two or more hemangioblastomas, a single hemangioblastoma associated with a characteristic visceral tumor, or a single hemangioblastoma or characteristic tumor associated with a family history of VHL [11].

The development of computed tomography (CT), ultrasound (US), and magnetic resonance imaging (MRI) in the 1970s and 1980s allowed radiographic diagnosis of silent tumors in asymptomatic individuals. These advances increased the number of identified VHL families worldwide and made detection of affected individuals within families more sensitive and reliable. During the 1970s, 1980s, and 1990s, advances in molecular biology, particularly the development of linkage analysis, made possible the identification of a location (or *position*) within the genome that is reliably co-inherited with specific, clinical phenotypes in autosomal-dominant diseases. The genomic position identified by linkage analysis is likely to harbor the disease gene responsible for the clinical phenotype. The disease gene can be retrieved by positional cloning. Linkage analysis requires (a) large families with many affected members and (b) sensitive and accurate means to assign clinical phenotype. These conditions for linkage analysis and positional cloning of the VHL disease gene were met only after the advent of modern imaging technology.

A hint as to the genomic location of the VHL gene first occurred in 1979 with the description of a family with hereditary clear cell cancer of the kidney [12]. Every family member who developed clear cell carcinoma had also inherited a karyotypic defect in which the short arm of chromosome 3 was disrupted by a translocation event. Subsequently, deletions of chromosome 3p were identified in sporadic clear cell carcinoma [13], further implicating the short arm of chromosome 3 as the position of a gene likely to be important for clear cell carcinoma tumorigenesis. VHL, as the most common syndrome of autosomal-dominant hereditary clear cell carcinoma, provided the best opportunity for positional cloning of a kidney cancer disease gene, and therefore research groups began studying patients from VHL families to begin the process of linkage analysis. The VHL gene was mapped to chromosome 3p [14], and in 1992, these efforts resulted in the identification of DNA probes that hybridized specifically to genomic positions very near the VHL gene on the short arm of chromosome 3 and that, for the first time, allowed accurate identification of VHL-affected patients before the formation of tumors [15]. In 1993, investigators positionally cloned the VHL gene itself (for a review, see [16]) and showed that the VHL gene was mutated not only in the hereditary cancer syndrome but also in most cases of sporadic clear cell carcinoma of the kidney [4,6,17,18]. Loss of heterozygosity of 3p and VHL mutations have been shown in other sporadic tumor types seen in VHL [19,20]. Recent molecular and cell biology studies have suggested that VHL may play a novel role in the regulation of transcription (see below).

Molecular biology

Loss of heterozygosity (LOH) studies using tumors from VHL patients have demonstrated that the VHL gene behaves as expected for a tumor suppressor gene. Using polymorphic markers from chromosome 3p, Tory et al. demonstrated that the genomic DNA of clear cell carcinoma tumors of VHL patients contained chromosomal deletions of regions in 3p [5]. In every tumor of VHL patients in whom parental lineage of the deleted 3p allele could be ascertained, the 3p region deleted was originally inherited from the unaffected parent, and thus presumably harbored a wild-type allele of the VHL disease gene. These finding fit Knudson's hypothesis that tumorigenesis in certain hereditary cancer syndromes (such as retinoblastoma) is initiated by a rate-limiting, two-step process [21]. The first step is the inheritance of a germline mutation in the disease-gene from the affected parent. (A germline mutation is a mutation present in the germ cells, i.e., sperm or ova, from the affected parent and gives rise to progeny with a constitutional mutation.) The second step occurs when an individual cell deletes or mutates the remaining wild-type copy of the disease-gene, completing the rate-limiting step needed for formation of tumors characterized by a clonal population of cells containing a germline mutation of one allele and newly acquired loss or mutation of the wild-type allele.

The *familial* clear cell kidney cancers of VHL patients are therefore thought to represent a consequence of the inheritance of only *one* functional copy of the VHL gene at the time of fertilization (figure 2-1). This situation allows a single mutational event, which inactivates the only functional copy of the VHL gene in a given cell, to free a cell from the tumor-inhibiting function of the VHL gene. Thus, cells acquiring a single mutation of the wild-type VHL gene, in certain tissues, have completed the presumed rate-limiting step required to enter a neoplastic pathway. The tendency to develop tumors in some tissues (eye, brain, viscera) but not others is not understood. In the case of *nonfamilial* (sporadic) clear cell kidney cancer, the individual inherits *two* normal, functional copies of the VHL gene (figure 2-1), both of which appear to be inactivated by two independent mutational events within a given cell

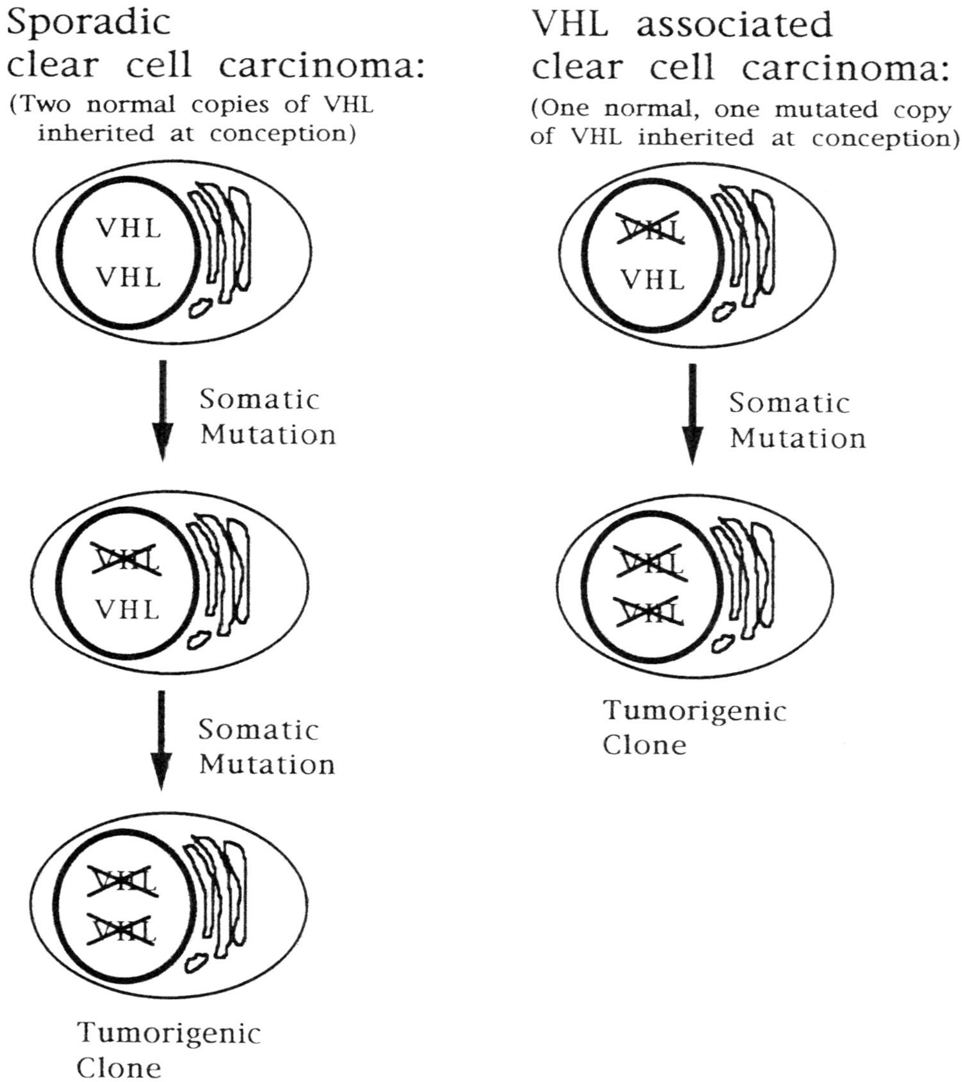

Figure 2-1. The two-mutations theory of tumor suppressor genes. According to the theory, inactivation of both functional VHL alleles within a single cell is associated with clear cell carcinoma in both nonfamilial (sporadic) and familial (VHL) cases. As diagrammed, normal patients who ultimately develop sporadic clear cell carcinoma require two independent mutational events occurring in the same cell to initiate tumorigenesis. By contrast, VHL patients are born with a constitutional germline mutation in every cell of their body and appear to require only one additional mutational event to initiate tumorigenesis in target organs. Tumors in VHL patients are more frequently multifocal, bilateral, and diagnosed at a younger age than corresponding sporadic tumors.

before tumor formation. Because only one additional mutational event is required for tumor formation in VHL patients, the tumors typically occur at a younger age and are more frequently bilateral than are corresponding sporadic tumors [22].

Clinical genetics

The VHL syndrome is inherited in an autosomal-dominant fashion. Thus, both men and women can be affected, and each child of an affected individual is predicted to have a 50% chance of inheriting the abnormal copy of the VHL gene from his or her affected parent. Rarely, a new mutation of the VHL gene occurs during oogenesis, spermatogenesis, or early embryogenesis and gives rise to an affected child whose parents are not affected by the VHL syndrome. Given the hereditary nature of the syndrome, relatives of a VHL patient should be screened for evidence of occult disease (see table 2-3 and discussion below).

During the linkage analysis efforts, DNA probes were discovered that identify polymorphic genomic positions typically inherited with the disease phenotype. These flanking probes can now be used clinically to identify with high probability asymptomatic family members carrying the VHL disease gene [15,23]. These probes detect restriction fragment length polymorphisms (RFLPs), which are frequently informative in identifying, with high probability, the inheritance of the region of 3p25–26 that carries the mutated VHL gene. More recently, microsatellite markers [24] and intragenic polymorphisms [25] (which are complementary methods of distinguishing inheritance of genomic positions) have been identified that may also prove helpful in determining VHL inheritance. Thus, asymptomatic members of an affected family can sometimes be screened for VHL disease with a blood test [15]. The testing is offered as a commercial service at two sites in the United States (see Resources). The testing is most informative when blood samples from multiple key family members are available for testing. Even then, many families will be 'uninformative' using the available DNA probes so that no determination regarding the inheritance of the disease gene can be made. Even in families for which the DNA probes are informative, recombination events may occur to produce infrequent false-negative and false-positive results. Even a true-positive test does not mean that the patient will inevitably become symptomatic. Because of these and other important subtleties, family members requesting DNA testing should be referred for counseling by a clinical geneticist or physician with experience in VHL, before testing, if possible.

Now that the precise sequence of the VHL gene is known, it is possible to test lymphocyte DNA, obtainable by a single blood draw from an individual, for the presence or absence of VHL mutations using single-stranded conformational polymorphisms (SSCPs), denaturing gradient gel electrophoresis (DGGE), or direct DNA sequencing. Likewise, the DNA of tumor samples can be tested for VHL aberrations. These research techniques are currently too cumbersome for testing of the general public, but theoretically allow determination of the sequence of the VHL gene in any tumor.

Clinical manifestations and general considerations

VHL is uncommon, with a minimum estimated birth frequency of 1 in 36,000 [23]. Patients can develop one or more tumors over the course of their lifetime, including clear cell renal carcinoma; hemangioblastomas of the CNS and retina; pheochromocytoma; and cysts of the kidney, pancreas, and epididymis (table 2-1). The degree of penetrance is age dependent: VHL infants are nearly all asymptomatic; patients are first diagnosed with VHL at a mean age of 26 years; and nearly all diagnosed cases present before age 65. Patients present with one or more characteristic tumors and/or a positive family history. The most frequent initial manifestations are retinal angiomatosis and cerebellar hemangioblastomatosis, with a mean age at first diagnosis in the mid- to late twenties. Approximately 10% present with clear cell carcinoma, with a mean age at first diagnosis of 44 years (table 2-1). Although individuals within a family often develop similar patterns of tumors, the disease expression is characteristically variable from patient to patient. Thus, primary relatives may develop tumors in different target tissues, in varying numbers, of varying aggressiveness, and with completely different complications from otherwise similar tumors (figure 2-2). Few patients develop all possible manifestations of VHL, and about half of VHL patients have only one manifestation of VHL. Many patients do not develop a disease manifestation until late in life, making lifelong screening of at-risk individuals necessary. Pheochromocytomas tend to cluster in certain families and not in others, a fact reflected in the classification of VHL disease [26] (see table 2-4 and figure 2-5 below).

Table 2-1. Manifestations of von Hippel–Lindau

Manifestation (n = 152)	Percentage of VHL patients affected	Mean age at diagnosis (years)	Presenting symptoms (%)[a]
Retinal angioma	59%	25	30%
Cerebellar hemangioblastoma	59%	29	39%
Spinal hemangioblastoma	13%	34	3%
Renal cell carcinoma	28%	44	9%
Pheochromocytoma	7%	20	5%
Asymptomatic (diagnosed by screening of at-risk individuals)	—	—	14% (19 retinal angiomas, 2 renal carcinomas, 1 pheochromocytoma)

[a] Initial manifestation diagnosed among all patients: 43% had retinal angioma, 39% had cerebellar hemangioblastoma, 3% had spinal hemangioblastoma, 10% had renal cell carcinoma, and 5% had pheochromocytoma.

From a single-institution study of 152 patients with at least one tumor, by Maher et al. [27].

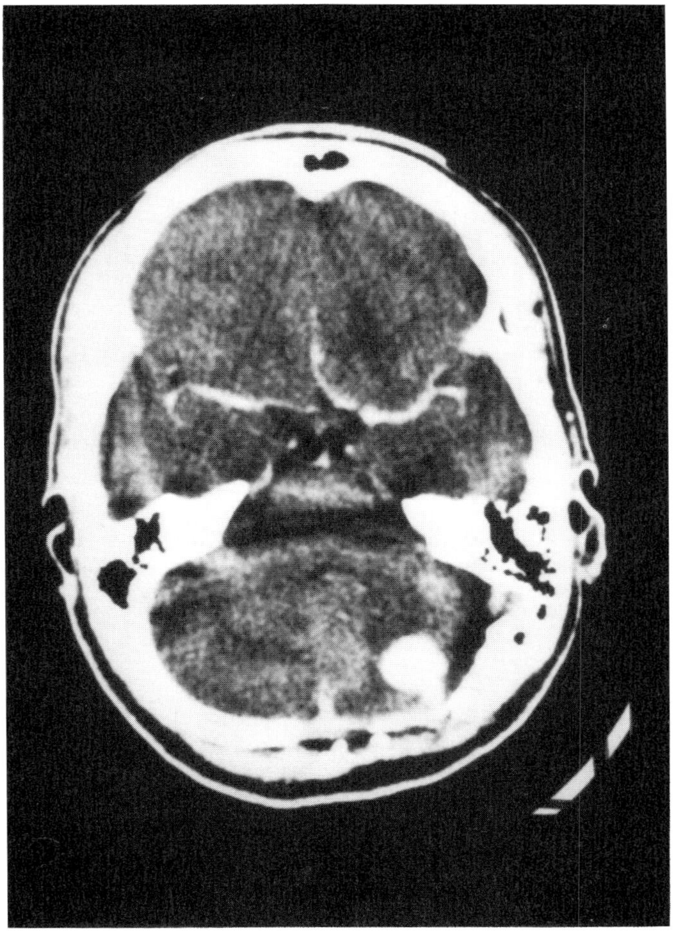

Figure 2-2. Head CT scan with intravenous contrast enhancement demonstrating a large cerebellar hemangioblastoma.

The disease has a broad spectrum of clinical severity. Clear cell carcinoma of the kidney and hemangioblastomas of the cerebellum or spine cause the majority of the morbidity and mortality of VHL. Clear cell carcinoma may invade locally and metastasize, primarily to bone, brain, and lung. CNS hemangioblastomas do not invade or metastasize, but may cause neurologic deficits and death by virtue of progressive growth within the confined space of the skull or spinal canal. Pheochromocytomas may episodically secrete catecholamines, resulting in hypertension, stroke, or unexpected perioperative complications, and retinal angiomas may cause retinal detachment and blindness. The symptoms experienced depend on the size, location, and growth rate of each tumor, yet a normal physical exam does not rule out the presence of extensive disease, and radiologic imaging of all target tissues must be performed to detect and track VHL tumors (tables 2-2 and 2-3). Clinical severity of VHL ranges from no symptoms to blindness, deafness, neurologic deficits, morbidity from surgical resection of solid tumors, renal failure or complications of renal transplant, and the complications of metastatic malignant disease.

Most clinicians feel that the most effective treatment is the prevention of tumor-related complications, often by surgical excision of tumors before symptoms or metastases. This approach requires presymptomatic diagnosis of tumors. Treatment may include genetic counseling; lifelong periodic screening; laser therapy of retinal angiomas; neurosurgical resection of CNS hemangioblastomas; resection of solid tumors and cysts of the kidney; medical management and surgical resection of pheochromocytomas, islet cell tumors, or adenocarcinomas of the pancreas; and management of depression, renal failure, deafness, blindness, or neurologic deficits. Optimal patient care may require a multidisciplinary approach tailored to the patient's needs. For individual patients, the skills of experienced geneticists, urologic oncologists, neurosurgeons, radiologists, ophthalmologists, otolaryngologists, medical oncologists, endocrinologists, social workers, clinical nurse specialists, and support staff may all be needed, and a single coordinator is often essential to orchestrate care. Early detection of tumors is critical in initiating effective treatment; therefore, periodic screening is important (table 2-3). Historically, VHL patients have a shortened lifespan, with a median age at death of 49 years; nearly half of patients were reported to die of complications from CNS hemangioblastomas or metastatic clear cell carcinoma [27]. These estimates are likely to improve with increased detection and improved management of presymptomatic disease.

Table 2-2. Clinical evaluation for diagnosis of von Hippel–Lindau disease (VHL)

Manifestation	Primary diagnostic procedure	Other tests and/or findings
Retinal angioma	Indirect ophthalmoscopy Fluorescein angiography	Tonometry
CNS hemangioblastoma	MRI of brain *and* spine with gadolinium	Careful, complete neurologic exam
Clear cell carcinoma and renal cysts	CT scan with and without contrast (age $>$ 20 yr) or US	Hematuria
Pancreatic cysts, islet cell tumors, adenocarcinoma	As above	Steatorrhea, endocrine effects of islet cell tumors
Pheochromocytoma	As above, plus 24-hr urinary catecholamines, VMA, Metanephrine	Abdominal MRI, MIBG scan, hypertension, anxiety attacks
Epididymal cysts and cystadenoma	US of scrotal contents	Palpable epididymal mass
Endolymphatic sac tumors	Thin-section MRI through the internal auditory canal	Unilateral tinnitus, deafness, audiologic testing

Adapted from Glenn [80].

Table 2-3. A screening regimen often used by clinicians managing VHL families. Screening of patients with known VHL disease must be individualized based on clinical judgment of risks

Ages	Screening tests
Infancy to 2 yrs	History and physical exam yearly Ophthalmoscopy yearly
Age 2 to 10 yrs	History and physical exam yearly Ophthalmoscopy yearly 24-hr urinary catecholamines every 1–2 yrs
Age 11 to 20 yrs	History and physical exam yearly Ophthalmoscopy yearly 24-hr urinary catecholamines every 1–2 yrs Abdominal US MRI of brain *and* spine with gadolinium every 2 yrs
Age above 20 yrs	History and physical exam yearly Ophthalmoscopy yearly 24-hr urinary catecholamines every 1–2 yrs Abdominal CT scan with and without IV contrast yearly (or every other year after age 60) US as needed to evaluate CT findings MRI of brain *and* spine with gadolinium every 2 yrs Thin-cut MRI and/or CT of the internal auditory canals as needed to evaluate symptoms of potential ELST

Adapted from Choyke [47].

Diagnosis and screening of affected and at-risk patients

A diagnosis of VHL should be entertained in patients with a family history of VHL, familial renal carcinoma, or familial pheochromocytoma. In the absence of a family history, VHL should be strongly suspected in patients who present with retinal angiomas; multiple cerebellar hemangioblastomas; one or more spinal hemangioblastomas; renal carcinoma that is multifocal, bilateral, or occurs before age 30; bilateral pheochromocytomas; or pancreatic cysts. Simple renal cysts and epididymal cysts occur too frequently in the general population to be reliable markers of VHL disease. Once a diagnosis of VHL is suspected, the patient should be extensively evaluated for typical VHL lesions (table 2-2). At the National Cancer Institute, this involves careful history and physical examination with emphasis on the family history and neurologic exam, ophthalmologic examination, MRI with gadolinium enhancement of the head and of the spine performed on separate days, CT exam with contrast and/or US of the abdomen, scrotal US, and quantitation of urinary catecholamine excretion.

Once VHL has been identified within a family, all at-risk family members are screened for occult disease (table 2-3). In some cases, genetic testing of family members can strongly suggest the presence or absence of the disease (see above). At-risk relatives and affected patients often avoid visits to the doctor for fear of unknown consequences. Nonjudgmental empathy, explanation of the potential benefits of screening, and gaining the trust of family members are important aspects of effective treatment. It may help to emphasize to an individual patient that serial screening may give him or her some control over the disease, allowing him or her to consider preventive interventions, such as surgery or laser therapy, before irreversible consequences occur; although VHL is currently incurable, individual tumors are frequently treatable when diagnosed early. The hereditary nature of VHL may precipitate a variety of issues, and complicated family relationships, denial, and assignment of blame for poor outcomes may complicate care. A VHL diagnosis carries lifelong financial, social, and psychological consequences and must be made cautiously.

Management of specific tumor types

Solid tumors and cysts of the kidney

A pathologic study of kidney tissue obtained from 16 VHL patients undergoing operative resection of kidney tumors and cysts revealed numerous, microscopic cystic and solid neoplasms in grossly normal renal tissue [28]. The numerous, microscopic solid neoplasms were seen only in tissue obtained from VHL patients, not in similar tissue obtained from patients with sporadic kidney cancer or from autopsy subjects without renal disease. Based on the number of observed lesions and the estimated volume examined, Walther et al. estimated each kidney from these 16 VHL patients to harbor an average of 1100 cysts and 600 clear cell neoplasms. This study clearly demonstrates the multifocal nature of neoplasms of the VHL kidney (figure 2-3).

Renal cysts are detected by CT and US in over 60% of VHL-affected patients beginning in the second decade and may be simple, complex (with both cystic and solid portions), or multiloculated [29]. The majority of renal cysts grow slowly over a period of years. Occasionally, simple cysts may regress and apparently disappear, or complex cysts may progress to a solid tumor. The cysts rarely affect renal function, may grow to very large size, and may be few or many number. Between 60% and 85% of VHL patients, with careful screening, are found to have cysts at some point. Some cysts show epithelial dysplasia, and in one study, malignant foci (cyst linings more than three clear-cells deep) were found in 25 of 116 (21%) resected cysts [30]. Of measurable cysts, larger cysts contained malignant foci more frequently, ranging from 3 of 12 (25%) for cysts less than 5 mm to 7 of 11 (64%) for cyst more than 2 cm. Using tissue immunohistochemistry, Kragel et al. provided evidence that simple cysts arose from distal tubular epithelium, compared with complex cysts and solid clear cell carcinoma masses, which arose from proximal tubular epithelium [31]. Rarely, extensive renal cystic disease in VHL patients may mimic autosomal-dominant polycystic kidney disease (ADPKD) and lead to renal failure [32]. Given the malignant potential of the VHL kidney, such nonfunctional kidneys should be surgically removed.

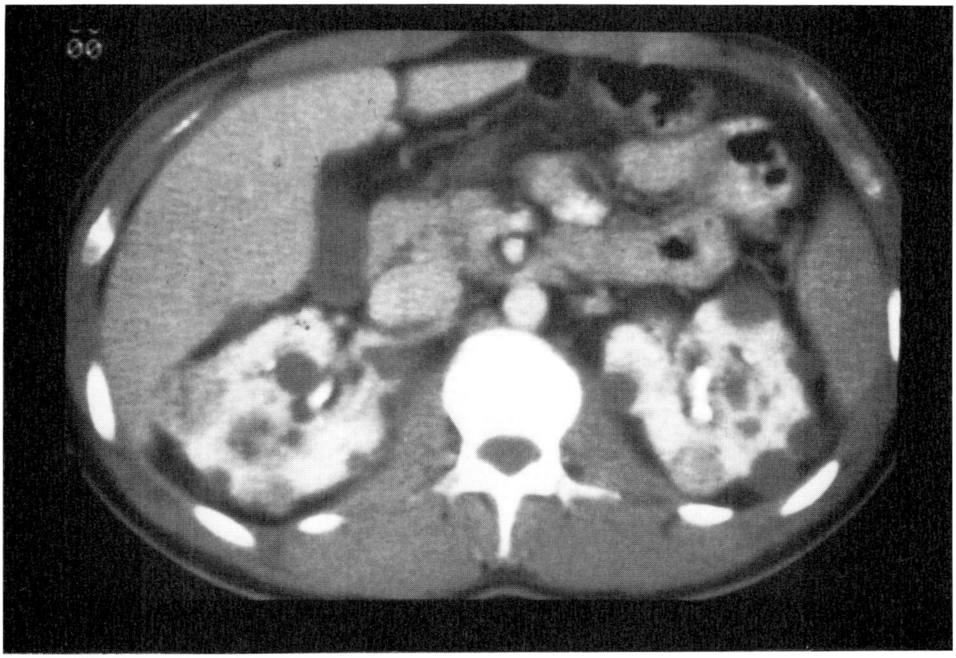

Figure 2-3. Abdominal CT scan with intravenous contrast enhancement demonstrating multiple, bilateral solid tumors of the kidneys.

Nearly all solid kidney tumors of VHL patients are malignant clear cell or predominantly clear cell carcinomas [29,30,33]. Solid (and cystic) lesions identified by prospective screening are usually surrounded by a well-circumscribed psuedocapsule. In 44 of 66 malignant lesions, tumor cells were seen invading the pseudocapsule, but in none of the 66 lesions did tumor extend through the pseudocapsule [30]. Nearly all solid tumors will enlarge over time, with a mean doubling time of 10 months, and have been observed to grow at rates of 0.2 to 2.2 cm/year (mean 1.6) [29]. Yearly or bi-yearly examination of kidney lesions with thin-section, contrast-enhanced CT allows an estimation of the tempo of growth. US is a useful, though less sensitive, adjunct used primarily to determine whether a lesion is cystic or solid. MRI may be helpful at times and can sometimes distinguish solid from cystic lesions.

Given the multifocal nature and lifelong risks, the optimal surgical strategy for management of cystic and solid kidney lesions must be developed on a case-by-case basis, preferably by urologic surgeons with experience in this disease. Options range from bilateral nephrectomy with subsequent dialysis and/or transplantation [34] to parenchymal-sparing surgery [35–37]. While bilateral nephrectomy removes the risk of metastatic disease, it adversely affects quality of life and introduces other potential complications. On the other hand, nephron-sparing surgery only lessens the lifetime risk of metastatic clear cell carcinoma. Several aspects of clear cell carcinoma in VHL guide surgical management of tumors of the VHL kidney, particular small, localized tumors detected by periodic screening. First, solid and cystic tumors are usually surrounded and contained within a well-circumscribed pseudocapsule of compressed tissue, thus permitting the option of enucleation with a margin of grossly normal tissue [38]. Second, the malignant lesions are multifocal, and grossly normal renal parenchyma may conceal microscopic malignant lesions. Third, nearly all tumors from VHL kidneys are low grade [30] and grow slowly. And lastly, although the natural history of VHL clear cell carcinoma has been carefully documented in only a small number of cases [29], sporadic renal carcinoma tumors measuring less than 3 to 5 cm have a low incidence of associated metastatic disease [39].

Given these considerations, M.M. Walther et al. reported on the use of parenchymal-sparing surgery in 19 VHL patients to control tumor growth, prevent metastasis, and maintain renal function [35]. All treatment options were discussed with patients. For patients electing nephron-sparing surgery, predetermined criteria were used to decide on the timing of operations. Patients with VHL and solid renal lesions were generally followed until the renal lesions were 3 cm in diameter. Smaller lesions centrally located or near vital structures were considered for earlier surgical resection. Patients were evaluated every 3 to 12 months by abdominal CT with and without intravenous contrast enhancement and by renal ultrasound, depending on documented rate of tumor growth and size of tumors. Given the predilection for multiorgan involvement, these patients were systematically evaluated preoperatively by 24-hour measurement of urinary catecholamine excretion, eye examination, MRI of the brain and spine with gadolinium enhancement, scrotal ultrasound, and chest radiography. Preoperative renal angiography was performed to provide a vascular road map of the kidney under consideration, and color Doppler intraoperative ultrasound was essential to aid in defining a plane of dissection [40] and to identify occult tumors, vascular structures, and the need for renal hypothermia and vascular occlusion during dissection of tumors. All cystic and solid lesions were removed, primarily by partial nephrectomy and enucleation of the tumor with a margin of normal tissue, yielding an average of 13 lesions removed per kidney. Renal function was preserved, and the majority of patients did not develop new solid lesions of the kidney over an average follow-up of two years. During this follow-up period, no patient opting for parenchymal-sparing surgery developed metastatic disease or required renal dialysis or transplantation. Subsequent to publication, one patient developed an isolated adrenal metastasis three years after partial nephrectomy, which was resected (M.M. Walther, personal communication).

Based on these and other findings [36], it may be possible to identify patients by serial screening who have indolent disease that can be managed by parenchymal-sparing surgery with removal of all lesions at the time of operation, as well as patients with aggressive or diffuse disease at much higher risk of metastasis who may require nephrectomy.

Metastatic clear cell carcinoma is resistant to standard chemotherapy and hormonal therapy [8]. Immunotherapy has shown promise [41]. New approaches may become apparent as the molecular function of the VHL gene product is defined.

Cerebellar, medullary and spinal hemangioblastomas

Unlike clear cell carcinoma, the cell of origin of CNS hemangioblastomas (HB) is not definitely known. HBs are highly vascular tumors comprosed of vascular channels lined by cuboidal endothelial cells and surrounded by stromal cells and pericytes [42,43]. A study of HB by northern blot, in situ hybridization analysis and immunohistochemistry provided evidence that the stromal cells secrete increased amounts of vascular endothelial growth factor (VEGF) compared to stromal cells from normal brain, and that tumor endothelial cells lining vascular channels express the cognate VEGF receptor [44]. This suggests that a paracrine mechanism involving VEGF may mediate neovascularization.

HB lesions occur in four radiologically distinct types: solid, cystic, cystic with a solid mural component, or, rarely, hemorrhagic. HBs do not invade locally and do not metastasize, but, by virtue of their unrestricted growth in confined spaces, they have the potential to cause hemorrhage, obstructive hydrocephalus, increased intracranial pressure, protean focal neurological deficits, and death.

Forty to seventy percent of patients diagnosed with VHL will have HBs [27,45]. The mean age at diagnosis of cerebellar and spinal cord lesions is 29 and 34 years, respectively (table 2-1). The three major sites of HB are the cerebellum (see figure 2-4), the spinal cord, and, less commonly, the brainstem. Even within these sites, there is a poorly understood predilection for tumor formation in certain areas such as the area postrema and the conus medullaris and craniocervical junction of the spinal cord [45]. Unusual sites include the pituitary and cerebrum. Unlike sporadic cases of HB, multiple tumors are common, and diagnosis occurs at a younger mean age.

Since many HBs are asymptomatic, periodic screening is important. The most common symptoms with cerebellar and brainstem lesions are headache, ataxia, nausea, and vomiting, and with spinal cord lesions are focal pain, sensory loss, or motor defect [46]. Positional vertigo, wide-based gait, nystagmus, dysmetria, papilledema, and ninth-cranial-nerve palsies have also been described as presenting symptoms. Erythrocytosis may occur as a result of erythropoetin secretion by the tumor and may require periodic phelbotomy. Erythrocytosis resolves with surgical excision of the tumor.

Cerebellar HB lesions occur within the parenchyma, frequently as cystic lesions with solid mural modules. Spinal HB can occur throughout the spinal cord, nerve roots, conus medullaris, and cauda equina. The tumors can be

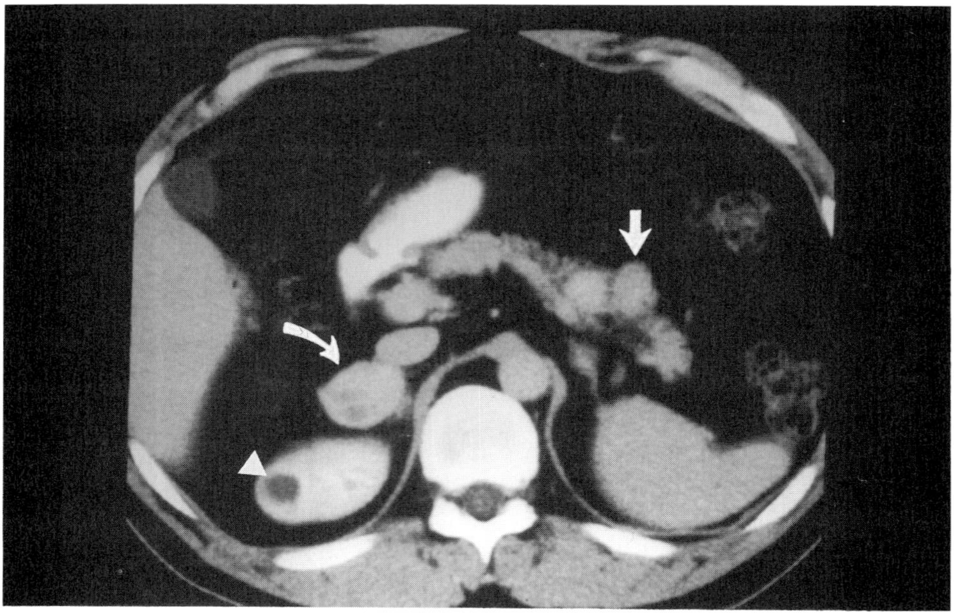

A

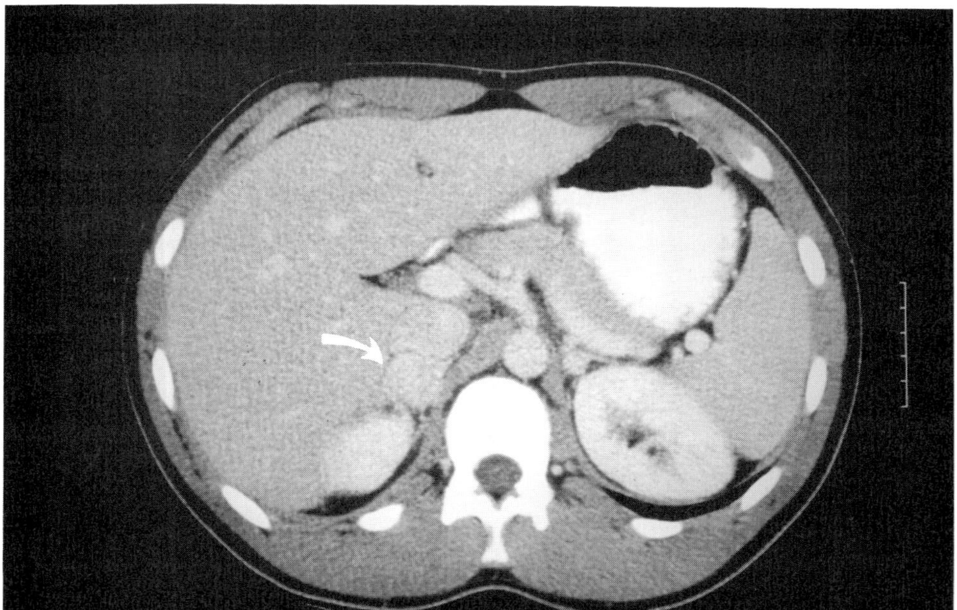

B

Figure 2-4. **A** Abdominal CT scan with contrast enhancement of a 45-year-old man demonstrating solid, enhancing tumors of the pancreas (straight arrows) and a large right adrenal tumor (curved arrows). A renal cyst is present (arrowhead). **B** His asymptomatic 15-year-old son was discovered to have a functional pheochromocytoma (curved arrow), as was his 12-year-old son (**C**, curved arrow).

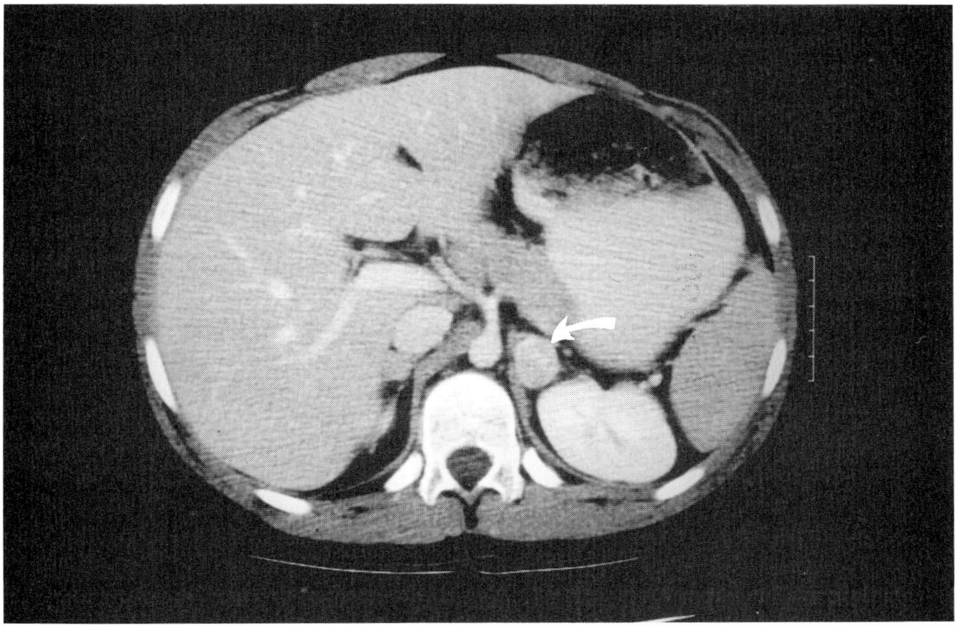

C

Figure 2-4. (Continued).

multiple, intramedullary, extramedullary, or partly both, sometimes resembling meningiomas. Syringomyelia occurs in up to 80% of cases of intramedullary spinal HB, producing local pain, sensory loss, propioceptive loss, paresis, and hypertonia.

Diagnosis of HB is best done by contrast-enhanced MRI, including a pre- and postcontrast T1-weighted imaging of the brain and spinal cord with thin sections through the posterior fossa and spinal cord. Neurologic sequelae of HB are frequently progressive and permanent, even after successful neurosurgical resection. Therefore it is important to diagnose HB at a presymptomatic stage, before tumors result in neurologic deficits. This can be done by initiation of biannual screening of at-risk individuals beginning at age 10 years (table 2-3). Like clear cell carcinoma, HB exists in both familial and sporadic form. Whereas only 5% to 30% of solitary cerebellar HBs are due to VHL, multiple cerebellar HB is diagnostic of VHL, and almost 80% of spinal HBs are due to VHL [47]. Solitary CNS HB in any site may be an initial manifestation of VHL and should prompt careful documentation of the patient's family history and screening studies. Treatment of HB in VHL patients requires neurosurgical expertise, and will not be discussed here, but may consist of resection of cysts or solid tumors that cause or threaten to cause obstructive hydrocephalus or other neurologic deficits [46,48]. External beam radiation therapy and stereotaxic radiosurgery have been used to treat inoperable lesions [49,50].

Retinal hemangioblastomas

These lesions have traditionally been called 'retinal angiomas' but are histologically identical of CNS hemangioblastomas [51]. The tumors do not metastasize; however, they can cause glaucoma and blindness by virtue of unchecked growth, retinal detachment, or extravasation of serum from the vasculature. They are among the earliest manifestation of VHL and have been diagnosed in individuals ages 1 to 90, with an average age at diagnosis of 25 years [27,52]. Diagnosis of subtle, preangiomatous lesions may require indirect ophthalmoscopy with or without flourescein angiography and tonometry. Established retinal hemangioblastomas are easily recognized by an experienced ophthalmologist on eye examination alone. Yearly ophthalmologic inspection of affected and at-risk patients is required, since multiple and bilateral angiomas may form at any time during the patient's lifetime [53]. Aggressive laser therapy of all detected angiomas may prevent complications. Occasionally, retinal angiomas are only discovered at a late stage, after blindness has occurred, necessitating enucleation for control of pain. A minority of VHL patients may also develop unusual retinal vasular hamartomas other than angiomas [54].

Pheochromocytomas

VHL appears to be the most common cause of hereditary pheochromocytoma: in one study, 16 of 82 (19.5%) patients with apparently sporadic pheochromocytoma actually had VHL [55]. Only 3 of the 82 patients had multiple endocrine neoplasia type 2, the next most common familial cause. Comparing patients with VHL versus those with sporadic pheochromocytomas, patients with VHL were diagnosed at a younger mean age, their tumors were more frequently multifocal in localization, and their tumors were less frequently invasive [55]. It is well recognized that pheochromocytomas are characteristic of some VHL families but not others [26,56]; this fact is recognized in the classification scheme of VHL (table 2-4), which distinguishes VHL without pheochromocytoma (type 1) from VHL with pheochromocytoma (type 2). Thus, in those families where pheochromocytomas do occur, they are frequently the presenting sign of the syndrome and often are diagnosed at a relatively young age [27] (figure 2-5). These adrenal tumors are frequently multiple, bilateral, and ectopic in VHL patients. They have a low metastatic potential; however, metastasis does rarely occur to regional lymph nodes or

Table 2-4. Proposed classification of VHL [26]

Type 1.	VHL *without* pheochromocytoma
Type 2.	VHL *with* pheochromocytoma
	2A. *without* renal cell carcinoma or pancreatic cysts
	2B. *with* renal cell carcinoma and/or pancreatic cysts

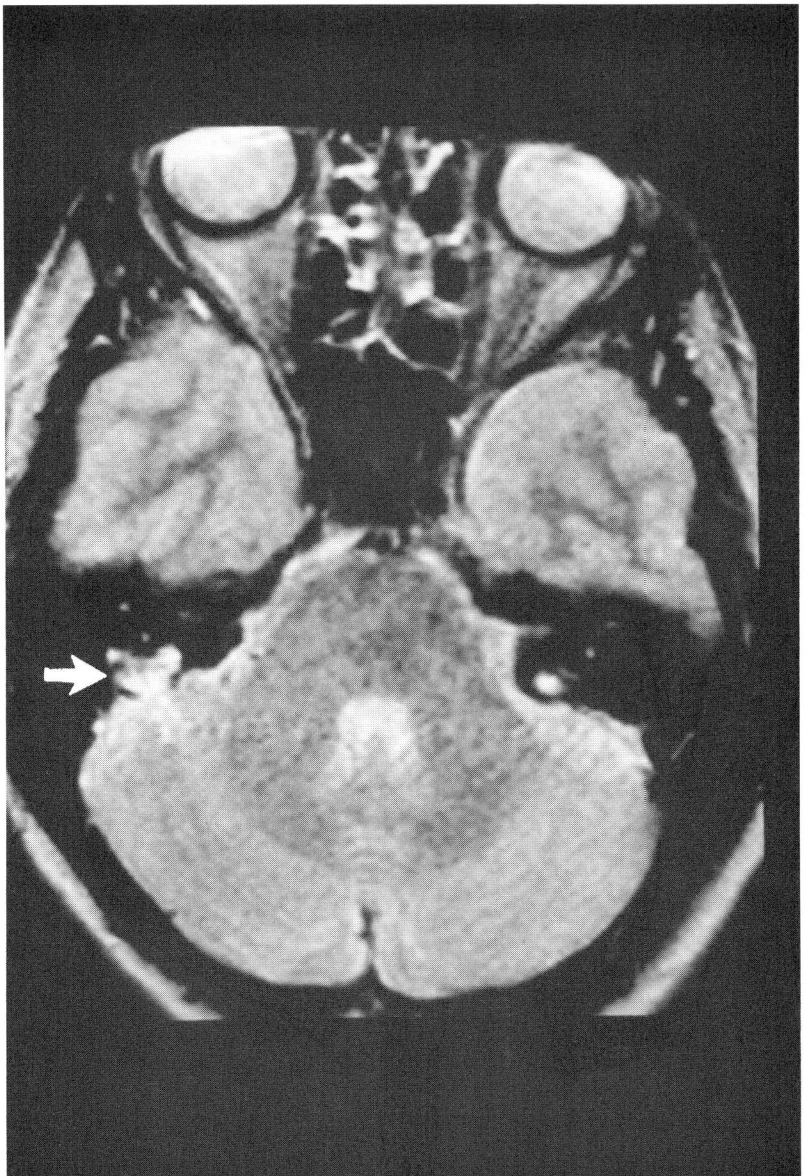

A

Figure 2-5. **A.** Head MRI with gadolinium enhancement of a 44-year-old woman with a 10-year history of left-sided hearing loss. Straight arrow marks large endolymphatic sac tumor (ELST). **B.** Head CT reveals erosion of the left temporal bone (curved arrow) by the patient's ELST.

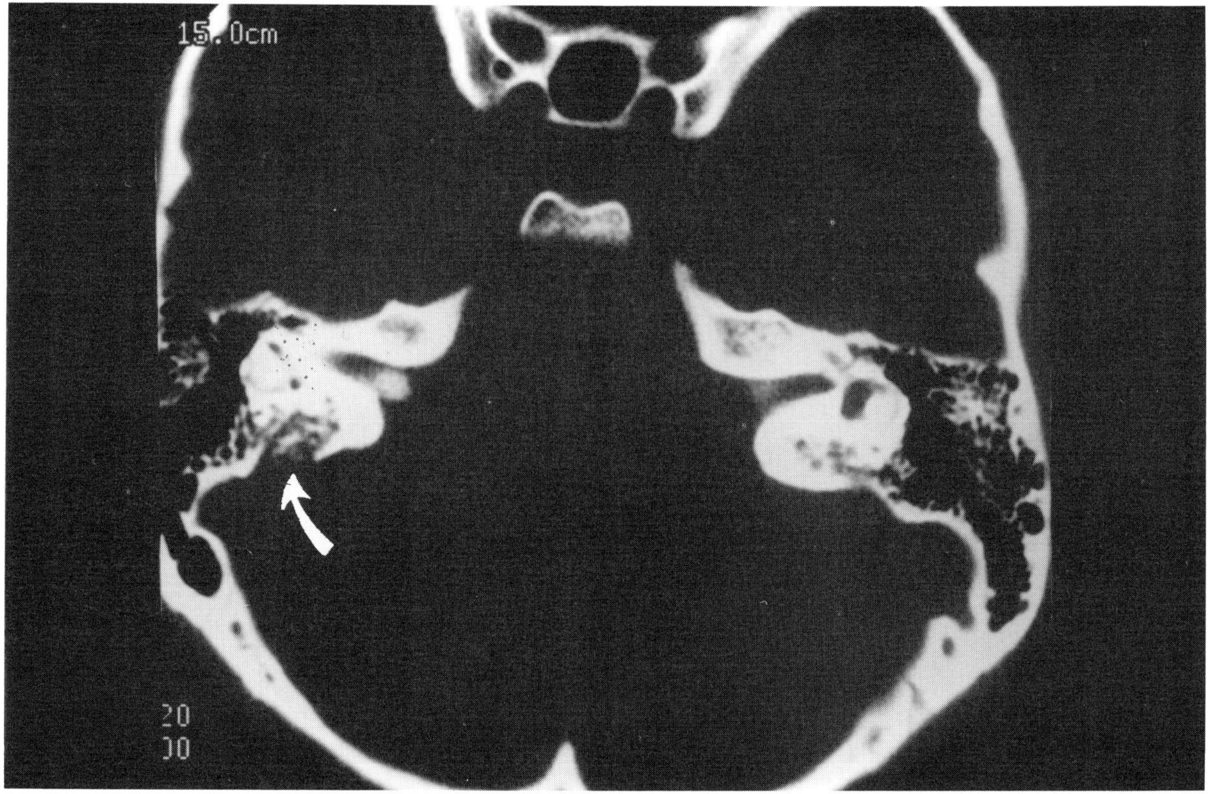

B

Figure 2-5. (Continued).

distant organs. Some adrenal tumors are nonfunctional, producing no symptoms or catecholamines, and may be followed prospectively without immediate intervention.

As in sporadic cases, pheochromocytomas may cause symptoms of episodic anxiety or sweating, paroxysmal or sustained hypertension, and headaches; however, the majority of adrenal tumors detected by screening are asymptomatic [57]. Diagnosis is made by 24-hour collection of urine for catecholamines including norepinephrine, epinephrine, dopamine, vanillylmandelic acid, and metanephrine. Very high levels of catecholamine (i.e., greater than twice the upper limits of normal) imply a functional pheochromocytoma, either within the adrenal gland or ectopically as a paraganglioma, which may then be imaged by CT scan with intravenous contrast, MRI imaging, or metaiodobenzylguanidine (MIBG) radioscintigraphy.

A functional pheochromocytoma must be excluded before elective surgery in a VHL patient to avoid anesthesia-induced hypertensive crisis. Functional pheochromocytomas identified preoperatively require alpha-adrenergic blockade using phenoxybenzamine or similar agents for at least two weeks before surgery and may be resected at the time of surgery. Bilateral adrenalectomy necessitates lifelong mineralocorticoid replacement with the addition of glucocorticoids during conditions of physiologic stress such as sepsis.

Interestingly, the germline mutations associated with families which develop pheochromocytomas have nearly always been missense mutations (i.e., one which results in the change of one amino acid in the final protein product of the gene) [26,57,58], a finding that may become more meaningful once the cell biology of the VHL protein is better defined.

Other tumors

Pancreatic cysts and tumors. Pancreatic cysts are rare in the general population. The presence of a pancreatic cyst in a patient with a family history of VHL is considered diagnostic of the syndrome. VHL patients can have several types of lesions of the pancreas, including pancreatic cysts, pancreatic cystadenomas, and islet cell tumors [59].

Pancreatic cysts are the most common pancreatic lesion in VHL. They form throughout the pancreas with no predilection for any particular site and vary in size up to several centimeters. These cysts are usually asymptomatic; however, rare cysts may cause biliary obstruction, pancreatitis, or symptoms of visceral compression necessitating biliary stent placement or percutaneous drainage [60]. In rare cases, replacement of pancreatic parenchyma may cause pancreatic insufficiency with steatorrhea or diabetes mellitus [61].

Serous cystadenomas appear as clusters of cysts within the pancreas, often with a central nidus of tumor (figure 2-2). As with simple cysts, these lesions are nonmetastatic and are usually asymptomatic unless they cause compression of the bile duct. Islet cell tumors, like pheochromocytomas, are thought to arise from neural crest. In VHL, these tumors are most frequently nonfunctional; however, they may be metastatic [62–64]. A study of 165 patients with VHL revealed 7 patients with pancreatic neuroendocrine tumors, each of whom had pheochromocytoma as the only other manifestation of the disease [57] (figure 2-5). Islet cell tumors may secrete peptide cytokines such as vasoactive intestinal polypeptide, calcitonin, insulin, glucagon, somatostatin, and gastrin.

Lesions of the pancreas are best imaged by CT scan of the abdomen with contrast. US is helpful in distinguishing cystic from solid lesions. No intervention is necessary for asymptomatic cysts or cystadenomas; however, pancreatectomy must be considered for solid tumors of the pancreas.

Epididymal and broad ligament cystadenomas. Although unilateral epididymal cysts occur in nearly one quarter of the general population [65], cysts and

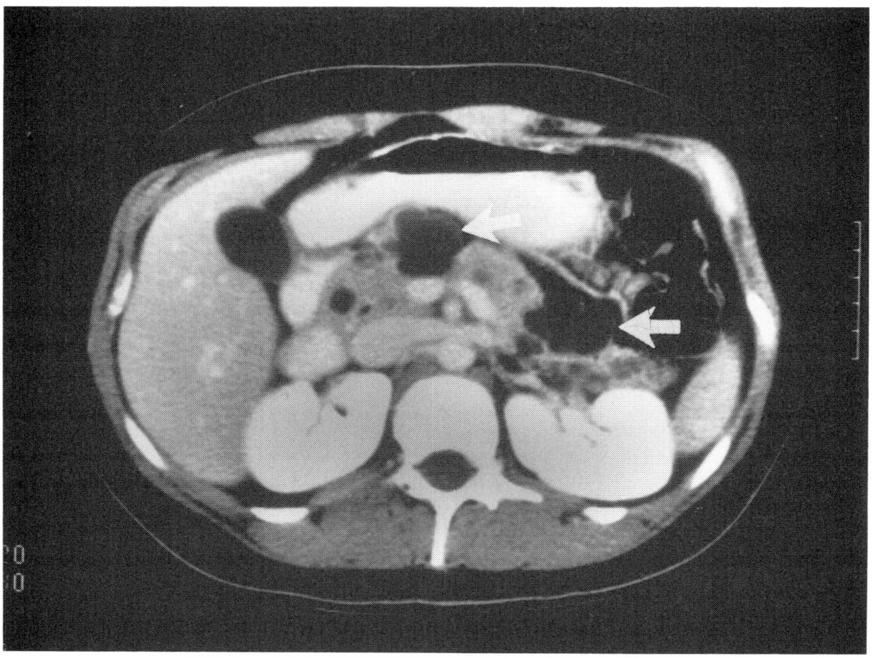

A

Figure 2-6. Clinical heterogeneity of VHL manifestations. **A.** Screening abdominal CT with IV contrast enhancement of an asymptomatic 16-year-old patient. Note extensive cysts of the pancreas, with normal kidneys. The clover-leaf appearance of the cysts is characteristic of cystadenomatous lesions (arrows). **B.** Screening abdominal CT with IV contrast demonstrating a solid tumor of the left kidney (arrow) in the asymptomatic 19-year-old sister of the patient shown in (A). These patients had one brother whose sole manifestation of VHL was retinal angiomas that had caused blindness in one eye. The patients' father had been recently diagnosed with VHL after presenting with massive hematuria, bulky bilateral renal carcinomas, and cerebellar hemangioblastomas.

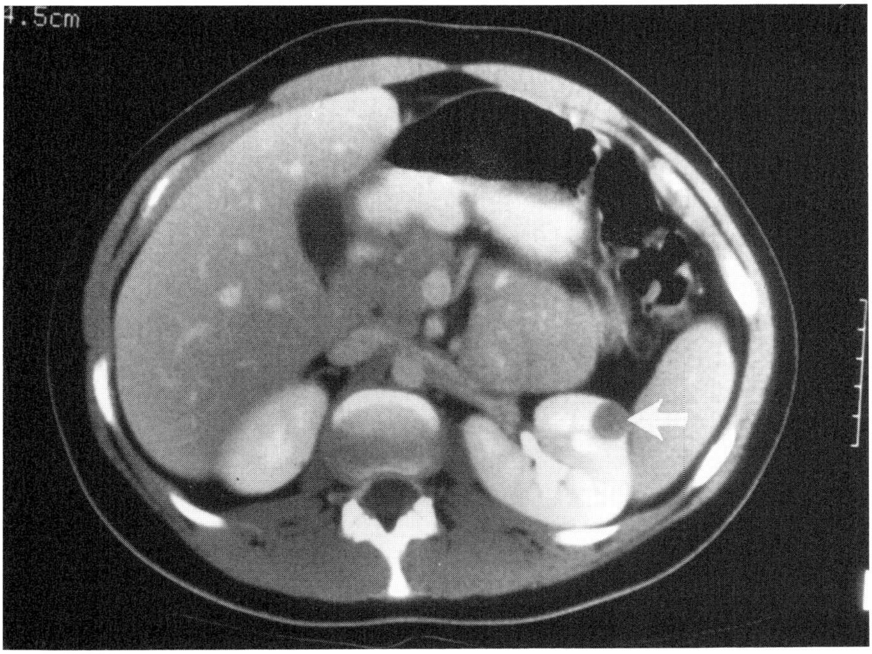

B

Figure 2-6. (Continued).

papillary cystadenomas occur bilaterally in 10% to 15% of VHL men, and bilateral epididymal papillary cystadenomas are virtually diagnostic of VHL. They do not metastasize and only rarely cause symptoms such as obstructive azoospermia. In men, the tumors may be easily palpable on physical exam and can be characterized as solid or cystic by ultrasound. These tumors do not normally require treatment, but may be useful in diagnosis.

In a very small percentage of women affected with VHL, tumors may arise from parauterine mesonephric duct remnants giving rise to broad ligament tumors known as benign adnexal papillary tumors of probable mesonephric origin (APMO) [66,67]. These tumors are analogous to epididymal papillary cystadenomas.

Endolymphatic sac tumor (ELST) of the middle ear. A small percentage of VHL patients develop papillary tumors of the temporal bone [67,68] (see figure 2-6). They are slow growing, with low metastatic potential, but are locally invasive, causing temporal bone destruction, hearing loss, tinitus, and vertigo. In one series, patients had a history of sensorineural hearing loss diagnosed an average of 10.6 years prior to diagnosis of the tumor [69]. The tumor may present with an external auditory canal mass, facial paralysis, and a destructive mass arising on the posterior fossa surface of the temporal bone.

Molecular and cell biology of the VHL protein

The VHL gene is a single-copy gene in man [4]. The human VHL gene directs transcription of messenger RNA detectable in all tissues by northern blot. The gene is remarkably conserved through evolution, and can be found by Southern blot in eukaryotic species as diverse as mammals, drosophila, and sea urchin, suggesting that VHL encodes a fundamental cellular function. VHL is not detected by Southern blot in the DNA of the unicellular eukaryote Saccharomyces cerevisiae (J. Gnarra, personal communication), which might suggest an evolutionary role in adaptation of single cells to multicellular life in an organism. Although the original cDNA cloned was thought to contain only a partial amino acid sequence, comparison of the DNA sequence of the original VHL clone to the mouse [70] and rat [71] homologues provides evidence that the original clone, g7, indeed contains the entire open reading frame (ORF) encoding the VHL protein, 213 amino acids long. The predicted amino acid sequence has no significant homology to other proteins and contains no functional amino acid motifs that might help explain its function. As might be expected of a tumor suppressor gene, the VHL gene, when transfected into a tumor cell line, suppressed the ability of the cell line to form tumors in nude mice [72].

The introduction of epitope-tagged versions of the VHL gene into cells in tissue culture established that the wild-type VHL protein, but not certain mutated VHL proteins, specifically complexed with other cellular proteins [69]. Two of these associated proteins were identified by protein microsequencing as Elongin B and Elongin C, regulatory subunits of a heterotrimeric transcription elongation factor known as Elongin [73,74]. Elongin was originally purified as a complex of three proteins that activated transcriptional elongation of RNA polymerase II, the major polymerase for messenger RNA [75–77]. The Elongin complex consists of an active subunit, Elongin A, and two regulatory subunits, Elongins B and C. Overexpressed VHL protein was shown to bind tightly and specifically to Elongins B and C and to prevent their assembly with Elongin A. This suggests a model in which VHL may compete with Elongin A for the binding of Elongins B and C, resulting in a transcriptionally active Elongin ABC complex, or a transcriptionally inactive VHL–Elongin BC complex in which the BC subunits may in effect be sequestered. Thus, the association of VHL with regulatory subunits of an activator of transcriptional elongation suggests that VHL may play a role in transcription. The binding site of Elongins B and C on VHL has been defined. The existence of naturally occuring VHL mutations that abrogate VHL–Elongin BC complex formation implicates the VHL–Elongin BC complex in the antitumorigenic function of VHL [71,74]. In one study of 67 VHL families with identified germline mutations, 42 families had mutations predicted to disrupt VHL binding to Elongins B and C [78].

After transient transfection into cells, the subcellular localization of the VHL protein varies from cell to cell [71]. In some cells, VHL stained the nucleus exclusively, in others the cytoplasm exclusively, and in yet others, both. Attempts to define specific environmental signals that might trigger changes in the subcellular localization of VHL have as yet been unsuccessful; however, a set of contrasting culture conditions, partly characterized by sparse versus confluent growth of the cells, was defined that results in a shift in predominant subcellular distribution of VHL [79]. Specifically, under conditions marked by sparse growth of the cells, the VHL gene product localized to a greater degree in the nucleus of cells. Under conditions marked by confluent growth of the cells, the VHL gene product localized to a greater degree to the cytoplasm. The change in predominant subcellular localization in response to changes in the culture conditions of cells, together with the evidence that the VHL protein may play a role in control of transcriptional elongation, suggests that VHL may respond to environmental signals to alter transcription of other genes, the net effect of which is to control normal growth in tissues.

Future questions

Efforts are underway to improve the genetic testing currently available. These efforts might allow VHL family members at minimal risk to avoid some of the cost, inconvenience, and anxiety associated with yearly screening. The continued medical care of and study of VHL patients at major academic centers provides the ongoing opportunity to refine the optimal approach to diagnosis and treatment of the multiple tumor types that occur in these patients. Intensive basic-science study of the function of the VHL gene product will hopefully provide insights into the early events of clear cell carcinoma tumorigenesis, as well as the early events in formation of the other tumor types present in VHL. These insights may identify new approaches to treatment of these tumors, both in VHL patients and in the general population.

Although the VHL gene is inactivated in sporadic and familial (VHL) clear cell renal carcinoma, it is not mutated in sporadic or familial papillary cancers of the kidney [6]. Familial papillary kidney cancer, like VHL, is an autosomal-dominant syndrome of predisposition to kidney cancer [81]. Families with hereditary papillary kidney cancer are currently under study at the National Cancer Institute in a search for other genes involved in renal neoplasias.

Resources

As of January 1996, there are two commercial services in the United States offering some form of DNA testing for a fee:

1. Ms. Corinne Boehm, DNA Diagnostics Laboratory, Center for Medical Genetics, Johns Hopkins Hospital, Baltimore, MD 21205, Tel: 1-410-955-0483; Fax 1-410-955-0484.
2. Lynn Godmilow, M.S.W., Director, Genetic Diagnostic Referral

Center, University of Pennsylvania, Department of Genetics, Philadelphia, PA 19104-6145, Tel: 1-215-573-9161; Fax: 1-215-573-7760; E-mail: godmilow@mail.med.upenn.edu

Support groups include:

1. VHL Family Alliance, 171 Clinton Rd, Brookline, MA 02146, Tel: 1-617-232-5946 or 1-800-767-4VHL). This organization publishes the 'VHL Family Forum' newsletter quarterly at a suggested subscription price of $25/year. They maintain an address on the World Wide Web: VHL@pipeline.com

2. The von Hippel–Lindau Syndrome Foundation, 35 Beaverson Blvd., Bldg 2, Suite B, Brick, NJ 08723 (voice mail only: 1-908-244-7635)

Acknowledgment

We thank J.R. Gnarra, S. Lee, A. Pause, D.Y.T. Chen, J. Wagner, and S. Zhou for helpful discussions and G.M. Glenn, M.M. Walther, K. Hagan, and R. Humphrey for critical reading of the manuscript. We thank C. Manolatos and K. Hurley for assistance in the care of these patients.

References

1. Glenn GM, Gnarra JR, Choyke PL, Walther MM, Zbar B, Linehan WM (1995). The molecular genetics of renal cell carcinoma. In Reghavan D, Scher H, Leibel S and Lange P (eds), *Principles and Practice of Genitourinary Oncology*. Philadelphia: JB Lippincott Company.
2. Gnarra JR, Lerman MI, Zbar BH, Linehan WM (1995). Genetics of renal cell carcinoma and evidence for a critical role for von Hippel–Lindau in renal tumorigenesis. Semin Oncol 22:3.
3. Knudson AG (1995). VHL gene mutation and clear-cell renal carcinomas. Cancer J Sci Am 1:180.
4. Latif F, Tory K, Gnarra J, et al. (1993). Identification of the von Hippel–Lindau disease tumor suppressor gene. Science 260:1317.
5. Tory K, Brauch H, Linehan MW, et al. (1989). Specific genetic change in tumors associated with von Hippel–Lindau disease. J Natl Cancer Inst 81:1097.
6. Gnarra J, Tory K, Weng Y, et al. (1994). Mutations of the VHL tumour suppressor gene in renal carcinoma. Natl Genet 7:85.
7. Herman JG, Latif F, Weng Y, et al. (1994). Silencing of the VHL tumor suppressor gene by DNA methylation in renal carcinoma. Proc Natl Acad Sci 91:9700.
8. Yagoda A, Abi-Rached B, Petrylak D (1995). Chemotherapy for advanced renal-cell carcinoma: 1983–1993. Semin Oncol 22:42.
9. Hippel EV (1904). Uber eine sehr seltene erkrankung der netzhaut. Klinische Beobachtungen Arch Opthalmol 59:83.
10. Lindau A (1926). Studien der kleinbirncysten bau: pathogenese und beziehungen zur angiomatosis retinae. Acta Radiol Microbiol Scandinavica 1:1.
11. Melman KL, Rosen SW (1964). Lindau's disease: review of the literature and study of a large kindred. Am J Med 36:595.
12. Cohen AJ, Li FP, Berg S, et al. (1979). Hereditary renal cell carcinoma associated with a chromosomal translocation. N Engl J Med 301:592.
13. Zbar BH, Brauch H, Talmadge C, Linehan MW (1987). Loss of alleles of loci on the short arm of chromosome 3 in renal cell carcinoma. Nature 327:721.

14. Seizinger BR, Rovlean GA, Ozelius LJ, et al. (1988). von Hippel–Lindau disease maps to the region of chromosome 3 associated with renal cell carcinoma. Nature 332:268.
15. Glenn GM, Linehan WM, Hosoe S, et al. (1992). Screening for von Hippel–Lindau disease by DNA polymorphism analysis. JAMA 67:1226.
16. Linehan WM, Lerman MI, Zbar B (1995). Identification of the von Hippel-Lindau (VHL) gene. Its role in renal cancer. JAMA 273:564.
17. Foster K, Prowse A, Berg Avd, et al. (1994). Somatic mutations of the von Hippel–Lindau tumor suppressor gene in non-familial clear cell renal carcinoma. Hum Mol Genet 3:2169.
18. Whaley JM, Naglich J, Gelbert L, et al. (1994). Germ-line mutations in the von Hippel–Lindau tumor-suppressor gene are similar to von Hippel–Lindau aberrations in sporadic renal cell carcinoma. Am J Hum Genet 55:1092.
19. Gilcrease MZ, Schmidt L, Zbar B, Truong L, Rutledge M, Wheeler T (1995). Somatic VHL mutations in clear cell papillary cystadenoma of the epididymis. Hum Pathol 26:1341.
20. Zeiger MA, Zbar B, Keiser H, Linehan WM, Gnarra JR (1995). Loss of heterozygosity on the short arm of chromosome 3 in sporadic, von Hippel–Lindau disease-associated, and familial pheochromocytoma. Genes Chromosomes Cancer 13:151.
21. Knudson AGJ (1971). Mutation and cancer: statistical study of retinoblastoma. Proc Natl Acad Sci 68:820.
22. Maher ER, Yates JRW, Ferguson-Smith MA (1990). Statistical analysis of the two stage mutation model in von Hippel–Lindau disease and in sporadic cerebellar hemangioblastoma and renal cell carcinoma. J Med Genet 27:311.
23. Maher ER, Iselius L, Yates JRW, et al. (1991). Von Hippel Lindau disease: a genetic study. J Med Genet 28:443.
24. Olschwang S, Boisson C, Richard S, Resche F, Thomas G (1995). DNA-based presymptomatic diagnosis for the von Hippel–Lindau disease by linkage analysis. Eur J Hum Genet 3:108.
25. Richards FM, Latif F, Lerman MI, Zbar B, Maher ER (1993). Taq1 and Pst1 RFLPs in the von Hippel–Lindau disease gene (VHL). Hum Mol Genet 2:1750.
26. Glenn GM, Lambert ND, Choyke P, et al. (1991). Von Hippel Lindau (VHL) disease: distinct phenotypes suggest more than one mutant allele at the VHL locus. Hum Genet 87:207–210.
27. Maher ER, Yates JRW, Harries R, et al. (1990). Clinical features and natural history of von Hippel–Lindau disease. Q J Med 77:1151.
28. Walther MM, Lubensky IA, Venzon D, Zbar B, Linehan WM (1995). Prevalence of microscopic lesions in grossly normal renal parenchyma from patients with von Hippel–Lindau disease, sporadic renal cell carcinoma and no renal disease: clinical implications. J Urol 154:2010.
29. Choyke PL, Glenn GM, Walther MM, et al. (1992). The natural history of renal lesions in von Hippel–Lindau disease: a serial CT imaging study in 28 patients. Am J Radiol 159: 1229.
30. Poston CD, Jaffe GS, Lubensky IA, Solomon D, Zbar B, Linehan WM, Walther MW (1995). Characterization of the renal pathology of a familial form of renal cell carcinoma associated with von Hippel–Lindau disease: clinical and molecular genetic implications. J Urol 153: 22.
31. Kragel PJ, Walther MM, Pestaner JP, Filling-Katz MR (1991). Simple renal cysts, atypical renal cysts and renal cell carcinoma in von Hippel–Lindau disease: a lectin and immunohistochemical study in six patients. Mod Pathol 4:210.
32. Lamiell JM, Stor RA, Hsia YE (1980). von Hippel–Lindau disease simulating polycystic kidney disease. Urology 15:287–290.
33. Nelson JB, Oyasu R, Dalton DP (1994). The clinical and pathologic manifestations of renal tumors in von Hippel–Lindau disease. J Urol 156:2221.
34. Steinbach F, Novick AC, Shoskes D (1994). Renal transplantation in patients with renal cell carcinoma and von Hippel–Lindau disease. Urology 44:760.
35. Walther MM, Choyke PL, Weiss G, et al. (1995). Parenchymal sparing surgery in patients with hereditary renal cell carcinoma. J Urol 153:913.

36. Steinbach F, Novick AC, Zincke H, et al. (1995). Treatment of renal cell carcinoma in von Hippel–Lindau disease: a multicenter study. J Urol 153:1995.
37. Nelson JB, Oyasu R, Dalton DP (1994). The clinical and pathologic manifestations of renal tumors in von Hippel–Lindau disease. J Urol 156:2221.
38. Walther MM, Thompson N, Linehan WM (1995). Enucleation procedures in patients with multiple hereditary renal tumors. World J Urol 13:248.
39. Curry NS, Shabel SI, WL Betsill J (1986). Small renal neoplasms: diagnostic imaging, pathologic features, and clinical course. Radiology 158:113.
40. Walther MM, Choyke PL, Hayes W, Shawker TH, Alexander RB, Linehan WM (1994). Evaluation of color Doppler intraoperative ultrasound in parenchymal sparing renal surgery. J Urol 152:1984.
41. Wirth M (1993). Immunotherapy for metastatic renal cell carcinoma. Urol Clin North Am 20:283.
42. Becker I, Paulus W, Roggendorf W (1989). Histogenesis of stromal cells in cerebellar hemangioblastoma. An immunohistochemical study. Am J Pathol 134:271.
43. Lodrini S, Lasio G, Cimino C, Pluchino F (1991). Hemangioblastoma: clinical characteristics, surgical results and immunohistochemical studies. J Neurosci 35:179.
44. Wizigmann-Voos S, Breier G, Risau W, Plate KH (1995). Up-regulation of vascular endothelial growth factor and its receptors in von Hippel–Lindau disease-associated and sporadic hemangioblastomas. Cancer Res 55:1358.
45. Filling-Katz MR, Choyke PL, Oldfield E, et al. (1991). Central nervous system involvement in von Hippel–Lindau disease. Neurology 41:41.
46. Neumann HPH, Eggerdt HR, Weigel K, Freidburg H, Wiestler OD, Schollmeyer P (1989). Hemangioblastomas of the central nervous system: a 10-year study with special reference to von Hippel–Lindau syndrome. J Neurosurg 70:24.
47. Choyke PL, Glenn GM, Walther MM, Patronas NJ, Linehan WM, Zbar B (1995). von Hippel–Lindau disease: genetic, clinical and imaging features. Radiology 194:629.
48. Symon L, Murota T, Pell M, Bordi L (1993). Surgical management of haemangioblastoma of the posterior fossa. Acta Neurochirurg 120:103.
49. Richardson RG, Griffin TW, Parker RG (1980). Intramedullary hemangioblastoma of the spinal cord: definitive management with irradiation. Cancer 45:49.
50. Page KA, Wayson K, Steinberg GK (1993). Stereotaxic radiosurgical ablation: an alternative treatment for recurrent and multifocal hemangioblastomas. Surg Neurol 40:424.
51. Grossniklaus HE, Thoma JW, Vigneswaran N, Jarrett WH III (1992). Retinal hemangioblastoma: a histologic, immunohistochemical ultrastructural evaluation. Ophthalmology 99:140.
52. Lamiell JM, Salazar FG, Hsia YE (1989). von Hippel–Lindau disease affecting 43 members of a single kindred. Medicine 68:1.
53. Moore AT, Maher ER, Rosen P, Gergor Z, Bird AC (1991). Ophthalmological screening for von Hippel–Lindau disease. Eye 5:723.
54. Schmidt D, Neumann HP (1995). Retinal vascular hamartoma in von Hippel–Lindau disease. Arch Ophthalmol 113:1163.
55. Neumann HP, Berger DP, Sigmund G (1993). Pheochromocytomas, multiple endocrine neoplasia type 2 and von Hippel–Lindau disease. N Engl J Med 329:1531.
56. Glenn GM, Lambert ND, Choyke P, et al. (1991). Von Hippel–Lindau (VHL) disease: distinct phenotypes suggest more than one mutant allele at the VHL locus. Hum Genet 87:207–210.
57. Walther MM, Reiter R, Keiser HR, et al. (submitted). Pheochromocytoma in von Hippel–Lindau disease: clinical and genetic characterization.
58. Richard S, Beigelman C, Duclos JM, et al. (1994). Pheochromocytoma as the first manifestation of von Hippel–Lindau disease. Surgery 116:1076.
59. Neumann HPH, Dinkel E, Brambs H, et al. (1991). Pancreatic lesions in the von Hippel–Lindau syndrome. Gastroenterology 101:465.
60. Deboever G, Dequif P, Maertens J (1992). Common bile duct obstruction due to pancreatic involvement in the von Hippel–Lindau syndrome. Am J Gastroenterol 87:1866.

61. Thompson RK, Peters JI, Sirinek KR, Levine BA (1989). von Hippel–Lindau syndrome presenting as pancreatic endocrine insufficiency: case report. Surgery 105:598.
62. Binkovitz LA, Johnson CD, Stephens DH (1990). Islet cell tumors in von Hippel–Lindau disease: increased prevalence and relationship to the multiple endocrine neoplasms. Am J Radiol 155:501.
63. Hull MT, Warfel KA, Muller J, Higgins JT (1979). Familial islet cell tumors in von Hippel–Lindau disease. Cancer 44:523.
64. Karsdorp N, Elderson A, Wittelbol-Post D, et al. (1994). von Hippel–Lindau disease: new strategies in early detection and treatment. Am J Med 97:158.
65. Chovil K, Thakore K, Choyke PL, Shawker TH, Linehan WM (1994). Scrotal sonography in normal subjects: prevalence of incidental findings. J Diagn Med Sonography 10:3.
66. Korn WT, Schatzki SC, DiSciullo AJ, Scully RE (1990). Papillary cystadenoma of the broad ligament in von Hippel–Lindau disease. Am J Obstet Gynecol 163:596.
67. Gaffey MJ, Mills SE, Boyd JC (1994). Aggressive papillary tumor of middle ear/temporal bone and adnexal papillary cystadenoma: manifestations of von Hippel–Lindau disease. Am J Surg Pathol 18:1254.
68. Palmer JM, Coker NJ, Harper RL (1989). Papillary adenoma of the temporal bone in von Hippel–Lindau disease. Otolaryngol Head Neck Surg 100:64.
69. Megerian CA, McKenna MJ, Nuss RC, et al. (1995). Endolymphatic sac tumors: histopathologic confirmation, clinical characterization, and implication in von Hippel–Lindau disease. Laryngoscope 105:801.
70. Gao J, Naglick JG, Laidlaw J, Whaley JM, Seizinger BR, Kley N (1995). Cloning and characterization of a mouse gene with homology to the human von Hippel–Lindau disease tumor suppressor gene: implications for the potential organization of the human von Hippel–Lindau disease gene. Cancer Res 55:743.
71. Duan DR, Humphrey JS, Chen DYT, et al. (1995). Characterization of the VHL tumor suppressor gene product: localization, complex formation, and the effect of natural inactivating mutations. Proc Natl Acad Sci 92:6459.
72. Iliopoulos O, Kibel A, Gray S, Kaelin WGJ (1995). Tumour suppression by the human von Hippel–Lindau gene product. Nat Med 1:822.
73. Duan DR, Pause A, Burgess WH, et al. (1995). Inhibition of transcription elongation by the VHL tumor suppressor protein. Science 269:1995.
74. Kibel A, Iliopoulos O, DeCaprio JA, Kaelin WGJ (1995). Binding of the von Hippel–Lindau tumor suppressor protein to Elongin B and C. Science 269:1444.
75. Garrett KP, Siyuan T, Bradsher JN, Lane WS, Conaway JW, Conaway RC (1994). Molecular cloning of an essential subunit of RNA Polymerase II elongation factor SIII. Proc Natl Acad Sci 91:5237.
76. Bradsher JN, Jackson KW, Conaway RC, Conaway JW (1993). RNA Polymerase II-transcription factor SII. I. Identification, purification and properties. J Biol Chem 268:25587.
77. Bradsher JN, Siyuan T, McLaury H-J, Conaway JW, Conaway RC (1993). RNA Polymerase II-transcription factor SIII. II. Functional properties and role in RNA chain elongation. J Biol Chem 268:25594.
78. Kishida T, Stackhouse TM, Chen F, Lerman MI, Zbar B (1995). Cellular proteins that bind the von Hippel–Lindau disease gene product: mapping of binding domains and the effect of missense mutations. Cancer Res 55:4544.
79. Lee S, Chen DYT, Humphrey JS, Gnarra JR, Linehan WM, Klausner RD (in press). Nuclear/cytoplasmic localization of the VHL tumor suppressor gene product is determined by cell density. Proc Natl Acad Sci.
80. Glenn GM, Choyke PL, Zbar B, Linehan WM (1990). Von Hippel–Lindau: clinical review and molecular genetics. Probl Urol 4:312.
81. Zbar B, Tory K, Merino M, et al. (1994). Hereditary papillary renal cell carcinoma. J Urol 151:561.

3. New pathologic techniques for diagnosing genitourinary malignancies

Kirk J. Wojno

As we enter the twenty-first century, early detection followed by surgical intervention is the basic paradigm for advances in cancer treatment strategies [1]. On the horizon are new therapeutic techniques incorporating our understanding about the molecular biology of cancer. Notions of gene therapy are already becoming reality, indicating the rapid advance in this area. At present, early detection and knowledge about the clinical and biologic significance of precursor states will dictate appropriate therapy, and will therefore be the focus of this chapter. For genitourinary (GU) malignancies, we will explore issues related to conventional as well as molecular screening and try to put them in perspective. This will involve a brief comment on the natural history of common neoplasms in each part of the genitourinary system (bladder, prostate, kidney, and testis), which will set the groundwork for further discussion regarding the significance of finding known genetic or molecular abnormalities. The statement by Dr. Sidransky in 1993, 'Regardless of the ultimate technique used or the precise gene markers, the identification of gene mutations in cytologic specimens will become an intimate part of cancer diagnosis and screening,' is rapidly becoming reality [2].

Neoplasia: molecular concepts

Cancer genetics

Cancer is the result of an accumulation of genetic alterations, either activation of proto-oncogenes or inactivation of tumor supressor genes which leads to a cascade of cellular events and results in abnormal cellular proliferation. An oncogene can be defined as a gene that when overexpressed contributes to carcinogenesis, progression, invasion, or metastasis, and a tumor supressor gene is a gene that when lost contributes to the same. Point mutations are commonly found in human neoplasms and involve both oncogenes and tumor supressor genes, including ras, p53, and APC, to name a few. The accumulation of such genetic changes provides a selective growth advantage to the cell population that contains them [3,4]. The goal of current tumor biology re-

Pienta, K.J., (ed.), DIAGNOSIS AND TREATMENT OF GENITOURINARY MALIGNANCIES.

search is to identify the key combination of genetic changes for each tumor type that leads to clinically significant events such as invasion or metastasis.

Tumor heterogeneity

Even though tumors are of clonal origin, by the time most are discovered or analyzed they contain tremendous heterogeneity. Heterogeneity within a single tumor exists at many levels, including cellular morphology, protein or mRNA expression, and alterations of the DNA template. Each of these levels is interrelated and dependent to a certain extent on the others. Heterogeneity is a two-edged sword: it contains tremendous information, but sampling the entire tumor is impossible. The results of any analysis of a neoplastic process are highly dependent on the sampling method and should take tumor heterogeneity into account. Doing so can be exceedingly difficult, however, because pathologic techniques examine only a minuscule fraction of the entire tumor. This is even more the case for molecular analysis than traditional histopathology. The heterogeneity found in advanced tumors is a sign of genetic instability, which in itself is an important marker of biologic behavior. It logically follows that the analysis of individual precursor lesions will not contain quite the heterogeneity of a malignant tumor that might facilitate their analysis. Also, many early genetic alterations are present in all subsequent subclones — a point exploited in many current molecular genetic analyses.

Multifocality

Synchronous head and neck tumors have been shown to have different p53 mutations, indicating that they were separate primaries rather than multifocal disease or local metastasis. Using this technique, it is possible to determine the primary origin of a lymph node metastasis [5]. Similar work is under way in bladder and prostate, both of which tend to be multifocal diseases. Work by Sakr et al. has shown that the metastases in prostate cancer are not always from the index (largest) tumor but can be from much smaller lesions with distinct genetic changes. This finding is good evidence that analysis of genetic alterations will have a role in predicting biologic behavior of tumors.

Screening and early detection

Screening definitions

Cancer screening can be defined as the process of examining a population (usually at high risk) to detect and diagnose cancer. Screening for malignancy can take place at many levels: history, physical exam, imaging, and pathologic analysis of fluids or tissues. This analysis of fluid or tissue can be at the level of the DNA template, the RNA transcript, the protein product, or the posttranslational modification. DNA analysis is now very sophisticated and can include techniques such as DNA fingerprint analysis (degree of methylation of a given gene). Molecular biology has become a leader in early cancer detection with the explosion of molecular techniques available to detect low levels of tumor markers and genetic alterations in very small samples. Mutations, translocations, amplifications, or deletions of genetic material can all be detected on very small quantities of material due to the advent of the polymerase chain reaction (PCR) and fluorescent in situ hybridization (FISH) technologies.

Pathologic screening

Screening until now has been the equivalent of diagnosis with the light microscope and the hemotoxylin and eosin or Papanicalou stain. The first neoplastic process amenable to widespread population-based screening was cervical cancer, the advent of cytologic cellular preparations made it possible to detect precancerous lesions, but only after a substantial body of evidence about the existence and progression rates of cervical precursor lesions had been established. Cervical cancer is still probably the only neoplastic process for which true asymptomatic pathologic screening is in place for the general population. This type of screening differs from the clinical screening advocated for other organ systems, such as breast (where the screening is based on imaging) or rectum (where screening boils down to a good annual digital rectal exam).

Molecular testing for elevated serum PSA is on the forefront of tumor markers that may be useful as a screening tool. This type of screening has led to increased analysis of pathologic specimens (tissue, serum, etc.) and has given rise to defined precursor lesions such as prostatic intraepithelial neoplasia (PIN) and bladder carcinoma in situ (CIS). The challenge to molecular biology is to try to define precursor lesions before they cause morphologic alterations, perhaps when these lesions are more amenable to low-risk therapeutic interventions or chemoprevention. Understanding the biology of precursor lesions at the molecular level will help determine the significance of finding certain genetic alterations in tumors and in screening specimens. Below we will discuss the major precursor lesions of the bladder (CIS), prostate (PIN), kidney (renal epithelial neoplasia/hyperplasia, and nephrogenic rests), and testis (intratubular germ cell neoplasia (ITGCN).

Molecular screening

The concept of molecular screening has been around for a while, but came to the forefront of genitourinary oncology after the publication of a New England Journal of Medicine article by Hruban et al. [6]. These authors looked at archival material from Hubert Humphrey and detected the same p53 mutation in cytologic material taken nine years before a tissue diagnosis of infiltrating carcinoma had been made [6].

Molecular screening is not restricted to tissue analysis since detection of circulating cells with reverse transcriptase polymerase chain reaction (RTPCR) may be of some value in screening for some malignancies at certain stages. New ideas for molecular screening based on host immune reactions have arisen with the finding that many patients with malignant neoplasms produce antibodies to p53 and that this seroconversion corresponds specifically to cancer with a sensitivity of 40%. Seropositivity has also been correlated with advanced disease [7].

Early detection

It is possible and even probable in the process of clonal evolution and malignant transformation that genetic alterations could precede morphologic changes [3]. To date, morphology has served well as a marker of malignant transformation, and there is evidence that changes in nuclear morphology accompany loss of tumor supressor genes [8]. However, the discrepancy between morphologic cancer and clinical behavior is extremely evident in prostate cancer, where a large proportion of the morphologic cancers will have an indolent course. Using primers made from the original tumor to screen for a specific mutation in the p53 gene, researchers have found such abnormalities in 60% of histologically benign surgical margins — a percentage that approximates the recurrence rate in head and neck cancers [9,10]. Molecular screening will need to use large numbers of oligomeric probes directed at key markers simultaneously to be able to detect a large proportion of the mutations in a certain gene that can be found in a given tumor [3]. Determining the temporal order of genetic alterations will be important in predicting the clinical behavior of neoplasms [11]. Future directions of molecular cancer screening will include newer automated techniques with pooled probes [1].

Microsatellite markers

Since many preinvasive lesions are small and therefore provide only minute samples for analysis, microsatellite markers to access allelic loss through PCR-based assays have been used instead of traditional southern blot analysis [11]. Microsatellites are tandem repeat DNA sequences that have a very high polymorphism rate in the human genome and therefore are very useful in gene mapping and linkage analysis [12]. They are also useful for the detection of a monoclonal population that has propagated a microsatellite alteration different from the germ line. This technique is simpler than characterizing and probing for mutations in tumor supressor genes, but is less sensitive by 2 to 3 orders of magnitude. This level of sensitivity may, however, prove to be enough for clinical samples. The major advantage of this technique is that it requires no knowledge about the primary tumor and is therefore more amenable to application as a screening test [12]. Multiplex PCR with additional markers may prove to enhance the sensitivity of this technique, which could then be applied as a screening technique to voided urine sample of an appropriate screening population.

Biomarker evaluation

All potential biomarkers should be shown to be independently correlated with patient outcome in a multivariate analysis of uniformly treated patients with long-term follow-up (at least five years). For prostate with a disease-specific mortality of only 7% at 10 years, such a correlation may be very difficult to show [13]. Therefore, the evaluation of biomarkers is highly dependent on the latency period of the neoplasm, which varies tremendously among genitourinary malignancies. Evaluation of precursor lesions is essential to the determination of latency period for malignant transformation. Studies of this type are highly dependent on the ease of obtaining surveillance biopsies with spatial correlation. This is difficult for solid organs such as kidney and prostate, a little more difficult for testis due to the lack of spatial information, and easiest for bladder, where detailed mapping is possible with cystoscopy.

Cost of screening

Cost and turnaround time will be the two most important factors in evaluating new methodologies for screening samples for genetic alterations. The time required for many procedures such as PCR is decreasing, and as tests become generally available, the turnaround time will only decrease further. Cost will follow shortly thereafter, but with currrent pressures to trim the cost of medical care, many tests will have to be proven to be cost effective and to improve not only diagnosis but also outcome.

Chemoprevention

Prostate carcinoma is unique in that it is one of the only GU tumors for which detection in the asymptomatic state is now possible via PSA testing (screening). With the advent of molecular biology, the door is now open for the development of new molecular assays for the detection of premalignant conditions before they are visible grossly or even by light microscopy [14,15]. The group of patients with only molecular evidence of carcinoma may derive some advantage from the employment of chemopreventative strategies [1]. Currently, several studies are under way that will examine the effect of chemopreventative agents on prostate cancer and precursor lesions such as PIN.

Mutations as screening tools

Point mutations by sequence of pooled clones

Point mutations in a specific gene can be detected by PCR amplification of a specific portion of the genome including the gene of interest, which can then be subcloned into a phage so that pooled clones can be sequenced to look for point mutations [16]. As mentioned above, this process is fairly time consuming, which may hamper its immediate implementation. The detection of mutations (i.e., p53 point mutations) with the polymerase chain reaction (PCR) not only may hold promise for screening but also may prove useful in the staging of tumors (i.e., assessment of margins) [17]. However, in order for this procedure to be of any value at the time of surgery, its turnaround time would need to be rapid enough to allow a decision to be made to alter the surgical procedure. At present, the significance of such a molecular positive margin is unknown. It will have to be determined whether the molecular positive margin in a morphologically normal sample carries with it the same risk for subsequent recurrence as the morphologically positive margin at the time of frozen section.

Point mutations as diagnostic markers of cancer

Although some researchers claim that the detection of certain point mutations is diagnostic of cancer [1], others argue that the summation of numerous genetic alterations defines the cancer phenotype [18]. Larger studies need to be done to determine the frequency with which people with point mutations in their p53 gene develop clinical tumors. The significance and timing of p53 mutations seems to be different for different cancers, being an early phenomenon in prostate cancer and a late phenomenon in colon cancer. Therefore, knowledge of the number and type of genetic alteration will be needed to prognosticate and better determine therapy. Tumor progression models will be needed for each type of cancer to prognosticate appropriately [1].

Oncogenes and tumor supressor genes as diagnostic tools

Oncogenes

Good general reviews have been written on the subject of oncogenes and tumor supressor genes [19]. These entities have been defined above. Many oncogenes have been discovered, including ABL, ERBB, GIP, GSP, MYC, RAS, RET, ROS, SAM, SIS, SRC, and TRK, to name a few [3]. The mechanisms of action for these oncogenes have been worked out to various degrees. Many are active as oncogenes when they are overexpressed by one of several mechanisms (double minutes, homogeneously staining regions, placement before another promoter). These are amenable to detection with current technology. Detection of oncogene overexpression has been shown to have prognostic value in certain tumor systems. Mutants of oncogenes that cause overexpression are uncommon and therefore are not useful as tumor markers.

Tumor supressor genes

Many tumor supressor genes have been identified, including RB, WT1, DCC, NF-1, NT-2, p53, and APC [3]. These cause tumors either by their loss or by their mutation, which causes inactivation of their normal function of keeping the potential malignant phenotype in check. Knowledge of the time course of their loss in a tumor progression model is important; i.e., p53 loss can be early or late, depending on the tumor. Mutations in some tumor supressor genes such as p53 result in the accumulation of protein due to defective clearance. This change makes them useful as diagnostic markers, because such overexpression is easily detected by immunoperoxidase technology.

Other new diagnostic techniques

Cell proliferation

Currently, several antibodies are available for the study of cell proliferation on either frozen or formalin-fixed paraffin-embedded material by standard immunohistochemical techniques. The Ki67 cell-cycle-associated antigen is present during the G1, S, G2, and M phases of the cell cycle and is therefore a useful marker of proliferation activity. Monoclonal antibody MIB1 and polyclonal antibody Ki67 recognize parts of the Ki67 antigen that survive formalin fixation. KiS1 recognizes a cell-cycle-associated antigen expressed during DNA synthesis. Currently, there is a wealth of other cell-cycle-associated antigens under development [20].

Apoptosis (programmed cell death) can be measured by the detection of fragmented DNA with the TUNEL assay (terminal deoxyribonucleotidyl-transferase-mediated dUTP-digoxigenin nick end labeling). However, this assay is not specific for apoptosis and will also stain necrosis. These findings may indicate that DNA fragmentation is a final common pathway for many forms of necrosis and not specific. Other methods, such as DNA ladders and electron microscopy, should remain the gold standard for now [21]. The apoptotic index is a useful prognostic indicator in certain tumor systems, but at present, tumor heterogeneity with respect to the rate of apoptosis and nonuniformity in enumeration methods have limited its overall utility. Although cumbersome and difficult to perform in paraffin-embedded material, flow cytometry has overcome problems of reproducibility and tumor heterogeneity by looking at a relatively large sample size. Its incorporation with other proliferation markers to determine an overall proliferation index offers promising results.

Angiogenesis

To date, measurement of angiogenesis has met with the same methodological problems in enumeration as has the proliferation index. Techniques such as flow cytometry are not amenable to counting blood vessels. Sophisticated computer-assisted counting methods have been used with some success, but they have not yet gained widespread acceptance. To date, correlation with tumor stage has been shown in prostate cancer by the work of several investigators, including work in our own laboratory. Of more interest is the mechanism by which tumors grow blood vessels and the potential benefit from inhibiting this blood vessel growth. Recent work by John Carroll and others (John Carroll, personal communication) has shown a possible relationship between angiogenesis and inflammatory cells such as mast cells. It has been shown that tumors produce increased cytokines (Interleukin B) that attract mast cells. Mast cells then are capable of degranulating and releasing basic fibroblast growth factor, which is a potent angiogenic factor. It is interesting to speculate that the tumor is using our normal wound-healing mechanism in a perverse manner to grow blood vessels that will allow it to have more aggressive behavior.

Complex adaptive systems and fractals

Recent work by Schwab and Pienta looking at chaos theory and complex adaptive systems such as multicellular organisms and neoplasia has shown that the application of chaos and antichaos theory to predict attractor states may be useful in trying to understand cancer biology and predict the key variables. This theory differs from other current theories in that it heavily relies on initial conditions to predict stable attractor states (Pienta, personal communication). We are currently exploring fractal analysis as a method of grading prostate neoplasia. Preliminary studies would indicate that the architectural pattern of prostate neoplasia has a fractal dimension, and since the current grading system (Gleason) is based solely on architectural pattern and is very predictive of tumor behavior, there is a good chance that fractal analysis by the box-counting method may provide a useful and reproducible grading method that would be inexpensive and cost effective. If prostate cancer is found to have a true fractal dimension, then this dimension should be independent of magnification and sample size and would therefore be of great utility in the interpretation of prostate needle biopsies, especially in predicting the pathologic grade of the tumor in the radical prostatectomy specimen.

Techniques

X inactivation. New techniques in the analysis of neoplasia have been uses in GYN oncology and may have a place in the analysis of GU tumors. In females, it can be determined which X chromosome is inactivated (inactivated X is highly methylated, therefore, using methylation-dependent restriction enzymes such as NOT1, one can determine which X chromosome is inactivated). In its normal state, the body is a mosaic of X chromosome inactivation. In a neoplasm (monoclonal proliferation), the same X chromosome is inactivated in all the cells. This finding may have a role in the analysis of low-grade papillary proliferations to determine whether they are true neoplasms or papillary hyperplasia.

Immunoperoxidase. Immunoperoxidase technology to detect protein expression at the cellular level has been widely available in diagnostic laboratories for well over a decade. Traditionally, one of the major problems with immunoperoxidase staining has been reproducibility of the staining technique. Now, however, with the advent of automated (robotic) immunoperoxidase staining instruments, the technique has become very reproducible. The main chanllenge ahead is to overcome tumor heterogeneity and to develop better quantitation. Currently, the lack of reproducible, well-defined criteria for the assessment of staining has impeded the development of new biomarkers that appear to be sensitive to tumor heterogeneity (i.e., c-erB-2) [22].

In situ. In situ hybridization and in situ RT PCR have arrived, and quantitative RT-PCR is on the way and will be developed shortly [23]. This approach will allow for the determination of the level of gene amplification in specific cell populations. Automated in situ instruments are just becoming available, and they should have the same impact as automated immunoperoxidase [24].

FISH. Automated fluorescent in situ hybridization (FISH) will also be possible on in situ instruments. This degree of automation should facilitate the development of assays that are reproducible on paraffin-embedded tissue sections. The main advantage of FISH is that genetic abnormalities can be localized to the exact cell population of interest.

Image analysis. Image analysis systems are constantly evolving and becoming better at semiquantitative analysis. The problem is that, in order to overcome tumor heterogeneity, large numbers of cells need to be analyzed. This generates a tremendous amount of data, which will be best analyzed with neural networks.

Neural networks. Neural networks will be needed to understand the large quantities of very complex data being generated with current automated instruments. In order for this approach to work, however, standards need to be developed, calibrated, and used by multiple institutions so that large quantities of data can be analyzed by these neural network systems.

Nuclear matrix. Embedment-free electron microscopy has opened the door to the study of nuclear matrix free from the artifacts of conventional plastic-embedded sections. Most of the non-protein-coding portion of the genome, which represents 90% of the genome, probably codes instructions for structure. At some level, structure and morphology are inexorably tied together. To quote Sheldon Penman, '. . . future cell scientists will marvel at the density and ingenuity of genomic instructions for structure while wondering how we could have overlooked them for so long' [25]. Immunoperoxidase techniques with antibodies directed at the nuclear matrix are currently being explored and may be useful as diagnostic markers. PC1 antibody appears to be a specific marker for prostate cancer, but currently it only works on frozen tissue. Additional study is needed, but this marker has the potential to be a very useful diagnostic tool (Allan Partin, personal communication).

Bladder

Outline of clinical issues

Of the over 50,000 new cases of bladder cancer diagnosed each year, 70% present with superficial disease, while 30% present with muscle-invasive disease or metastasis. Of the localized superficial disease, approximately 70% will recur, with 30% showing grade and stage progression. About half of those with muscle-invasive disease will develop metastasis, even with aggressive local therapy [26]. Therefore, markers that could identify the 50% of high-grade superficial tumors that are prone to muscle invasion would be useful [27]. Developing good screening tools to identify all patients with localized superficial disease and being able to predict which of these patients will progress and with what time course are the main diagnostic goals in this area. Recent work in molecular biology and cancer genetics, along with the automation of many techniques like immunoperoxidase, in situ hybridization, and PCR, has allowed major progress in this area.

Precursor lesions

Flat transitional cell carcinoma in situ is thought to be a major precursor lesion in the urinary bladder. There is more debate about the possible role of low-grade papillary neoplasia (papilloma and grade 1 papillary TCC) as precursor lesions; these proliferative states may only indicate that the patient is at higher risk for development of invasive carcinoma. Utilizing current biomarkers (genetic and other) to determine which of these lesions will be clinically significant is a laudable goal. The following sections will describe the current state of the art with regard to clinically useful biomarkers and diagnostic tools.

Heterogeneity

Although the concept of monoclonality is important to an understanding of neoplasia at a certain level, it is now clear that tumors are heterogeneous when examined at the molecular level. It is the genetic instability itself that gives tumors an advantage and is responsible for their diversity. Heterogeneity exists at many levels: morphology, patterns of recurrence, and progression. Conventional histology is not able to tell the whole story, and therefore additional markers (genetic, molecular, etc.) can provide additional information.

Molecular genetics

Genetic analysis can take place at several levels: from course to fine and from the chromosome to the gene. The results of numerous such investigations have provided enough information to model the genetic alterations of neoplastic progression to malignancy. Microsatellite alterations are frequent events in bladder neoplasia and therefore provide easy access to look for genetic loss in a given region [28]. Deletions have been reported in chromosomes 3p, 6q, 9q, 9p21, 11p, 13q, 17p, and 18q. Such genetic loss suggests that these locations may harbor tumor supressor genes. These locations may also serve as useful diagnostic markers. Several correlations of genetic loss with morphologic progression (e.g., 9q is present early in bladder cancer, 17p LOH is important in invasion [29], and 3p and 6q LOH correlate with progression [26]) have led to the following genetic model of progression [39]:

Superficial noninvasive	9q
Invasion	3p, 5q, 17p, 9p
Late/progression	4p, 6q, 8p, 11p, 13q, 14q, 18q

Some important facts about some of the above-noted genetic alterations and about others that do not fit well into this model are briefly described below. In most bladder cancers, there is loss of all of chromosome 9 [30]. Several lines of evidence suggest that the tumor supressor gene CDKN2 located at 9p21 is not the only tumor supressor gene in this region [31,32]. Noninvasive lesions seem to have 9q loss, while invasive lesions have 9p loss. Inactivation of a gene on chromosome 9q appears to be important in bladder cancer initiation [33,34]. Other important regions of loss include 14q12, which is lost in 25% of bladder tumors [35], and 8p deletions in invasive bladder tumors [36] MDM2 protein abnormalities (gene location 12q13–14) are associated with bladder cancer, but there is no evidence of gene amplification [37]. Frequent genetic losses occur on 9q, 11p, and 17p, which would indicate that these sites contain putative tumor supressor genes [17]. Papillary tumors are different than carcinoma in situ with reference to p53 mutation and chromosome 9 alterations, and therefore these tumors may reflect different pathways of progression. Detecting these differences may be useful diagnostically, since chromosome 9 abnormalities occur early in papillary neoplasms and p53 abnormalities occur early in CIS [38].

Interphase cytogenetics with FISH have been useful in identifying numerical abnormalities, which correlate with progression on chromosomes 1, 7, 9, 11, and 18 [39].

X inactivation studies have shown that multiple tumors in the same bladder were of the same clone, i.e., came from the same cell [33]. This finding has implications for interpretation of bladder neoplasia in general, since some cases are more likely spread from a primary rather than from a field effect.

Tumor supressor genes

Tumor supressor genes code for elements involved in the regulation of the cell cycle or of cell growth and differentiation [26]. The term *tumor suppressor genes* arose because the loss of cell cycle regulation gives rise to uncontrolled cell proliferation and hence, potentially, to a tumor. Two key tumor supressor genes in bladder cancer are Rb and p53.

Rb (13q14) encodes a nuclear phosphoprotein (DNA binding domain) that plays a central role in the control of cell division and differentiation. It is inactivated by phosphorylation, which occurs in S phase and G2/M. LOH and altered protein expression (immunoperoxidase) are prognostic indicators in bladder cancer [26]. Altered Rb expression by immunoperoxidase is a late event in the progression of human bladder cancer [40]. Tumors with altered Rb protein expression (decreased staining) have a more aggressive behavior [41].

p53 (17p13.1) encodes a nuclear phosphoprotein involved in transcriptional control of cell proliferation. It serves as a regulatory checkpoint, arresting cells in the G1 phase to allow the cell to undertake DNA repair. Mutations cause nonfunctional protein accumulation that has a prolonged half life and can be measured by immunoperoxidase. There is a good correlation between increased p53 expression and worse prognosis [26]. Not all mutations result in overexpression [45] Nuclear immunoreactivity correlates with intragenic mutations. Some mutations cause truncation of the protein with loss of the signal for nuclear localization. Immunoperoxidase with PAb1801 and PAb240 showed 90% accuracy in detecting p53 mutations when compared to the combination of RFLP, SSCP, and sequencing. From these findings, it can be concluded that the vast majority of p53 mutations can be detected with immunoperoxidase staining in a reliable reproducible manner [42]. p53 mutations in bladder cancer are typically GC $\rightarrow$ CG and AT $\rightarrow$ GC and are thought to result from aromatic amines present in the bladders of cigarette smokers [43]. p53 nuclear overexpression has independent prognostic value for survival in patients with invasive bladder cancer treated with neoadjuvant chemotherapy. Randomized clinical trials stratified by p53 status in the neoadjuvant setting are under way [44]. In one study, grade was better than the p53 immunoperoxidase status for predicting progression. However, immunoperoxidase has many problems with objective, reproducible interpretations, as does nuclear grading [45].

Oncogenes

c-erB-2 is closely related to epidermal growth factor receptor, which has been shown to be overexpressed in bladder tumors [65,46]. c-erB-2 expression seems to correlate with stage and grade of bladder tumors [47], but this point is controversial; some studies state that it does not correlate with stage or grade [48]. Correlation of gene amplification by differential PCR (which involves amplification of a reference gene (a known single copy) and a target gene (unknown copies) within the same reaction tube) correlated with progression, but protein overexpression measured by immunoperoxidase could not be correlated with progression. In a multivariate analysis, stage and grade were still more powerful predictors of recurrence or progression. c-erB-2 may be useful as a diagnostic marker but not as a prognostic marker, since only 47% of tumors stained [49]. Problems with differential PCR to detect amplification include tumor heterogeneity and stromal contamination.

H-ras was cloned from the T24 bladder cancer cell line, and even though the hope was that this oncogene would play an important role in bladder cancer, H-ras has subsequently been found in only 10% of bladder tumors examined [50,51]. A recent prospective study found H-ras mutations in 44% of urine cytology specimens — a finding that was able to add significant sensitivity to cytology alone [52].

More genetics

Five-year survival varies tenfold, from 90% to 9%, for localized vs. distantly metastatic disease [53]. Clonal p53 mutations detected in urothelium to date are conceptually thought to be specific for bladder neoplasia. However, reports of sensitivity have hovered around 60% [17,54]. When present in the primary tumor, these p53 mutations can be detected in the urine in a large proportion of patients [55]. The large number of reported mutations would make it difficult to employ screening with this technique unless pooled probes were developed [17]. Even though molecular biology is rapidly advancing, light microscopic examination still remains the gold standard to which all other techniques must be compared [56].

Microsatellite alterations in the tetranucleotide sequence (AAAG) occur in 15% of transitional cell carcinomas of the bladder. The finding of this abnormality would indicate a clonal population of cells and therefore a neoplasm. However, other repeat sequences studied had a much lower yield in the bladder than in other organs. The combination of seven markers would be able to detect 28% of neoplasms by this technique [12]. Multiplex PCR with a mixture of many primers may also be useful.

Comparative genomic hybridization uses DNA from normal and tumor samples labeled with two different fluorochromes to probe the genome (normal karyotype) looking for gain or loss of genetic material. When this technique was applied to bladder cancer, amplification of 16q21–q22, and 6p22 were noted [57,58].

DNA content and cell cycle

Ninety-seven percent of flat CIS is aneuploid, and patients with multiple aneuploid populations have a worse prognosis [59]. The high rate of aneuploid in CIS makes it difficult to construe this as a useful prognosticator. However, DNA ploidy may have a role in predicting the behavior of grade 2 tumors.

Cell surface antigens

Blood-group antigens have received some attention in bladder cancer. The glactosyltransferase coding for the A and B blood-group antigens resides on 9q34. Loss of 9q is an early event in bladder carcinogenesis and occurs in 60% of cases [39]. Lewis X is not present on normal adult urothelium. The finding of Lewis X on the urothelium is a good indicator of neoplasia. However, this finding is only good in secretors, who make up 75% of the population. It appears to be useful for cancer detection and does correlate with stage. One potential pitfall is that some nonneoplastic umbrella cells can be positive [60]. Use of P12 monoclonal antibody to detect Lewis X can increase the sensitivity of cytology for the detection of noninvasive bladder cancer. This approach may also be useful in follow-up of therapeutic response and tumor recurrence [61].

Tumor-associated antigens

Monoclonal antibodies directed against bladder-tumor-associated antigens OM5, 19A211, and M344 have been associated with superficial tumors and only OM5 staining for normal. T43, T138, and G4-E7 preferentially stain invasive tumors. Mano4/4 and 486P3/12 stain only neoplasms but cannot distinguish invasive from noninvasive lesions [62].

Differentiation antigens T43 and T138 are monoclonal antibodies to bladder-cancer-related antigens that are not expressed in the benign urothelium or low-grade tumors [63].

E-cadherin has decreased expression in invasive bladder tumors [64]. Integrins are important in cellular adhesion [65], and Integrin a6b4 has increased expression in bladder cancer.

Growth factors

Cathepsin D loss correlates with grade and stage in univariate analysis, but was not significant in multivariate analysis of survival where only stage was significant for overall survival [66]. Epidermal growth factor level is significantly reduced in bladder cancer patients and may serve as a marker of malignancy [67].

At this time, only a few molecular markers — namely, EGFR, Rb, and p53 — seem to have definite prognostic value and need to be studied in prospective trials [68].

Receptor

The cell-surface receptor for hyaluronic acid, CD44, is expressed by both normal and malignant urothelial cells. Numerous CD44 isoforms have recently been identified that are derived by alternative ribonucleic acid splicing.

Individual variant exons in and of themselves are not specific for carcinoma, but retention of introns seems to be specific for bladder neoplasia [69,70]. PCR-based assays or in situ hybridization with riboprobes may be a powerful diagnostic tool, as well as a means to follow recurrence.

Angiogenesis

Tumor angiogenesis correlates with lymph node status in invasive bladder cancer. Maximum vascular density counts of 186/mm^2 were noted as the mean for cases with metastatic disease, while counts of 75/mm^2 were noted for nonmetastatic cases [71].

Urine screening

Urine chemical screening for CA 19.9 can be a very sensitive marker for bladder cancer in high-risk populations. However, before this technique can gain general acceptance, it needs to have Bayes' theorem applied [72]. High levels of CA 19.9 and TPA correlate with poor prognosis and could be useful in follow-up of bladder cancer patients [73]. Beta-glucuronidase activity is higher in those with TCC and renal cell carcinoma and is much higher than in renal cytologies [74]. Cadherin levels can be detected in the urine by immunoblot technique [75] and may be increased in cancer patients, but further study including quantitation is needed.

Ten percent of bladder cancer patients have elevated serum BHCG, but there are confilcting results about the predictive value of this measure with reference to stage [76,77]. Altered transcription patterns of BHCG by RT-PCR have been shown in bladder cancer compared to normal bladder [78].

Prostate

Clinical issues

In 1995, 244,000 U.S. men were diagnosed with prostate cancer [79]. Recently, it has been estimated that prostate cancer has a 479-day doubling time. Therefore, it would take 40 years for one cell to become a pathologically detectable 1-cm tumor [80]. Prostate cancer is diagnosed in 1 of 11 males in the U.S., with 65% having clinically organ-confined disease amenable to surgical therapy. However, of those who undergo surgery, only 50% are found to have organ-confined disease [81]. Which patients have tumors that will become clinically significant in their lifetime and will need radical treatment, and which patients are potentially amenable to a watchful waiting strategy? Which patients treated with surgery will progress and may benefit from early adjuvant therapy? Although tumor grading with the Gleason system has made initial inroads into some of these questions, we currently need a better way to predict prognosis for the 75% of cases with a Gleason grade between 5 and 7, where this system has little prognostic power [81].

Prognostication can take place at many levels, all of which may be interlinked. Morphologic changes occur with the development of neoplasia, and better assessment of these changes in a reproducible manner may lead to better prognostication. These include changes at the nuclear, cellular, glandular, and stromal levels. Partin et al. see cell motility, growth rate, nuclear shape, DNA content, and membrane charge as areas that have been shown to be of some utility and that therefore deserve to be tested in large clinical trials [81]. New molecular techniques now allow for detection of changes in the DNA template, RNA transcript, and protein expression, these are also fruitful areas that need further investigation in large trials, and they will be discussed further below.

Precursor lesions

High-grade PIN has been associated with cancer at the biologic, morphologic, and genetic levels. There is good evidence that this lesion is the precursor to adenocarcinoma of the prostate, and therefore some researchers have suggested it as a good target for chemoprevention studies [82].

Hereditary and genetic aspects of prostate cancer

Molecular biology of prostate cancer. The molecular biology of prostate cancer has been well reviewed [83]. Between 5% and 10% of all prostate cancer and 40% of early onset prostate cancer are familial, with a Mendelian inheritance pattern proposed to be autosomal dominant [84,89]. Use of this familial information will aid the search for prostate-specific genetic alterations (germline and somatic) that will allow screening for prostate cancer. These markers may also help define which tumors will be clinically significant — especially those that occur in a younger age group, where a great proportion are likely to be clinically significant in the lifetime of the patient.

Comparative genomic hybridization has determined that losses are five times more common than gains and most often involved 8p, 13q, 6q, 16q, 18q, and 9p [85]. This technique has proven valuable in determining areas of the genome that deserve further investigation. In conjunction with other techniques such as microsatellite markers looking for LOH, this technique has also documented chromosome abnormalities in prostate cancer, including loss on chromosomes 1, 2, 5, 7, 7q, 8p, 10q, and 16q and gains on chromosomes 7, 14, 20, and 22 [86–89]. Tumors that recur have frequent gains in 7, 8q, and X [85]. Recent studies have shown a deletion in 8p22 in 70% of prostate cancers in both early and late disease — evidence that strongly suggests the presence of a tumor supressor gene in this region. Looking for this common deletion could be very useful in the staging of prostate cancer and potentially in the evaluation of margins [90]. Molecular probing after nonsurgical treatment such as radiation therapy may aid us in the evaluation of postradiation biopsies.

According to the molecular progression schema that have been proposed based on the summary of genetic alterations to date, germline mutations and hypermethylation of 17 and 8p loss are early events and contribute to histologic prostate cancer, but 16 loss, RB loss, p53 loss, and decreased e-cadherin are late events as tumors acquire metastatic potential [91].

Altered DNA methylation patterns have been noted in a majority of cases [81], a finding that may prove to yield valuable information.

Coupling information on genetic instability and on clonal selection for a given tumor has great potential to yield prognostic information [92]. For example, if the important genetic alterations for prostate cancer progression were known, and the rate at which additional alterations were acquired was also known (estimate of genetic instability), then one could predict at which time the tumor would acquire significant biologic potential. With this information, an appropriate treatment strategy could be planned.

Oncogenes. Oncogenes studied in prostate cancer include ras, myc, c-sis, bcl-2, and c-erB-2. ras and myc oncogenes have been most extensively studied in prostate cancer. Infrequent structural alterations have been noted, with the most common scenario being altered transcription [93].

Ras is a signal-transduction G protein that transfers information from outside the cell to the nucleus. Mutations in ras stimulate proliferation, even in the absence of external signals. Racial differences exist in mutation rates (low in U.S. and high in Japan — a difference of 25%) [94]. ras expression has been studied with immunoperoxidase and found to be correlated with tumor grade [93,95]. However, ras p21 immunoperoxidase staining lacks specificity for cancer and therefore will not be useful as a diagnostic tool [96,97].

The c-myc protein product is involved in cell growth and differentiation. The protein product is expressed in 70% of BPH and T1a cancers [98]. c-myc copy-number gains can be detected by FISH, and protein overexpression can be detected by immunoperoxidase. Altered protein expression has been found in low-stage and low-grade prostate cancer. myc expression appears to have an inverse correlation with differentiation [99]. Gene amplifications is a rare cause of protein overexpression [100].

c-erB-2 is located on chromosome 17q21. c-erbB-2 overexpression and changes in subcellular distribution appear to be an early event in prostate cancer. Both metastasis and primary tumors have similar staining patterns [101]. These alterations have also been identified in PIN [102–104]. c-erbB-2 needs further study to define its role in the prognostication of prostate cancer [105].

Altered c-met proto-oncogene expression is frequently detected in PIN and high-grade cancer [106]. Again these findings are only preliminary, and further study is needed to determine whether this marker will be useful in the diagnosis and management of prostate cancer.

bcl-2 will be discussed in the section on apoptosis.

Tumor supressor genes. The tumor supressor genes most studied in prostate cancer are RB, p53, and e-cadherin [107–111]. Whereas mutations of oncogenes are common in some tumors, genetic loss is much more common in prostate cancer.

RB phosphoprotein product acts as a brake on the cell cycle: it prevents cells in G1 from entering S phase. The discordance of Rb LOH with protein expression loss by immunohistochemistry suggests another tumor supressor gene in the region of 13q14 [112,113]. Forty-five percent of clinically localized prostate cancer has evidence of allelic loss on 13q. Lack of correlation with Rb protein expression is evidence for a novel tumor supressor gene in the region distal to RB [114].

p53 (17p) phosphoprotein arrests cells in G1. This gene is frequently mutated (point mutations). Mutations are associated with abnormal cellular metabolism and resultant cellular accumulation, which can be detected by immunoperoxidase techniques. p53 overexpression occurs in 28% of prostate cancers and correlates with grade and presence of metastatic disease [115].

The most frequent sites of genetic loss are 7, 8p22, 10, and 16q; these are also possible sites of novel tumor supressor genes [93,116]. There also appears to be a novel tumor supressor gene centromeric to brca1 on 17q21 [117].

FISH has proven to be a valuable tool in prostate cancer. As technology advances and automated systems become available, this trend will continue. FISH has detected genetic abnormalities in prostate cancer on chromosomes 7, 8, 10, 11, 12, and 22 [118,119].

Although several tumor supressor genes have been characterized and several more have been postulated, no prostate-specific tumor gene has yet been identified. As our knowledge increases about the interrelationships of these genetic alterations, we will be able to use them as diagnostic and prognostic tests in our battle against prostate cancer.

Metastasis supressor gene. Knowledge of the cellular and molecular changes associated with acquisition of metastatic potential will allow appropriate substaging so that appropriate decisions can be made about therapy [120]. Although local extraprostatic extension is important and correlates with risk of progression, it is the ability of the tumor to metastasize that is the clinically significant event that will eventually lead to the patient's demise. The e-cadherin gene located on 16q22.1 has been found to have alterations in half of prostate cancer cases. Low or altered expression of e-cadherin correlates with higher grade and metastasis [92,121,122]. KAI1 appears to be a metastasis supressor gene [79]. Tumors that express KAI1 are much less metastatic than those that do not. These markers may be useful predictors of a tumor's metastatic potential.

Ploidy

Ploidy by traditional methods (Fulgen staining) is crude at best. It has provided insight into the fact that information is available in numerical chromosome abnormalities. The major factor limiting its utility is the fact that 80% of prostate cancer is diploid, and at present there are no grounds to make clinical decisions (i.e., deny radical therapy) based on the finding of aneuploid status. New, more sensitive methods such as FISH with alpha satellite probes for centromere counting, directed at hot spots such as 7 and 8, may be much more powerful biomarkers for prognostication [123]. At present, ploidy is only useful for determining which T3 or higher lesion is likely to be hormone responsive [13].

Proliferation markers

MIB1 has been shown to be the antibody of choice for the determination of cell proliferation activity in formalin-fixed prostate tissue [124]. Staining with this method has the best chance to be a useful and widely used marker when used as a component of a proliferation index.

Apoptosis

Apoptosis is defined as programmed cell death. It is an active, energy-requiring process that requires the activation of several genes. c-fos is involved in signal transduction and is thought to play a regulatory role in apoptosis. Bcl-2 is the most widely studied regulator of apoptosis; it inhibits apoptosis, which is important in follicular lymphomas, and has been shown to be overexpressed in hormone refractory prostate cancer [125]. Both sis and fos expression are turned on by androgens, which may be a clue to the regulation of apoptosis by the cell [126].

Nuclear matrix protein

Nuclear matrix protein PC-1 stains only prostate cancer. It is currently only available for frozen tissue but may soon be available for formalin-fixed material [127]. pp32 is a newly described marker that stains a nuclear phosphoprotein expressed in cells competent for self-renewal. It stains PIN and high-grade cancers, but further study is needed to access its utility as a diagnostic or prognostic marker. An antibody that works on formalin-fixed tissue will soon be available [128].

Multivariate analysis

Multivariate analysis of nuclear shape, Gleason grade, and her2/neu and PCNA (immunoperoxidase) correlate with progression. Multivariate analyses such as this need to be carried out, because a combination of markers will be required to correctly predict the progression status of patients [129,130]. We should be looking not just at biochemical progression but also at metastasis and disease-specific mortality.

Univariate analysis is important in identifying potential biomarkers, but these need to be combined with others and tested in a multivariate analysis against standard prognosticators such as stage and grade to determining their ability to prognosticate. We must also be mindful of the cost of these new tests in this era of cost containment. Many of these markers may help us understand the disease, but few will have clinical utility.

Growth factors

The major growth factor studied in prostate cancer is EGFR, but to date there are conflicting data regarding its prognostic utility [131,132].

Other markers

Cathepsin D is important in invasion and metastasis, and increased expression correlates with grade and stage in prostate cancer [133]. Elevated 12-Limmunoperoxidaseygenase mRNA correlates with advanced stage and poor differentiation [134]. PTH-LP is expressed in neuroencocrine cells and in the majority of cancers and PIN such that its altered expression and its autocrine function is an early event in prostate cancer tumorogenesis (Dr. Cheryl Lee, personal communication).

Microdissection

Microdissection is essential, especially in a heterogeneous tumor like prostate cancer. This procedure is especially necessary when one is looking for genetic loss, because contaminating normal tissue, PIN, or another morphology of cancer may mask potentially meaningful results [135]. Tumor heterogeneity is the biggest problem to the genetic study of prostate cancer. Both separation of tumor from stroma and the inherent genetic heterogeneity present in tumors that are often multifocal are currently hampering efforts in this area.

Altered glycolsylation

Other evidence of altered glycosylation in prostate cancer is offered by work on Lewis-X, which has altered expression in prostate cancer [136].

Best possible biomarkers for chemoprevention studies

There is no clear-cut consensus as to the relative importance of the vast array of biomarkers in tumorogenesis or progression [137]. A consensus panel statement has recommended nuclear roundness, MIB-1, ploidy, c-erbB-2, angiogensis, and high-grade PIN as surrogate endpoint biomarkers [82]. A proliferation index may be useful with incorporation of MIB-1 staining and apoptosis [138].

Angiogenesis

Tumor growth and metastasis are dependent on the development of blood vessels, therefore, a switch to a highly angiogenic phenotype is important in the development of large-volume tumors and the ability to metastasize [120]. Preliminary evidence indicates that angiogenesis may be a useful prognostic marker for prostate cancer. Current research is hampered by sampling issues. Methods of counting vessels have included an average of randomly chosen fields versus finding the area of maximal angiogenesis and counting that region. This area of investigation has much potential as a potential therapeutic target.

Kidney

Clinical issues

Renal cell carcinoma makes up 3% of adult malignancies, and Wilm's tumor makes up 8% of childhood solid malignancies. Due to the widespread use of improved imaging techniques, many renal tumors are diagnosed incidentally. While renal tumors are much less common than prostate cancer and bladder cancer, they are usually very aggressive tumors at the time of diagnosis. As we find more and more small (0.3–3 cm) tumors by imaging, we will need to have methods to correctly diagnose and classify these tumors. Molecular genetic analysis of fine needle aspirates of these lesions may in the future be able to correctly classify these tumors prior to resection due to characteristic patterns of genetic alteration currently being observed in the research laboratory.

Precursor lesions

Renal epithelial hyperplasia and small renal epithelial tumors of low malignant potential (formally called adenomas) are the best candidates for precursor lesions to renal cell carcinoma; however, this hypothesis will be difficult to prove, since this retroperitoneally located solid organ is not easily sampled for pathologic analysis. Nephrogenic rests are the best candidate for precursor lesion of Wilm's tumor.

Molecular biology

Loss of any 3p alleles occurs in 96% of evaluable cases of renal cell carcinoma. Genetic alterations of 5q and 17p occur in only 53% and 35% of cases, respectively [139]. Loss of 17p and 18 along with increased dosage of 5q and 7 is correlated with advanced disease and poor prognosis [140,141]. LOH at 3p appears to be specific to clear cell nonpapillary renal cell carcinoma. As opposed to 90% of renal cell carcinomas that have deletions on 3p, papillary tumors have retained this genetic material. Papillary tumors have triploidy of chromosomes 7 and 17 and loss of Y [141]. FISH for chromosome 7 has been used to differentiate papillary form nonpapillary tumors. The biologic significance of papillary renal cell carcinoma as diagnosed by light microscopy is unclear, since there have been conflicting reports as to the biologic significance of these lesions. Since this group of tumors is genetically distinct, it will be important to determine if these genetic findings have true biologic significance [142].

Screening and diagnosis by linkage analysis may be appropriate for von Hippel–Lindau (VHL) kindreds so that those who are carriers may be screened and followed appropriately, and so that the cost and bother of screening noncarriers within kindreds may be relieved [143].

Tumor supressor genes

The VHL tumor supressor gene on chromosome 3p26 is lost in the vast majority of sporadic kidney cancers (85%) [144]. Since this abnormality is so in kidney cancer, it may be useful as a diagnostic marker on FNA and urine specimens to screen for sporadic renal cell carcinomas.

Oncogenes

There is little evidence that oncogene mutations will be useful as diagnostic or prognostic markers, in contrast to their value in other tumor systems.

Other tumor markers

Expression of basic fibroblast growth factor correlates with poor prognosis in kidney tumors [145]. bFGF, which is found in mast cell granules, has been correlated with angiogenesis in certain tumor systems.

Collecting duct cancer

Collecting duct carcinoma does not have 3p loss but instead losses of 8p and 13q, each in about 50% of cases. In this group of tumors, 8p LOH is associated with higher stage and poorer prognosis. Both these losses may represent sites of tumor supressor genes; in fact, the chromosomal loss in 13 has been shown to be the RB gene [146]. This may be a useful marker for prognostication in this group of tumors.

Oncocytomas

Oncocytomas show no loss at 3p, a finding that would be useful in the analysis of oncocytic lesions on needle biopsy. No genetic alterations are known [141].

Studies of the mitochondrial genetics of these lesions, characterized by accumulation of mitochondria in the cytoplasm, may shed light in this area.

Chromophobe cell carcinomas

Chromophobe cell carcinoma has genetic alterations in 3p, 5q, and 17 in a combination that does not occur in other kidney tumors [147].

Proliferation activity

Proliferation-activity labeling with Ki67 adds prognostic information in renal cell carcinoma [148,149].

Wilm's tumor

Wilm's tumors have genetic loss on 11p13, where the transcription-factor genes WT-1 and WIT-1 reside [150]. Both 11p13 and 11p15 are important in Wilm's tumor; WT-1 is thought to function like a tumor supressor gene [151]. The WT-2 gene on chromosome 11p15 is also thought to be of importance in Wilm's tumor biology. Genomic imprinting is important for WT-2, because it is almost always the maternal gene that is lost [152]. Since mutation of the WT gene is rare (%), the fact that several genes seem to be important in tumorogenesis screening for mutations may not be useful. There may be some predictive value in the diversity of genetic alterations in a given tumor. These alterations may also be useful in a pooled format when surgical washing fluids are looked at as part of operative staging.

Serum and urine markers may be of some value in the diagnosis and management of Wilm's tumor, but further study is needed to clarify their role. Serum renin is a marker of nephroblastoma and correlates with stage of disease [153]. Urinary hyaluronic acid is elevated in patients with Wilm's tumor and is correlated with stage [154].

Future diagnostics for kidney

There is a need for improvement in the diagnosis and prognostication of renal cell carcinoma, especially because a greater proportion of tumors are being identified at a small size. It is these tumors that are most amenable to this new technology. If one could biopsy a small lesion and determine whether it had any of several identified genetic defects, then one could predict cell type and possibly behavior in many cases. For example, it would be valuable to know if a 2-cm tumor were an oncocytoma, which could then be amenable to more conservative therapy, i.e., partial nephrectomy or even watchful waiting. An FNA that shows oncocytic cells currently cannot distinguish between an oncocytoma and renal cell areas of oncocytic change. No genetic loss on 3p would be strong evidence in favor of an oncocytoma. If 3p losses were identified on cells from an FNA by FISH analysis, this finding would exclude an oncocytoma and establish the diagnosis of renal cell carcinoma. Since the therapies for these lesions are markedly different, knowledge of the diagnosis prior to nephrectomy would be of great value.

Testis

Clinical issues

In no other organ is tumor heterogeneity as great as in testicular germ cell tumors. Although these are most common neoplasm in the young adult male population, there are only 6000 cases and 350 deaths of testicular cancer annually in the U.S. However, the incidence appears to be rising [155]. Markers to better define clinical stage and progression are needed to better determine which patients need aggressive therapy after diagnosis. The diagnosis and therapy of testicular tumors are very good for an otherwise aggressive neoplasm. Cure rates well above 90% are achievable in most instances. New diagnostics have the potential to make the most difference in identifying germ cell tumors in other locations and in differentiating them from other malignancies, most of which have a poor prognosis and are not amenable to therapy. Also, since the morphologic diversity of testis germ cell tumors is great, with very little in the way of prognostic information related to this morphologic diversity, perhaps there is prognostic information in the genetic alterations harbored in this group of neoplasms.

Precursor lesions

Intratubular germ cell neoplasia (ITGCN) is the best candidate for a precursor lesion of germ cell tumors (GCTs) of the testis. ITGCN carries a five-year, 50% risk of developing a GCT of the testis. It is interesting that ITGCN does not have the characteristic isochromosome 12p, as do most GCTs. This is evidence that i12p is an early and specific event in testis cancer.

Genetics

i12p occurs in 80% of GCTs [156,157]. All GCTs contain some level of chromosomal abnormality on 12p, i.e., supranumary 12p sequences of uniparental origin are present in all cases [158,159]. FISH probes of the alpha satellite region are capable of detecting i12p [160]. Fish or PCR technology can currently be applied on fresh or frozen tissue and soon reliably on formalin-fixed material, which may make this procedure easier and more cost effective [161]. Applications such as to monitor margins or peritoneal wash specimens after RPLD are on the horizon. Aside from chromosome 12, altered dosage has been noted on chromosomes 5 and 7 [162].

DCC is located on chromosome 18q21 and shows LOH in 45% of all types of GCTs. This finding indicates that this genetic alteration is an early event in GCT development [163].

Oncogenes

Mutations of oncogenes are fairly common in germ cell tumors. N-ras mutations occur in 57% of seminomas and 60% of nonseminomatous GCTs [164,165]. ki-ras or another tumor supressor gene on 12 has been shown to be altered in some germ cell tumors [166,171]. The c-kit oncogene has altered expression in 80% of seminomas and 7% of nonseminomas. This finding may have some diagnostic utility in determining whether a tumor is a seminoma or the solid variant of embryonal carcinoma — a distinction that can be difficult to make on morphologic grounds alone. c-kit is also expressed in intratubular germ cell neoplasia. A polyclonal antibody is available for immunoperoxidase analysis [167]. hst-1 has altered expression in 63% of nonseminoma and 4% of seminomatous germ cell tumors [171].

Differential expression of oncogenes has been explored, and there is a difference in well differentiated and undifferentiated tumors. This area needs further study to see if it will yield any prognostic information [168].

Tumor supressor genes

Rb has altered expression in testis tumors. At present, this finding is not useful as a prognostic or diagnostic marker for the evaluation of testicular neoplasms.

Proliferation markers

Low MIB-1 staining with immunoperoxidase, i.e., a low proliferation index, predicts a low-risk group for stage A testis tumor patients [169]. Proliferation index may have a role in defining low-stage patients who should be followed by close observation.

Other tumor markers

NME genes have LOH in teratomas but not in embryonal carcinoma. NME is a nucleotide diphosphate kinase (NDPK), and a critical level of NDPK must be present to suppress somatic differentiation [170].

There is some evidence that glutathione s-transferase pi (GSTP) alterations may be important as a prognostic or diagnostic marker in testis tumors [166].

The use of these alterations as clinically significant biomarkers is yet to be determined.

Tumor markers hCG, AFP, LDH, and PLAP, which are now standard markers, can now be detected with ultrasensative RIAs, which can detect nanogram amounts. None of these tumor markers is specific for testis cancer, and all can be elevated in other cancers [171].

Altered glycosylation patterns have been commonly found in human cancers. Loss of galactosylgloboside Gb5 correlates with metastasis in seminoma. The loss of this band can be observed by TLC and detection with monoclonal antibodies [172], which may aid in the preoperative staging of testis cancer and in selecting patients for observation protocols.

Midline carcinomas

Since poorly differentiated carcinomas of unknown primary do poorly with systemic chemotherapy, and since germ cell tumors respond well to cisplatin-based chemotherapy, it is critical to identify patients with these diseases even if their numbers are small. Histology and immunohistochemistry are not always useful in this regard. In one study, half the patients with midline poorly differentiated carcinomas had abnormalities of chromosome 12 by southern blot analysis consistent with germ cell origin. These abnormalities included i12p, del12q, and add12p [173].

Conclusion

As the molecular techniques described above gain more widespread use, the cost per test should come down, making them practical for use as screening, diagnostic, and prognostic tools. These new techniques are still not as cost-effective as the hemotoxylin- and eosin-stained slide for the diagnosis of malignancy at the current stage of detection, but they may prove useful in the future, if we detect and treat precursor lesions that are not detectable with the light microscope. Even the current molecular probes are most useful when they can be localized to a certain cell, as with in situ hybridization or insitu reverse transcriptase PCR.

The application of laboratory techniques in a clinical setting requires a non-labor-intensive and reproducible assay, widely available with quality control, and readily interpretable results (NIH Consensus Conference, 1991). Future research needs to focus both on improving therapy and on understanding putative biomarkers so that the relevant ones can be incorporated into the everyday practice of medicine.

Mathematical modeling, such as that used by The Memorial Sloan Kettering group for germ cell tumors, should be applied to all GU malignancies so that the use of biomarkers can be optimized. This is absolutely necessary in this era of cost containment [165].

References

1. Sidransky D, Boyle J, Koch W (1993). Molecular screening. Prospects for a new approach. Arch Otolaryngol Head Neck Surg 119(11):1187–1190.

2. Sidransky D (1993). ene mutations in cytologic diagnosis (Meeting abstract). Proc Annu Meet Am Assoc Cancer Res 34:615–616, 1993.
3. Mao L, Sidransky D (1994). Cancer screening based on genetic alterations in human tumors. Cancer Res 54(7 Suppl):1939s–1940s.
4. Sidransky D (1995). Molecular markers in cancer: can we make better predictions? Int J Cancer 64(1):1–2.
5. Koch WM, Boyle JO, Mao L, Hakim J, Hruban RH, Sidransky D (1994). p53 gene mutations as markers of tumor spread in synchronous oral cancers. Arch Otolaryngol Head Neck Surg 120(9):943–947.
6. Hruban RH, van der Riet P, Erozan YS, Sidransky D (1994). Brief report: molecular biology and the early detection of carcinoma of the bladder — the case of Hubert H. Humphrey. N Engl J Med 330(18):1276–1278.
7. Muller M, Volkmann M, Zentgraf H, Galle PR (1994). Clinical implications of the p53 tumor supressor gene. N Engl J Med 330:865.
8. Boyd J, Pienta KJ, Getzenberg RH, Coffey DS, Barrett JC (1991). Preneoplastic alterations in nuclear morphology that accompany loss of tumor suppressor phenotype. J Natl Cancer Inst 83(12):862–866.
9. Brennan JA, Mao L, Boyle JO, Hruban RH, Koch WM, Sidransky D (1994). Reassessment of histopathology based on molecular analysis. Proc Annu Meet Am Assoc Cancer Res 35:A1319.
10. Brennan JA, Mao L, Hruban RH, Boyle JO, Eby YJ, Koch WM, Goodman SN, Sidransky D (1995). Molecular assessment of histopathological staging in squamous-cell carcinoma of the head and neck. N Engl J Med 332(7):429–435.
11. Sidransky D (1994). Genetic alterations in preinvasive lesions and mucosal margins of HNSC patients (Meeting abstract). Proc Annu Meet Am Assoc Cancer Res 35:685.
12. Mao L, Lee DJ, Tockman MS, Erozan YS, Askin F, Sidransky D (1994). Microsatellite alterations as clonal markers for the detection of human cancer. Proc Natl Acad Sci USA 91(21):9871–9875.
13. Hammond EH, Grignon DJ (1995). Current status of tissue markers as prognostic factors in prostatic adenocarcinoma. Int J Radiat Oncol Biol Phys 31(2):419–422.
14. Sidransky D, Tokino T, Hamilton SR, et al. (1992). Identification of ras oncogene mutations in the stool of patients with curable colorectal tumors. Science 256:102–105.
15. Tobi M, Lou F-C, Ronai Z (1994). Detection of K-ras mutations in colonic effluent samples from patients without evidence of colorectal carcinoma. J Natl Cancer Inst 86:1007–1010.
16. Sidransky D (1994). Molecular screening — how long can we afford to wait? J Natl Cancer Inst 86(13):955–956.
17. Sidransky D, Von Eschenbach A, Tsai YC, et al. (1991). Identification of p53 gene mutations in bladder cancers and urine samples. Science 252:706–709.
18. Vogelstein B, Fearon ER, Hamilton SR, et al. (1992). Genetic alterations during colorectal tumor development. N Engl J Med 319:525–532.
19. Furmanski P, Herman CJ, Padarathsingh M (1993). Molecular mechanisms of tumor development and progression: new targets for prevention, diagnosis, and therapy — a pathology B study section workshop. Working report from the Division of Research Grants, National Institutes of Health. Cancer Res 53(20):5055–5059.
20. Barnes DM, Gilbert CE (1995). Determination of cell proliferation. J Clin Pathol Mol Pathol 48:M2–M5.
21. Grasil-Kraupp B, et al. (1995). Insitu detection of fragmented DNA (TUNEL Assay) fails to discriminate among apaptosis, necrosis and autolytic cell death: A cautionary note. Hepatology 21:1465–1468.
22. Kay EW, Walsh CJ, Cassidy M, Curran B, Leader M (1994). C-erbB-2 immunostaining: problems with interpretation. J Clin Pathol 47(9):816–822.
23. Saloman RN (1995). Introduction to quantitative reverse transcriptase polymerase chain reaction. Diagn Mol Pathol 4:82–84.

24. Pan LX, Diss TC, Isaacson PG (1995). The polymerase chain reaction in histopathology. Histopathology 256:201–217.
25. Penman S (1995). Rethinking cell structure. Proc Natl Acad Sci USA 92:5251–5257.
26. Bosl GJ, Fair WR, Herr HW, Bajorin DF, Dalbagni G, Sarkis AS, Reuter VE, Cordon-Cardo C, Sheinfeld J, Scher HI (1994). Bladder cancer: advances in biology and treatment. Crit Rev Oncol Hematol 16(1):33–70.
27. Fradet Y, Cordon-Cardo C (1993). Critical appraisal of tumor markers in bladder cancer. Semin Urol 11(3):145–153.
28. Orlow I, Lianes P, Lacombe L, Dalbagni G, Reuter VE, Cordon-Cardo C (1994). Chromosome 9 allelic losses and microsatellite alterations in human bladder tumors. Cancer Res 54(11):2848–2851.
29. Dalbagni G, Presti JC Jr, Reuter VE, Zhang ZF, Sarkis AS, Fair WR, Cordon-Cardo C (1993). Molecular genetic alterations of chromosome 17 and p53 nuclear overexpression in human bladder cancer. Diagn Mol Pathol 2(1):4–13.
30. Ruppert JM, Tokino K, Sidransky D (1993). Evidence for two bladder cancer suppressor loci on human chromosome 9. Cancer Res 53(21):5093–5095.
31. Cairns P, Tokino K, Eby Y, Sidransky D (1994). Homozygous deletions of 9p21 in primary human bladder tumors detected by comparative multiplex polymerase chain reaction. Cancer Res 54(6):1422–1424.
32. Cairns P, Eby Y, Tokino K, Sidransky D (1995). Evidence for a suppressor locus at 9p21 distinct from CDKN2 in bladder cancer (meeting abstract). Proc Annu Meet Am Assoc Cancer Res 36:A1170.
33. Sidransky D, Frost P, Von Eschenbach A, Oyasu R, Preisinger AC, Vogelstein B (1992). Clonal origin bladder cancer. N Engl J Med 326(11):737–740.
34. Cairns P, Shaw ME, Knowles MA (1993). Initiation of bladder cancer may involve deletion of a tumour-suppressor gene on chromosome 9. Oncogene 8(4):1083–1085.
35. Chang WY, Cairns P, Schoenberg MP, Polascik TJ, Sidransky D (1995). Novel suppressor loci on chromosome 14q in primary bladder cancer. Cancer Res 55(15):3246–3249.
36. Knowles MA, Shaw ME, Proctor AJ (1993). Deletion mapping of chromosome 8 in cancers of the urinary bladder using restriction length polymorphisms and microsetellite polymorphisms. Oncogene 8:1357–1364.
37. Lianes P, Orlow I, Zhang ZF, Oliva MR, Sarkis AS, Reuter VE, Cordon-Cardo C (1994). Altered patterns of MDM2 and TP53 expression in human bladder cancer. J Natl Cancer Inst 86(17):1325–1330.
38. Spruck CH III, Ohneseit PF, Gonzalez-Zulueta M, Esrig D, Miyao N, Tsai YC, Lerner SP, Schmutte C, Yang AS, Cote R, et al. (1994). Two molecular pathways to transitional cell carcinoma of the bladder. Cancer Res 54(3):784–788.
39. Cordon-Cardo C, Dalbagni G, Sarkis AS, Reuter VE (1994). Genetic alterations associated with bladder cancer. Important Adv Oncol ••:71–83.
40. Presti JC Jr, Reuter VE, Galan T, Fair WR, Cordon-Cardo C (1991). Molecular genetic alterations in superficial and locally advanced human bladder cancer. Cancer Res 51(19):5405–5409.
41. Cordon-Cardo C, Wartinger D, Petrylak D, Dalbagni G, Fair WR, Fuks Z, Reuter VE (1992). Altered expression of the retinoblastoma gene product: prognostic indicator in bladder cancer. J Natl Cancer Inst 84(16):1251–1256.
42. Cordon-Cardo C, Dalbagni G, Saez GT, Oliva MR, Zhang ZF, Rosai J, Reuter VE, Pellicer A (1994). p53 mutations in human bladder cancer: genotypic versus phenotypic patterns. Int J Cancer 56(3):347–353.
43. Brennan JA, Boyle JO, Koch WM, Goodman SN, Hruban RH, Eby YJ, Couch MJ, Forastiere AA, Sidransky D (1995). Association between cigarette smoking and mutation of the p53 gene in squamous-cell carcinoma of the head and neck. N Engl J Med 332(11):712–717.
44. Sarkis AS, Bajorin DF, Reuter VE, Herr HW, Netto G, Zhang ZF, Schultz PK, Cordon-Cardo C, Scher HI (1995). Prognostic value of p53 nuclear overexpression in patients

with invasive bladder cancer treated with neoadjuvant MVAC. J Clin Oncol 13(6):1384–1390.
45. Thomas DJ, Robinson MC, Charlton R, Wilkinson S, Shenton BK, Neal DE (1994). P53 expression, ploidy and progression in pT1 transitional cell carcinoma of the bladder. Br J Urol 73(5):533–537.
46. Sidransky D, Messing E (1992). Molecular genetics and biochemical mechanisms in bladder cancer. Oncogenes, tumor suppressor genes, and growth factors. Urol Clin North Am 19(4):629–639.
47. Sandberg AA, Berger CS (1994). Review of chromosome studies in urological tumors. II. Cytogenetics and molecular genetics of bladder cancer. J Urol 151(3):545–560.
48. Berner A, Jacobsen AB, Fossa SD, Nesland JM (1993). Expression of c-erbB-2 protein, neuron-specific enolase and DNA flow cytometry in locally advanced transitional cell carcinoma of the urinary bladder. Histopathology 22(4):327–333.
49. Underwood M, Bartlett J, Reeves J, Gardiner DS, Scott R, Cooke T (1995). C-erbB-2 gene amplification: a molecular marker in recurrent bladder tumors? Cancer Res 55(11):2422–2430.
50. Jones PA, Droller MJ (1993). Pathways of development and progression in bladder cancer: new correlations between clinical observations and molecular mechanisms. Semin Urol 11(4):177–192.
51. Knowles MA, Williamson M (1993). Mutation of H-ras is infrequent in bladder cancer. Cancer Res 53:133.
52. Fitzgerald JM, Ramchurren N, Rieger K, Levesque P, Silverman M, Libertino JA, Summerhayes IC (1995). Identification of H-ras mutations in urine sediments complements cytology in the detection of bladder tumors. J Natl Cancer Inst 87(2):129–133.
53. Boring CC, Squires TS, Tong T (1993). Cancer statistics. J Clin Cancer 43:7–26.
54. Fujimoto K, Yamada Y, Okajima E, et al. (1992). Frequent association of p53 gene mutations in invasive bladder cancer. Cancer Res 52:1393–1398.
55. Sidransky D, Von Eschenbach A, Tsai YC, Jones P, Summerhayes I, Marshall F, Paul M, Green P, Hamilton SR, Frost P, et al. (1991). The p53 gene is frequently altered in primary invasive bladder carcinoma and can be identified in urine sediment. Proc Annu Meet Am Assoc Cancer Res 32:A1865.
56. Reuter VE (1990). Pathology of bladder cancer: assessment of prognostic variables and response to therapy. Semin Oncol 17(5):524–532.
57. Kallioniemi A, Kallioniwmi OP, Sudar D, Rutovitz D, Gray JW, Waldman F, Pinkel D (1992). Comparative genomic hybridization for molecular cytogenetic analysis of solid tumors. Science 258:818–821.
58. Voorter C, Joos S, Bringuier P, et al. (1995). Detection of chromosomal imbalances in transitional cell carcinoma of the bladder by comparative genomic hybridization. Am J Pathol 146:1341–1354.
59. Norming U, Tribukait B, Gustafson H, Nyman CR, Wang N, Wijkstrom V (1992). DNA profile and tumor progression in primary carcinoma insitu of the bladder. J Urol 147:11–15.
60. Sheinfeld J, Reuter VE, Sarkis AS, Cordon-Cardo C (1992). Blood group antigens in normal and neoplastic urothelium. J Cell Biochem Suppl 16I:50–55.
61. Golijanin D, Sherman Y, Shapiro A, Pode D (1995). Detection of bladder tumors by immunostaining of the Lewis X antigen in cells from voided urine. Urology 46(2):173–177.
62. Aprikian AG, Sarkis AS, Reuter VE, Cordon-Cardo C, Sheinfeld J (1993). Biological markers of prognosis in transitional cell carcinoma of the bladder: current concepts. Semin Urol 11(3):137–144.
63. Fradet Y, Tardif M, Bourget L, Robert J (1990). Clinical cancer progression in urinary bladder tumors evaluated by multiparameter flow cytometry with monoclonal antibodies. Cancer Res 50:432–437.
64. Bringuier PP, Umbas R, Schaafsma HE, et al. (1993). Decreased E-cadherin immunoreactivity correlates with poor survival in patients with bladder tumors. Cancer Res 53:3241–3245.

65. Grossman HB, Washington RW, Carey TE, Liebert M (1992). Alterations of antigen expression in superficial bladder cancer. J Biochm Suppl 161:63–68.
66. Dickinson AJ, Fox SB, Newcomb PV, Persad RA, Sibley GN, Harris AL (1995). An immunohistochemical and prognostic evaluation of cathepsin D expression in 105 bladder carcinomas. J Urol 154(1):237–241.
67. Messing EM, Murphy-Brooks N (1994). Recovery of epidermal growth factor in voided urine of patients with bladder cancer. Urology 44(4):502–506.
68. Vet JA, Debruyne FM, Schalken JA (1994). Molecular prognostic factors in bladder cancer. World J Urol 12(2):84–88.
69. Matsumura Y, Sugiyama •• et al. (1995). Universal retension of introns in CD44 gene transcripts in bladder cancer provides new diagnostic and clinical oncologic opportunities. J Pathol 177:11–20.
70. Hong RL, Pu YS, Hsieh TS, Chu JS, Lee WJ (1995). Expressions of E-cadherin and exon v6-containing isoforms of CD44 and their prognostic values in human transitional cell carcinoma. J Urol 153(6):2025–2028.
71. Jaeger TM, Weidner KC, Moore DH, Kerschmann RI, Waldman FM, Carroll PR (1995). Tumor angiogenesis correlates with lymph node metastasis in invasive bladder cancer. J Urol 154:69–71.
72. Mansour OA, Shouman SA, Khafagy M, Basma H, Liebmann PM, Schauenstein K, el-Ahmady O (1995). Urinary CA 19.9 as marker for bladder cancer. Lancet 346(8973):512–513.
73. Casetta G, Piana P, Cavallini A, Vottero M, Tizzani A (1993). Urinary levels of tumour associated antigens (CA 19-9, TPA and CEA) in patients with neoplastic and non-neoplastic urothelial abnormalities. Br J Urol 72(1):60–64.
74. Ho KJ, Kuo SH (1995). Urinary beta-glucuronidase activity as initial screening test for urinary tract malignancy in high risk patients. Cancer 76:473–478.
75. Banks RE, Porter WH, Whelan P, Smith PH, Selby PJ (1995). Soluble forms of the adhesion molecule E-cadherin in urine. J Clin Pathol 48(2):179–180.
76. Smith DJ, Evans HJ, Newman J, Chapple CR (1994). Ectopic human chorionic gonadotrophin (HCG) production: is the detection by serum analysis of HCG of clinical relevance in transitional cell carcinoma of the bladder? Br J Urol 73(4):409–412.
77. Dobrowolski ZF, Byrska B, Dolezal M (1994). Prognostic value of beta human chorionic gonadotrophin in blood serum of patients with urinary bladder tumours. Int Urol Nephrol 26(3):301–306.
78. Lazar V, Diez SG, Laurent A, Giovangrandi Y, Radvanyi F, Chopin D, Bidart JM, Bellet D, Vidaud M (1995). Expression of human chorionic gonadotropin beta subunit genes in superficial and invasive bladder carcinomas. Cancer Res 55(17):3735–3738.
79. Marx J (1995). New clue to prostate cancer spread. Science 268(5212):799–800.
80. Berges RR, Vukanovic J, Epstein JI, CarMichel M, Cisek L, Johnson DE, Veltri RW, Walsh PC, Isaccs JT (1995). Implication of cell kinetic changes during the progression of human prostate cancer. Clin Cancer Res 1:473–480.
81. Partin AW, Coffey DS (1994). Benign and malignant prostatic neoplasms: human studies. Recent Prog Horm Res 49:293–331.
82. Bostwick GG, Burke HB, Wheeler TM, et al. (1994). The most promising surrogate endpoint biomarkers for screening candidate chemopreventative compounds for prostatic adenocarcinoma in short term phase II clinical trials. J Cell Biochem Suppl 19:283–289.
83. Netto GJ, Humphrey PA (1994). Molecular biologic aspects of human prostatic carcinoma. Am J Clin Pathol 102(4 Suppl 1):S57–S64.
84. Carter BS, et al. (1993). Hereditary prostate cancer: Epidemiologic and clinical features. J Urol 150:797–802.
85. Visakorpi T, Kallioniemi AS, Hyytinen ER, et al. (1995). Genetic changes in primary and recurrent prostate cancer by comparative genomic hybridization. Cancer Res 55:342–347.
86. Brothman AR, Peehl DM, Patel AM, McNeal JM (1990). Frequency and pattern of karyotypic abnormalities in prostate cancer. Cancer Res 50:3795–3803.

87. Sandberg AA (1992). Chromosomal abnormalities and related events in prostate cancer. Hum Pathol 23:368–380.
88. Sakr WA, Macoska JA, Benson P, Grignon DJ, Wolman SR, Pontes JE, Crissman JD (1994). Cancer Res 54:3273–3277.
89. Carter BS (1993). Studies of the genetic epidemiology and molecular genetics of human prostate cancer. Diss Abstr Int [B] 53(8):3927.
90. Bova GS, et al. (1993). Homozygous deletion and frequent allelic loss of chromosome 8q22 loci in prostate cancer. Cancer Res 53:3869–3873.
91. Isaacs WB, Bova GS, Morton RA, Bussemakers MJ, Brooks JD, Ewing CM (1995). Molecular biology of prostate cancer progression. Cancer Surv 23:19–32.
92. Rinker-Schaeffer CW, Isaacs WB, Isaacs JT (1993). Molecular and cellular markers for metastatic prostate cancer. Cancer Metastasis Rev 12(1):3–10.
93. Effert PJ, Strohmeyer TG (1994). Basic research in prostate cancer: molecular biology. Acta Urol Belg 62(1):15–21.
94. Watanabe M, Shiraishi T, Yatain R, Nomura A, Stemmermann GN (1994). International comparison of ras gene mutations in latent prostate carcinoma. Int J Cancer 58:174–178.
95. Carter BS, Epstein JI, Isaacs WB (1990). ras gene mutations in human prostate cancer. Cancer Res 50:6830–6832.
96. Viola MV, Fromowitz F, Oravez S, et al. (1986). Expression of ras oncoprotein p21 in prostate cancer. N Engl J Med 314:133.
97. Varma VA, Austin GE, O'CFonnell AC (1989). Antibodies to ras oncoprotein p21 lack immunohistochemical specificity for neoplastic epithelium in human prostate tissue. Arch Pathol Lab Med 113:16.
98. Fox SB, Persad RA, Royds J, Kure RN, Silcocks PB, Collins CC (1993). p53 and c-myc expression in stage A1 prostate adenocarcinoma: useful prognostic determinants? J Urol 150:490–494.
99. Buttyan R, Sawczuk MC, Benson MC, Siegal JD, Olsson CA (1987). Enhanced expression of the c-myc proto-oncogene in high grade prostatic cancers. Prostate 11:327–337.
100. Sauter G, Corroll P, Moch H, et al. (1995). c-myc copy number gains in bladder cancer detected by FISH. Am J Pathol 146:1131–1139.
101. Myers RB, Srivastava S, Oelschlager DK, Grizzle WE (••). Expression of p160 erbB-3 and p185 erbB-2 in prostatic intraepithelial neoplasia and prostatic adenocarcinoma. J Natl Cancer Inst 86:1140–1145.
102. Bostwick GB (1994). c-erbB-2 oncogene expression in prostatic intraepithelial neoplasia; mounting evidence for a precursor role. J Natl Cancer Inst 86:1108–1110.
103. Ware JL, Maygarden SJ, Knoontz WW, Strom SC (1991). Immunohistochemical detection of c-erbB-2 protein in human benign and neoplastic prostate. Human Pathol 22:254–258.
104. Ross JS, Nazeer T, Church K (1993). Contribution of Her-2/nu oncogene expression to DNA content analysis in prediction of prognosis of prostate carcinoma. Mod Pathol 6:68A.
105. Zhau HE, Pisters LL, Hall MC, Troncoso P, et al. (1994). Biomarkers associated with prostate cancer progression. J Cell Biochem Suppl 19:208–216.
106. Pisters LL, Troncoso P, Zhau HE, et al. (1995). C-met protooncogene expression in benign and malignant human prostate tissue. J Urol 154:293–298.
107. Moul JW (1995). The clinical relevance of oncogenes and tumor supressor genes in prostate cancer. Monogr Urol 16 (4).
108. Prendergast NJ, Walther PJ (1995). Genetic alterations in prostatic adenocarcinoma. Surg Oncol Clin N Am 4(2):241–255.
109. Sakar F, Sakr W, Li Y-W, Macoska J, Ball K, Crissman J (1992). Analysis of Rb gene deletion in human prostatic adeoncarcinomas. Mod Pathol 6:59A.
110. Castagnaro M, Yandell D, Hiort O, et al. (1993). p53 and androgen receptor genes analysis in human prostate cancer. Mod Pathol 6:57A.
111. Fan K, Smith D (1993). Correlative analysis of normal and mutant p53 gene products in human prostate adenocarcinoma. Mod Pathol 6:59A.
112. Yoo GH, Xu HJ, Brennan JA, Westra W, Hruban RH, Koch W, Benedict WF, Sidransky D

(1994). Infrequent inactivation of the retinoblastoma gene despite frequent loss of chromosome 13q in head and neck squamous cell carcinoma. Cancer Res 54(17):4603–4606.
113. Cooney K, Wetzel J, Mariver S, Singleton T, Wojno KJ (in press). Distinct regions of allelic loss on chromosome 13 in prostate cancer. Cancer Res.
114. Cooney KA, Wetzel JC, Merajver SD, Macoska JA, Wojno KJ (in press). Distrinct regions of allelic loss on chromosome 13q in prostate cancer. Cancer Res.
115. Hughes JH, Cohen MB, Robinson RA (1995). p53 immunoreactivity in primary and metastatic prostate adenocarcinoma. Mod Pathol 8:462–466.
116. Bova GS, Carter BS, Bussemakers MJ, Emi M, Fujiwara Y, Kyprianou N, Jacobs SC, Robinson JC, Epstein JI, Walsh PC, et al. (1993). Homozygous deletion and frequent allelic loss of chromosome 8p22 loci in human prostate cancer. Cancer Res 53(17):3869–3873.
117. Gao X, Zacharek A, Grignon DJ, Sakr W, Powell IJ, Porter AT, Honn KV (1995). Localization of potential tumor supressor loci to a <2 Mb region on chromosome 17q in human prostate cancer. Oncogene 11:1241–1247.
118. Takahashi S, Qian J, Brown JA, Alcaraz A, Bostwick DG, Lieber MM, Jenkins RB (1994). Potential markers of prostate cancer aggressiveness detected by fluorescence insitu hybridization in needle biopsies. Cancer Res 54:3574–3579.
119. Macoska JA, Trybus TM, Sakr WA, Wolf MC, Benson PD, Powel IJ, Pontes JE (••). Fluorescent insitu hybridization analysis of 8p allelic loss and chromosome 8 instability in human prostate cancer. Cancer Res 54:3824–3830.
120. Rinker-Schaeffer CW, Partin AW, Isaacs WB, Coffey DS, Isaacs JT (1994). Molecular and cellular changes associated with the acquisition of metastatic ability by prostatic cancer cells. Prostate 25(5):249–265.
121. Isaacs WB, Bova GS, Morton RA, Bussemakers MJ, Brooks JD, Ewing CM (1994). Molecular biology of prostate cancer. Semin Oncol 21(5):514–521.
122. Giroldi LA, Bringuier PP, Schalken JA (1994–95). Defective E-cadherin function in urological cancers: clinical implications and molecular mechanisms. Invasion Metastasis 14(1–6):71–81.
123. Lieber MM (1994). DNA ploidy in prostate cancer: potential measurement as a surrogate endpoint biomarker. J Cell Biochem Suppl 19:246–248.
124. Hepburn PJ, Glynne-Jones E, Goddard L, Gee JM, Harper ME (1995). Cell proliferation in prostatic carcinoma: comparative analysis of Ki-67, MIB-1 and PCNA. Histochem J 27(3):196–203.
125. Raffo AJ, Perlman H, Chen M, Day M, Streitman JS, Buttyan R (1995). Overexpression of bcl-2 protects prostate cancer cells from apoptosis in vitro and confers resistance to androgen depletion in vivo. Cancer Res 55:4438–4445.
126. Smith RG, Nag A (1987). Regulation of c-cis expression in tumors of the male reproductive tract. Prog Clin Biol Res 239:113–122.
127. Partin AW, Getzenberg RH, Carmichael MJ, Vindivich D, Yoo J, Epstein JI, Coffey DS (1993). Nuclear matrix protein patterns in human benign prostatic hyperplasia and prostate cancer. Cancer Res 53(4):744–746.
128. Walensky LD, Coffey DS, Chen TH, Wu TC, Pasternack GR (1993). A novel M(r) 32,000 nuclear phosphoprotein is selectively expressed in cells competent for self-renewal. Cancer Res 53(19):4720–4726.
129. Veltri RW, Partin AW, Epstein JE, Marley GM, Miller CM, Singer DS, Patton KP, Criley SR, Coffey DS (1994). Quantitative nuclear morphometry, Markovian texture descriptors, and DNA content captured on a CAS-200 image analysis system, combined with PCNA and HER-2/neu immunohistochemistry for prediction of prostate cancer progression. J Cell Biochem (Suppl) 19:249–258.
130. Veltri RW, Partin AW, Epstein JI, Criley SR, Wright GL Jr, Marley GM, Miller MC, Singer DP, Patton KP, Coffey DS (1994). Prognostic value of multivariate analysis of biomarkers for prostate cancer progression and staging following radical prostatectomy. Proc Annu Meet Am Assoc Cancer Res 35:A1211.

131. Morris GL, Dodd JG (1990). Epidermal growth factor receptor mRNA levels in human prostate tumors and cell lines. J Urol 143:1272–1274.
132. Maygarden SJ, Strom S, Ware JI (1992). Localization of EGFR by immunohistochemical methods in human prostate carcinoma, prostatic intraepithelial neoplasia and benign hyperplasia. Arch Pathol Lab Med 116:269–273.
133. Kuczyk M, Serth J, Denil J, Hofner K, Allhoff E, Jonas U (1994). Cathepsin D expression and the possible role of lysosomal proteases as a prognostic factor in prostate cancer. J Urol 151:286A.
134. Gao X, Grignon DJ, Chbihi T, Zacharek A, Chen YQ, Sakr W, Porter AT, Crissman JD, Pontes JE, Powell IJ, et al. (1995). Elevated 12-limmunoperoxidaseygenase mRNA expression correlates with advanced stage and poor differentiation of human prostate cancer. Urology 46(2):227–237.
135. Berthon P, Dimitrov T, Stower M, Cussenot O, Maitland NJ (1995). A microdissection approach to detect molecular markers during progression of prostate cancer. Br J Cancer 72:946–951.
136. Martensson S, Bigler SA, Brown M, Lange PH, Brawer MK, Hakomori S (1995). Sialyl-Lewis(x) and related carbohydrate antigens in the prostate. Hum Pathol 26(7):735–739.
137. Maygarden SJ (1994). Applications of immunohistochemistry to the diagnosis and prognostication of prostate carcinoma and prostatic intraepithelial neoplasia. Pathol Annu 29(Pt 1): 303–320.
138. Spires SE, Bankes ER, Davey DD, Jennings CD, Wood DP, Cibull ML (1994). Proliferating cell nuclear antigen in prostatic adenocarcinoma; correlation with established prognostic factors. Urology 43:660–666.
139. Brauch H, Pomer S, Hieronymus T, Schadt T, Lohrke H, Komitowski D (1994). Genetic alterations in sporadic renal-cell carcinoma: molecular analyses of tumor suppressor gene harboring chromosomal regions 3p, 5q, and 17p. World J Urol 12(3):162–168.
140. Presti JC Jr, Reuter VE, Cordon-Cardo C, Mazumdar M, Fair WR, Jhanwar SC (1993). Allelic deletions in renal tumors: histopathological correlations. Cancer Res 53(23):5780–5783.
141. Presti JC Jr, Rao PH, Chen Q, Reuter VE, Li FP, Fair WR, Jhanwar SC (1991). Histopathological, cytogenetic, and molecular characterization of renal cortical tumors. Cancer Res 51(5):1544–1552.
142. Lager DJ, Huston BJ, Timmerman TG, Bonsib SM (1995). Papillary renal tumors: morphologic, cytochemical, and genotypic features. Cancer 76:669–673.
143. Gnarra JR, Glenn GM, Latif F, Anglard P, Lerman MI, Zbar B, Linehan WM (1993). Molecular genetic studies of sporadic and familial renal cell carcinoma. Urol Clin North Am 20(2):207–216.
144. Karp JE, Broder S (1995). Molecular foundations of cancer: new targets for intervention. Nature Med 4:309–320.
145. Nanus DM, Schmitz-Drager BJ, Motzer RJ, Lee AC, Vlamis V, Cordon-Cardo C, Albino AP, Reuter VE (1993). Expression of basic fibroblast growth factor in primary human renal tumors: correlation with poor survival. J Natl Cancer Inst 85(19):1597–1599.
146. Schoenberg M, Cairns P, Brooks JD, Marshall FF, Epstein JI, Isaacs WB, Sidransky D (1995). Frequent loss of chromosome arms 8p and 13q in collecting duct carcinoma (CDC) of the kidney. Genes Chromosome Cancer 12(1):76–80.
147. Kovacs G (1993). Molecular cytogenetics of renal cell tumors. Adv Cancer Res 62:89–124.
148. Delahunt B, Bethwaite PB, Thornton A, Ribas JL (1995). Proliferation of renal cell carcinoma assessed by fixation-resistant polyclonal Ki-67 antibody labeling. Correlation with clinical outcome. Cancer 75(11):2714–2719.
149. de Riese WT, Crabtree WN, Allhoff EP, Werner M, Liedke S, Lenis G, Atzpodien J, Kirchner H (1993). Prognostic significance of Ki-67 immunostaining in nonmetastatic renal cell carcinoma. J Clin Oncol 11(9):1804–1808.
150. Huang A (1994). Molecular characterization of the Wilms' tumor locus on chromosome 11p13. Diss Abstr Int [B] 55(3):721.

151. Baird PN, Pritchard J, Cowell JK (1994). Molecular genetic analysis of chromosome 11p in familial Wilms tumour. Br J Cancer 69(6):1072–1077.
152. Coppes MJ, Williams BR (1994). The molecular genetics of Wilms tumor. Cancer Invest 12(1):57–65.
153. Elder JS (1995). Renin in Wilms' tumor: prorenin as an indicator. J Urol 154(1):325–326.
154. Lin RY, Argenta PA, Sullivan KM, Stern R, Adzick NS (1995). Urinary hyaluronic acid is a Wilms' tumor marker. J Pediatr Surg 30(2):304–308.
155. Sheinfeld J (1994). Nonseminomatous germ cell tumors of the testis: current concepts and controversies. Urology 44(1):2–14.
156. Rodriguez E, Mathew S, Reuter V, Ilson DH, Bosl GJ, Chaganti RSK (1992). Cytogenetic analysis of 124 prospectively ascertained male germ cell tumors. Cancer Res 52:2285–2291.
157. Bosl GJ, Ilson DH, Rodriguez E, Motzer RJ, Reuter VE, Chaganti RS (1994). Clinical relevance of the i(12p) marker chromosome in germ cell tumors. J Natl Cancer Inst 86(5):349–355.
158. Geurts van Kessel A, Suijkerbuijk RF, Sinke RJ, Looijenga L, Oosterhuis JW, de Jong B (1993). Molecular cytogenetics of human germ cell tumours: i(12p) and related chromosomal anomalies. Eur Urol 23(1):23–29.
159. Rodriguez E, Houldsworth J, Reuter VE, Meltzer P, Zhang J, Trent JM, Bosl GJ, Chaganti RS (1993). Molecular cytogenetic analysis of i(12p)-negative human male germ cell tumors. Genes Chromosome Cancer 8(4):230–236.
160. Mukherjee AB, Murty VV, Rodriguez E, Reuter VE, Bosl GJ, Chaganti RS (1991). Detection and analysis of origin of i(12p), a diagnostic marker of human male germ cell tumors, by fluorescence in situ hybridization. Genes Chromosome Cancer 3(4):300–307.
161. Rodriguez E, Mathew S, Mukherjee AB, Reuter VE, Bosl GJ, Chaganti RS (1992). Analysis of chromosome 12 aneuploidy in interphase cells from human male germ cell tumors by fluorescence in situ hybridization. Genes Chromosome Cancer 5(1):21–29.
162. Peltomaki PT (1993). Molecular genetic alterations in human testicular cancer. Diss Abstr Int [C] 54(1):198.
163. Murty VV, Li RG, Houldsworth J, Bronson DL, Reuter VE, Bosl GJ, Chaganti RS (1994). Frequent allelic deletions and loss of expression characterize the DCC gene in male germ cell tumors. Oncogene 9(11):3227–3231.
164. Ganguly S, Murty VV, Samaniego F, Reuter VE, Bosl GJ, Chaganti RS (1990). Detection of preferential NRAS mutations in human male germ cell tumors by the polymerase chain reaction. Genes Chromosome Cancer 1(3):228–232.
165. Bosl GJ (1993). Prognostic factors for metastatic testicular germ cell tumours: the Memorial Sloan-Kettering cancer model. Eur Urol 23(1):182–187.
166. Strohmeyer T (1994). Urothelial cancers. Cytogenetic and molecular biology principles. Urologe A 33(2):122–127.
167. Rajpert-De Meyts E, Skakkebaek NE (1994). Expression of the c-kit protein product in carcinoma-in-situ and invasive testicular germ cell tumours. Int J Androl 17(2):85–92.
168. Shuin T, Misaki H, Kubota Y, Yao M, Hosaka M (1994). Differential expression of protooncogenes in human germ cell tumors of the testis. Cancer 73(6):1721–1727.
169. Albers P, Orazi A, Ulbright TM, Miller GA, Haidar JH, Donohue JP, Foster RS (1995). Prognostic significance of immunohistochemical proliferation markers (Ki-67/MIB-1 and proliferation-associated nuclear antigen), p53 protein accumulation, and neovascularization in clinical stage A nonseminomatous testicular germ cell tumors. Mod Pathol 8(5):492–497.
170. Baker JM, Murty VV, Potla L, Mendola CE, Rodriguez E, Reuter VE, Bosl GG, Chaganti RS (1994). Loss of heterozygosity and decreased expression of NME genes correlate with teratomatous differentiation in human male germ cell tumors. Biochem Biophys Res Commun 202(2):1096–1103.
171. Klein EA (1993). Tumor markers in testis cancer. Urol Clin North Am 20(1):67–73.

172. Ohyama C, Orikasa S, Kawamura S, et al. (1995). Galactosylgloboside expression in seminoma; inverse correlation with metastatic potential. Cancer 76:1043–1050.
173. Motzer RJ, Rodriguez E, Reuter VE, Samaniego F, Dmitrovsky E, Bajorin DF, Pfister DG, Parsa NZ, Chaganti RS, Bosl GJ (1991). Genetic analysis as an aid in diagnosis for patients with midline carcinomas of uncertain histologies. J Natl Cancer Inst 83(5):341–346.

4. Reverse transcriptase- polymerase chain reaction (RT-PCR) to detect prostate cancer micrometastasis in the blood

Kai-Ling Yao, Mary Josephine Pilat, and Kenneth J. Pienta

Since the high mortality rate of prostate cancer is directly associated with the incidence of cancer metastasis, early detection of metastasizing prostate cancer cells in the blood has very important clinical implications. Conventional screening and staging modalities often fail to identify patients who may have prostate cancer that is already metastatic [1], and it has been estimated that 60% of new patients may have asymptomatic micrometastasis. It is therefore of great importance to be able to define which patients are at risk for the development of further metastatic disease [2,3]. It has been suggested that the detection of circulating prostate cancer cells in the peripheral blood may allow assessment of disease state [4], although the exact clinical significance of circulating cancer cells remains unclear. Animal experiments using solid tumors have shown that only two cells per milliliter of blood may be enough for tumor metastasis from hematogenous dissemination [5–7]. Based on these studies, a technique to detect circulating cells must be highly sensitive, detecting ten tumor cells in a five milliliter blood sample. Although immunohistochemical and other immunological techniques that use antibodies against tumor-associated antigens or tissue-specific antigens are helpful in detecting the primary site of metastatic disease and the presence of small foci of metastatic disease, these techniques are not sensitive enough to detect such a small number of cancer cells in a large quantity of nonneoplastic cells. It is through the development of Reverse Transcriptase- Polymerase Chain Reaction (RT-PCR) and new tumor markers that the desired sensitivity for this approach becomes possible. The high sensitivity and specificity obtained from this technique as well as the small quantity of test material required makes RT-PCR a definite front runner in the race for early detection of micrometastasis in prostate cancer.

PCR

It would be difficult to understand RT-PCR without first understanding the polymerase chain reaction (PCR). PCR is a technique used to identify and amplify specific DNA sequences. It was first invented by Kary Mullis in 1985

Pienta, K.J., (ed.), DIAGNOSIS AND TREATMENT OF GENITOURINARY MALIGNANCIES.

[8,9], and after subsequent improvement and the introduction of thermostable DNA polymerases [10], PCR has become a standard molecular biology procedure widely used in research and clinical applications. PCR has revolutionized the way molecular experiments are performed and is expected to be the main technique for routine clinical testing for genetic, infectious, and neoplastic diseases in the next 15 years [11].

PCR is a surprisingly simple technique that requires a much smaller amount of target DNA than previously used techniques. The minimum amount of DNA sample necessary for a PCR reaction is roughly 200 nanograms in comparison to 10 micrograms needed for Southern analysis of genomic DNA. The purpose of PCR is to amplify target DNA (figure 4-1). There are five basic components of a PCR reaction: 1) target DNA (genomic DNA from a sample or complementary DNA (cDNA) synthesized from RNA samples), 2) two primers (18–25-base-pair synthetic single-stranded DNA molecules that specifically share the same sequences as each end of target DNA, called sense and antisense, respectively), 3) DNA polymerase, 4) deoxy-nucleotide-triphosphates (dNTPs, dATP, dCTP, dGTP, dTTP), and 5) a reaction buffer. All these components are mixed in a reaction tube that is then incubated in an automated thermocycler, and the reaction proceeds through four steps in a cyclic fashion (figure 4-1). First, double-stranded target DNA is denatured at 95°C, with the two strands separating from each other (denaturation step). Two primers anneal to the target DNA at each end of the sequence (annealing step), and the DNA is extended from the primers in a 5′ to 3′ direction mediated by DNA polymerase and using dNTPs as sources for the added bases. This completes the first cycle of target DNA duplication. The process is then repeated a number of times, and in a matter of a few hours, a segment of target DNA can be specifically amplified by a factor of 10^6 or more. The PCR products can then be electrophoresed with molecular weight markers on an agarose gel and visualized by ethidium bromide staining under UV light.

The mechanism of the PCR reaction is well understood, and one can easily optimize the reaction to a desired specificity and sensitivity. Conditions that can be adjusted include PCR primers, buffer composition, annealing temperature, the duration of the extension step, and the number of cycles. Two other PCR manipulations that are widely used to increase sensitivity and specificity are nested PCR and Southern blotting of PCR products. In nested PCR, after the first set of PCR reactions has been completed, a second PCR is performed using the first PCR product as a template and a second pair of specific primers located within the region of the first PCR product (figure 4-2). This technique increases detection sensitivity and also greatly enhances specificity. Southern blotting analysis [12] of PCR products involves resolving the products by electrophoresis on an agarose gel and subsequently transferring these fragments onto a nucleotide-binding membrane (figure 4-3). This membrane is then hybridized with a chemically (fluorescein) or radioactively (usually ^{32}P or

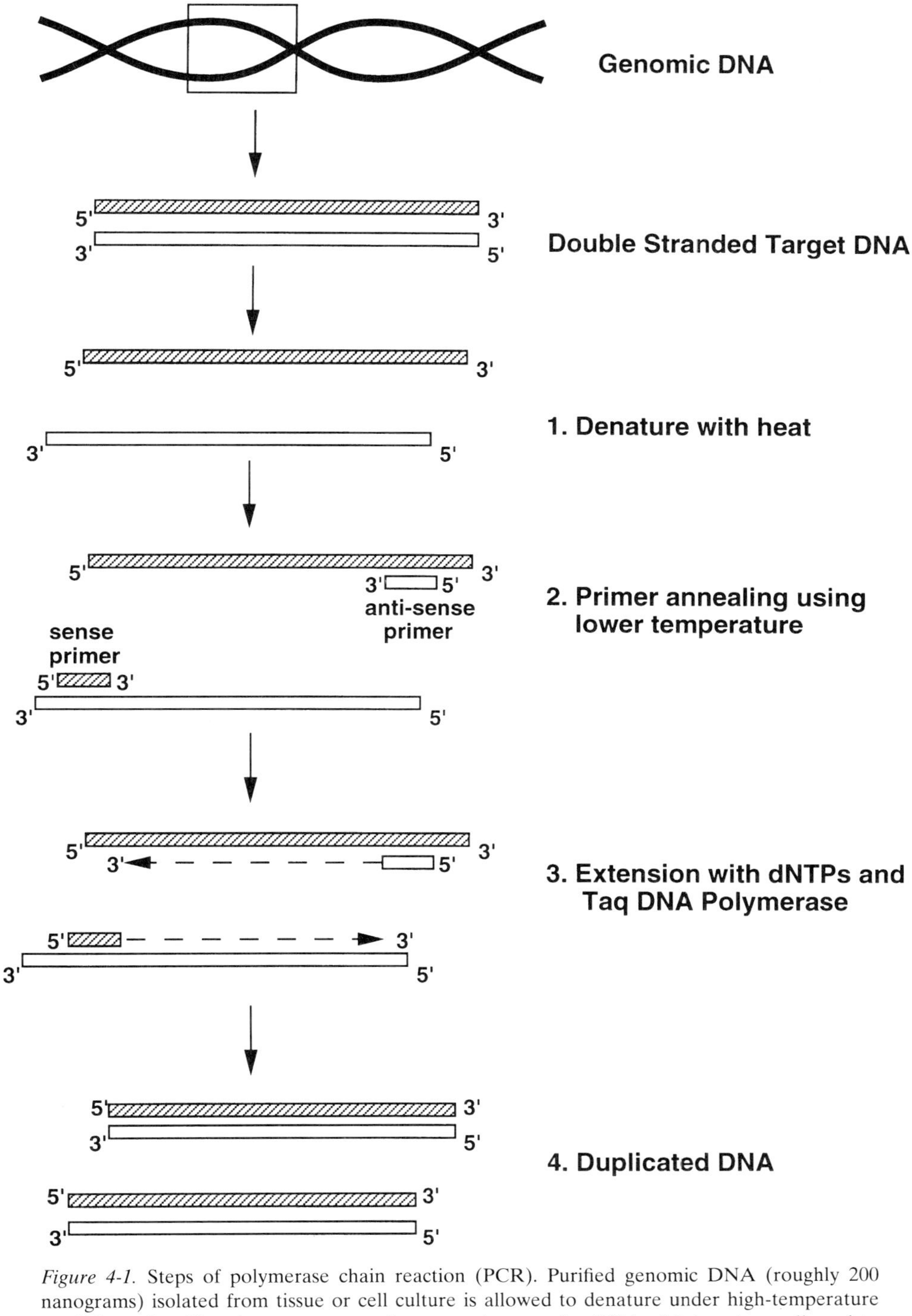

Figure 4-1. Steps of polymerase chain reaction (PCR). Purified genomic DNA (roughly 200 nanograms) isolated from tissue or cell culture is allowed to denature under high-temperature conditions. Specific primers corresponding to regions on the DNA of interest are allowed to anneal at a lower temperature. Using these primers, the new strands of DNA are extended using dNTPs and Taq DNA polymerase. At the end of the cycle, amplification of the target DNA is achieved and the process repeats for a number of cycles, amplifying the DNA of interest by a factor of 10^6 or more.

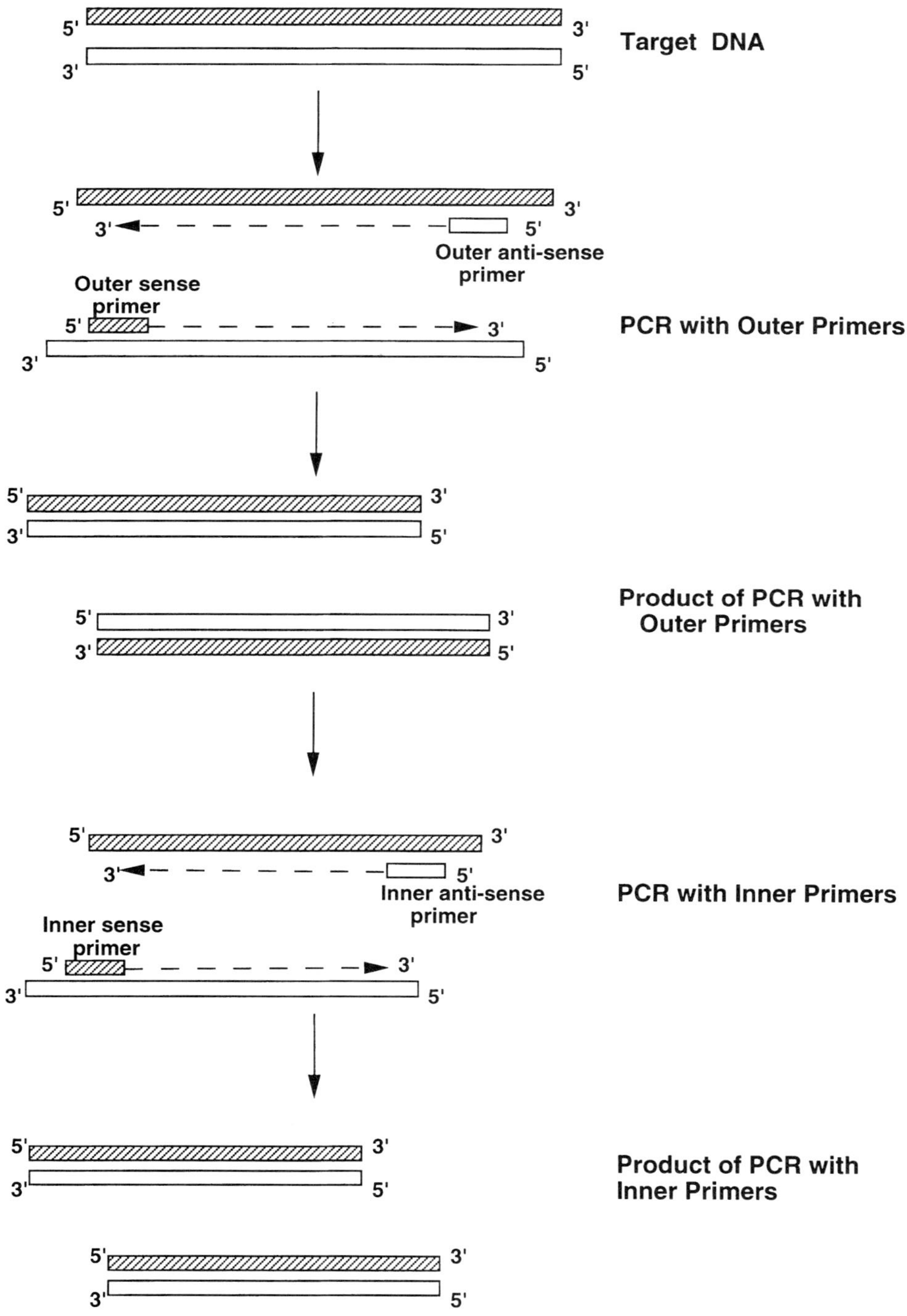

Figure 4-2. Steps of nested PCR. Target DNA isolated from tissue or cell culture is allowed to denature, specific primers to the DNA of interest are allowed to anneal, and the DNA is extended as described in the legend to figure 4-1. The PCR product using the first set of primers is then subjected to another series of PCR reactions using a second set of primers that anneal to an area of DNA interior to the annealing site of the first set of primers. Using this technique, the DNA of interest is amplified to a higher degree, increasing the detection sensitivity as well as specificity of the reaction.

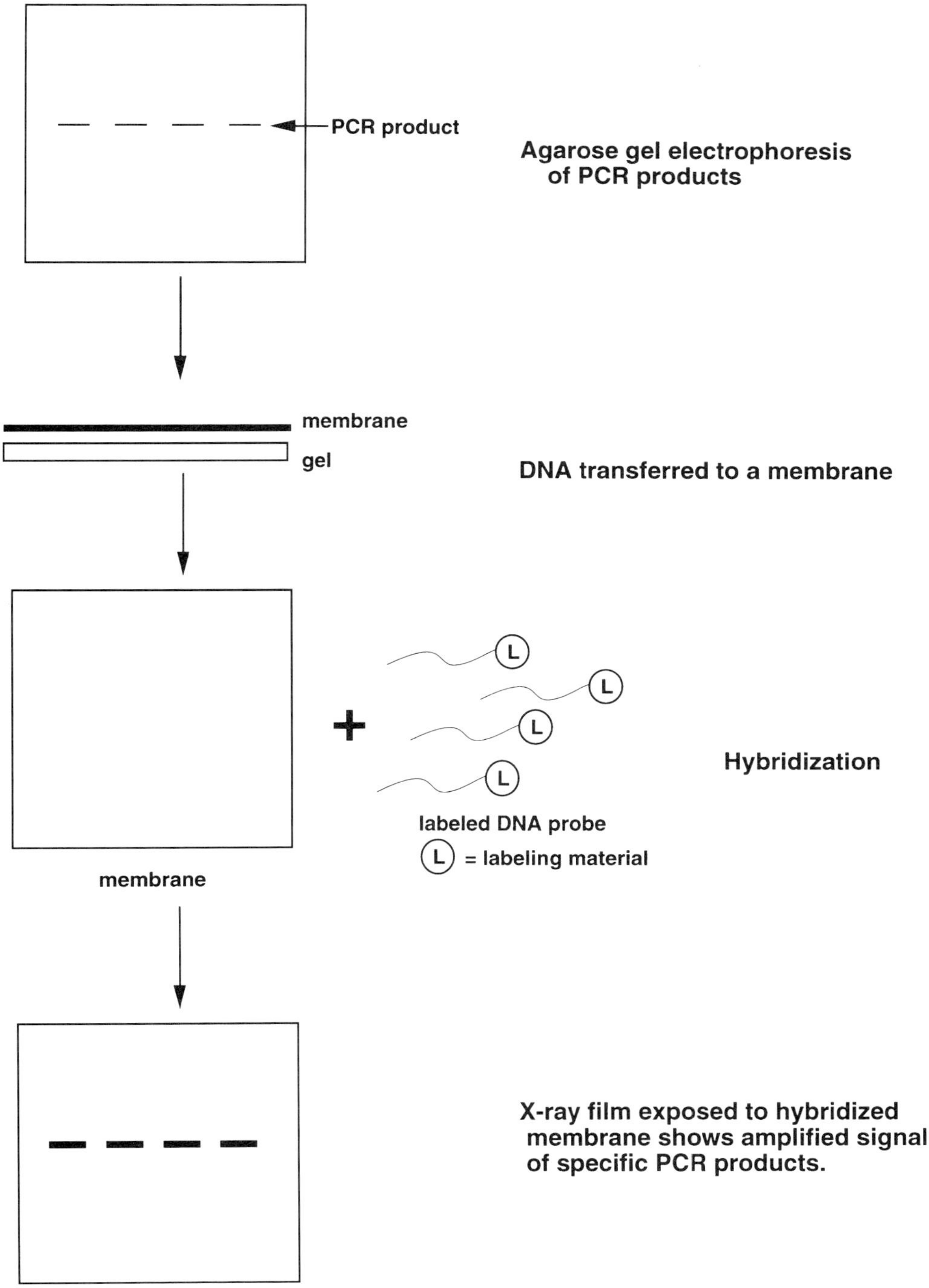

Figure 4-3. Southern blot analysis. DNA of interest (i.e., PCR product) is subjected to agarose gel electrophoresis. The DNA is then transferred via capillary action onto a nucleotide-binding membrane. A radioactively or chemically labeled probe specific to the DNA of interest is incubated with the membrane under appropriate conditions. This probe will hybridize to the DNA on the membrane that corresponds to the target DNA. After the membrane is washed to reduce nonspecific binding, it is exposed to X-ray film, which upon development shows the amplified signal of the PCR product.

^{35}S) labeled DNA fragment (oligo DNA probe) that shares the same sequence as a region within the PCR product. After incubation with the labeled probe, the membrane is washed to decrease nonspecific binding of the probe and then exposed to X-ray film to visualize the signal. The use of a specific DNA probe to the product of interest excludes possible nonspecific products, which are often observed in PCR reactions.

RT-PCR

Reverse transcriptase-PCR is used to detect the expression of specific genes. Specific mRNA species in a small amount of a total cellular RNA sample (roughly 100 nanograms) are used as templates for a first-strand cDNA synthesis using the enzyme reverse transcriptase (figure 4-4). This cDNA is then used directly as a template for the subsequent PCR reaction [8,9]. This allows direct detection of the expression of a particular gene product of interest as well as quantitation of this expression under the proper reaction conditions.

As one can imagine, RT-PCR is a powerful tool, allowing the detection of a single mRNA species in a complex mixture of thousands of other mRNAs. In comparison to the amount of RNA required for Northern analysis (10 micrograms), RT-PCR requires only one microgram of total cellular RNA. Furthermore, if the mRNA of interest is specific to one particular cell type, one can easily identify the presence of this cell in a heterogeneous cell population with minimal sample required. Therefore, one should be able to detect circulating tumor cells in peripheral blood, provided that these tumor cells have a specific marker. It should be noted that RNA is very unstable in the extracellular environment and degrades quickly. Consequently, a positive result from a blood sample would suggest the presence of tumor cells, not merely their RNA.

Although immunological techniques have historically been used in the detection of tumor metastasis, RT-PCR, in theory, appears to be a better assay, since it yields higher specificity and sensitivity along with being a more straightforward technique. In most cases, if one has good access to DNA sequence information plus a service for gene analysis and oligo DNA synthesis, it is possible to develop a RT-PCR assay that can be easily adjusted for sensitivity and specificity. In comparison to immunological techniques, where problems with antibody production and antibody–antigen interactions often cause difficulties in technical prediction and data interpretation, RT-PCR is more sensitive in detection as well as much more straightforward technically. Furthermore, immunological assays detect proteins, the final product of gene expression. True detection of gene expression may be difficult when analyzing protein products, since a number of molecular events may occur before this final step [13,14].

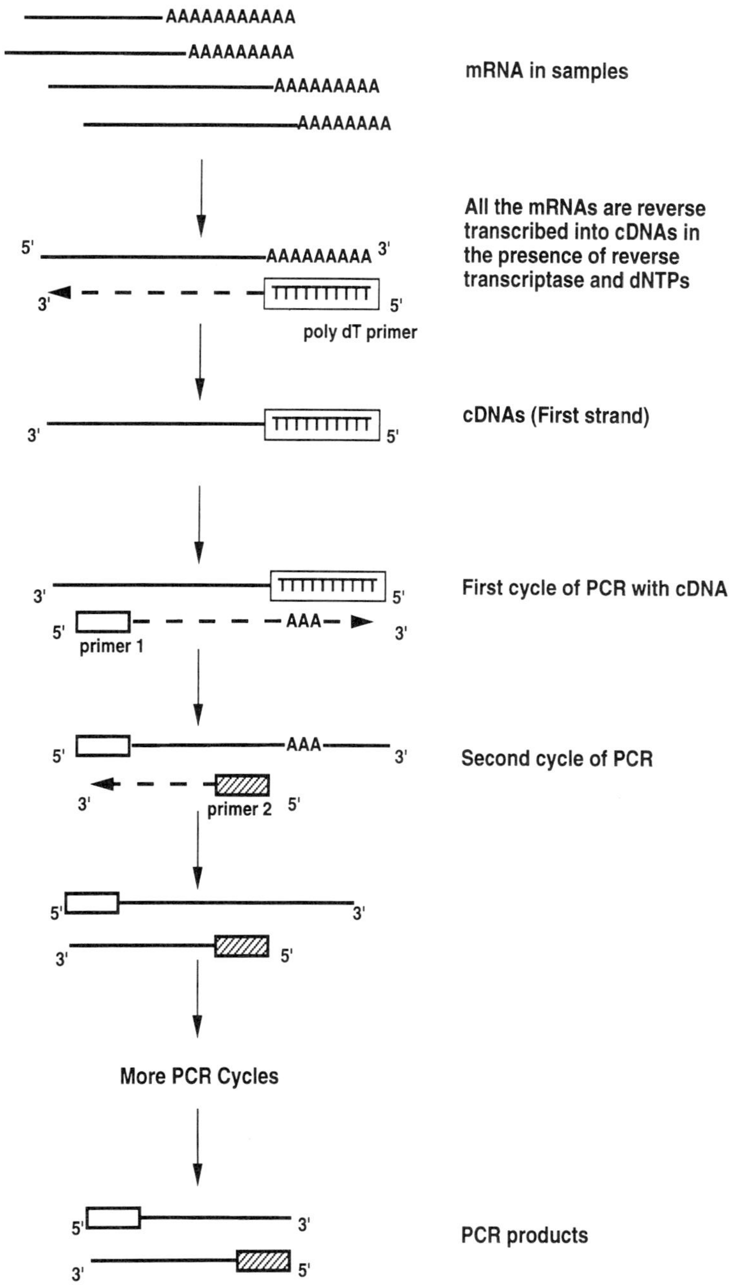

Figure 4-4. Steps of reverse transcriptase-polymerase chain reaction (RT-PCR). Total cellular RNA is isolated from tissue sample or cell culture. mRNA in the sample (roughly 1 microgram of total RNA) is then reverse transcribed into complementary DNA using reverse transcriptase and dNTPs. This cDNA strand is then allowed to anneal to a primer sequence specific to the mRNA of interest, and a new DNA strand is synthesized from this primer sequence using dNTPs and Taq polymerase as described in the legend to figure 4-1. This double-stranded DNA molecule then undergoes several cycles of PCR (described in figure 4-1) until amplification of a DNA segment corresponding to a target mRNA molecule is achieved.

Detection of prostate cancer cells in the blood

RT-PCR is more specific and sensitive than immunohistochemistry for detecting minute amounts of tumor cells mixed in normal cells in blood or lymph nodes, as demonstrated by previous studies in leukemia [15–17], melanoma [18], neuroblastoma [19], and prostate cancer [20]. Encouraged by the technical advantage of RT-PCR and aware of the urgent need of the clinical community for an effective way to detect and better understand micrometastasis in prostate cancer, investigators have been actively searching for an RT-PCR-based assay in detecting circulating prostate cancer cells in blood for the past 5 years.

The development of a clinically useful assay takes a combination of a good detecting system in terms of sensitivity and specificity as well as a good tumor marker in terms of level of expression and cell-type specificity. In prostate cancer, two markers have been actively pursued for RT-PCR detection of circulating cells: prostate-specific antigen (PSA) and prostate-specific membrane antigen (PSM). PSA, a 33-kDa protein, was originally thought to be produced exclusively by prostatic epithelial cells [21] and has been used extensively as a prostate cancer marker to monitor progression of disease. More recently, elevated PSA has been seen in other tumor tissues such as breast, although it appears that PSA is mainly localized to the tumor and not secreted into the peripheral system [22]. PSM is a 100-kDa integral transmembrane glycoprotein recently cloned from the human prostate cancer cell line LNCaP by Israeli et al. [23] and has thus far been detected only in prostate cells [24]. The following is a synopsis of the results obtained from several groups using PSA and PSM mRNA-based RT-PCR in detecting circulating prostate tumor cells (summarized in table 4-1).

RT-PCR for PSA mRNA

Three main facts have been established when examining the literature addressing PSA mRNA-positive cells in the blood of prostate cancer patients

Table 4-1. General comparison of PSM vs PSA mRNA-based RT-PCR

	Sensitivity (%)					
	MET	LA	OC	HR	LS-PSA	Specificity (%)
PSM	60–80	>60	30–70	80–100	50–60	95–100
PSA	0.9–50[a]	6–20	0–16[a]	50–60	0–3	97–100

[a] An interesting exception to this data is the work by Katz et al. [26] described in the text.
Abbreviations: MET, patients with metastatic prostate carcinoma; LA, patients with locally advanced ($T3^{+}$) prostate cancer; OC, patients with organ-confined prostate cancer; HR, patients with hormone-refractory prostate cancer; and LS-PSA, patients with low or negative serum PSA after treatment.

[25–29]. First, it is clear that PSA mRNA-positive cells exist only in the blood of prostate cancer patients. Detection of PSA mRNA-positive cells appears to be much more specific than the immunological detection of PSA protein. This finding can be attributed to immunological methods involving antibodies that often have some degree of cross-reactivities with antigens from other cell types. Furthermore, flow cytometry studies demonstrate a high amount of PSA-positive cells (i.e., false positives) due to uptake of PSA antigen by host immunocytes rather than circulating prostatic epithelial cells [30].

In general, the sensitivity of the methods reported so far in the literature have been rather low. Even in patients with metastatic diseases, the sensitivity is lower than 50%. It should be noted, however, that the actual percentage of patients who have circulating cells in their peripheral blood is unknown. Some investigators [27–29] have tried to enhance the sensitivity by using nested PCR and/or Southern blot analysis. By using the prostate carcinoma cell line LNCaP as a positive control, they were able to detect as few as 3 to 10 PSA mRNA-positive cells in $3–6 \times 10^6$ non-PSA-expressing cells, depending on the method used. When utilizing patient samples, however, they failed to show a corresponding sensitivity. An exception to these results was a study reported by Katz [26]. This group was able to increase the sensitivity of their RT-PCR based assay by the addition of a digoxigenin-modified nucleotide to the PCR reaction. After transfer of PCR products from an agarose gel to a membrane, an enzyme labeled anti-digoxigenin antibody detection system was added to observe the presence of PCR product. With this method, the researchers were able to detect PSA mRNA-positive cells in 14 of 18 (77.8%) patients with metastatic prostate cancer and 25 of 65 (38.5%) patients with clinically localized disease (T1-2b). Furthermore, this study established a strong correlation between RT-PCR positivity and the presence of capsular tumor penetration as well as between RT-PCR positivity and the detection of carcinoma at the surgical margin. Their method was statistically shown to be remarkably superior to the commonly used staging modalities, such as computed tomography scan, endorectal coil magnetic resonance imaging, PSA density, or Gleason score. The sensitivity of this method is the highest thus far of all reported detection methods for prostate cancer circulating cells.

Another consistent finding amongst the reported studies on PSA mRNA detection in circulating cells was the inconsistency of PSA expression with different disease states. Although detection sensitivity of the methods reported was generally low in patients with clinically diagnosed metastatic prostate cancer, there were a number of cases in which PSA mRNA-positive cells were detected with up to 20% positivity (with the exception of the data reported by Katz et al. [26]) in patients with clinically localized prostate cancer (table 4-1). These results suggest that the detectabilities of PSA-positive cells between the two groups were not as proportionally related as one would expect.

Several questions arise from these reports. The first is why, utilizing the same RT-PCR technique that had such high sensitivity in detecting PSA mRNA-positive cells in vitro with the LNCaP prostate cancer cell line, does one obtain such low sensitivity examining circulating cells in the blood even from patients with metastatic prostate cancer? Furthermore, why, with the same methods, is the relationship between detectability of tumor cells in patients with localized prostate cancer and those with metastatic disease not proportional?

The RT-PCR assay alone cannot be the reason for this generally low detection sensitivity of PSA mRNA in blood samples. It has been well documented that the combination of RT-PCR and Southern blotting methods are very sensitive for the detection of PSA mRNA in tissues other than blood, including lymph nodes [20] and bone marrow [31]. Both of these studies reported 100% sensitivity in detection of PSA mRNA-positive cells in patients having metastatic prostate cancer in these tissues, with their detection being much superior to concomitant immunohistochemical analysis for PSA protein. In the study with lymph nodes [20], Deguchi et al. were able to further demonstrate a detection limit of 1 LNCaP cell in 10^6 peripheral mononuclear cells. Thus far, however, no group has been able to obtain this degree of sensitivity for PSA mRNA in circulating cells from the peripheral blood of patients in vivo.

Since methodology does not appear to be the only answer, it would seem that one would have to examine the process of circulating tumor cells in the blood. There have been several suggestions to explain the lower detection limits obtained in vivo. Mereno et al. has suggested that circulating tumor cells may be poorly differentiated, expressing low levels of PSA that may not be detected [25]. Furthermore, patients with high Gleason-grade tumors may also be less likely to have circulating tumor cells that express PSA mRNA [27]. It has also been proposed that prostate tumor cells may shed intermittently into the circulation, and one would detect tumor cells only if the blood were examined during the proper time period [28]. Finally, as PSA is upregulated by androgens [32], prostate cancer patients receiving androgen-deprivation treatment may test negative for PSA mRNA-positive cells, since PSA expression is suppressed [29]. Based on the above results and explanations, it would appear that several problems may arise when utilizing a PSA mRNA-based RT-PCR to detect circulating prostate cancer cells in vivo. Inconsistency and poor detection limits must be alleviated before this assay would be beneficial to the clinical community.

RT-PCR for PSM mRNA

The recently cloned PSM molecule has been reported to be a better marker than PSA in the detection of circulating prostate cancer cells at a molecular level [4,33–35]. Three separate investigations have been reported in which detection of circulating prostate cancer cells positive for PSM and PSA mRNAs were studied in a comparison fashion [33–35]. These studies increased their detection limits and specificity by using nested PCR and Southern analysis. Their results demonstrate that assays for PSM mRNA-positive circulating cells were more sensitive than PSA mRNA-positive cells in both metastatic and localized prostate cancer patients.

In a study reported in 1994 by Israeli et al. [33], the sensitivity of both PSM and PSA mRNA-based RT-PCR was reported as one cancer cell in 10^6 nonneoplastic cells. When comparing the sensitivity obtained on actual patient samples, however, the sensitivities of the two assays were significantly different. Of 77 prostate cancer patients examined, 62.5% were positive for PSM mRNA, while only 9.1% were positive for PSA mRNA. In stage D patients receiving androgen ablation therapy, 66.7% were positive for PSM mRNA in comparison to 25% positive for PSA mRNA. In patients with clinically localized prostate cancer following radical prostatectomy, 60% of the patients were positive for PSM mRNA versus 6.1% for PSA mRNA. Finally, in postradical prostatectomy patients with negative serum PSA values, PSM mRNA was detected in 67.7% of patients, while PSA mRNA was detected in only 3% of those examined. Interestingly, 4 of 40 control patients were positive for PSM mRNA cells. Two of these patients were later found to have previously undetected prostate cancer. Similar results have been obtained utilizing a different set of PCR primers by Israeli et al. in a more recent study [34].

Loric et al. was able to detect five prostate cancer LNCaP cells in 5.5×10^6 nucleated blood cells in vitro using either PSM or PSA mRNA based RT-PCR [35]. When analyzing 60 prostate cancer patients, however, the results obtained with PSM and PSA primers were quite different. Forty patients (67%) were positive for PSM mRNA-containing cells, while only 20 (33%) were positive for PSA mRNA. Eighty-five percent of metastatic patients were positive for PSM mRNA, in comparison to 51% of the patients having detectable PSA mRNA. There was also a higher rate of detection of PSM mRNA (35%) than PSA mRNA (1%) in patients with clinically localized prostate cancer. Furthermore, of nine patients receiving androgen deprivation therapy, who later were seen to have hormone-refractory prostate cancer, 100% were positive for PSM mRNA cells, while 60% were positive for PSA mRNA-containing cells. Of 53 controls examined, none were positive for either marker.

The consistent sensitivity of PSM mRNA-based RT-PCR has never been achieved by PSA mRNA-based RT-PCR techniques. This higher sensitivity may be partially explained by the observation that PSM mRNA appears to be upregulated after androgen deprivation [24,35]. Furthermore, since PSM is overexpressed in anaplastic cells, and since metastatic cells represent a more aggressive and poorly differentiated cell type, circulating prostate cancer cells may express a higher level of PSM mRNA per cell than PSA mRNA [33]. As in the PSA mRNA detection data, however, results were not directly proportional to clinical staging of the disease, with some patients with early disease having a higher frequency of positivity than patients with more advanced disease. Regardless, although results vary between methods and studies, the sensitivity of the PSM mRNA-based RT-PCR in general has proved to be superior to PSA mRNA-based RT-PCR as well as conventional staging modalities.

Clinical usefulness

Based on the review presented above, PSM mRNA-based RT-PCR appears to be more sensitive and a promising new technique for detecting circulating prostate cancer cells in the peripheral blood of patients. Although PSA mRNA-based RT-PCR detection limits have generally been low, the methods of Katz et al. have increased the sensitivity of this assay, and further work should be done to evaluate its clinical implications. Its clinical usefulness, however, may be questioned because of the inconsistent expression of PSA mRNA, the low expression of PSA in poorly differentiated tumors, and the downregulation of PSA mRNA upon androgen withdrawal. A further advantage that the PSM mRNA-based assay has over the PSA mRNA-based assay is its enhanced detection rate in patients undergoing hormone therapy. More clinically relevant at this point, however, is the ability of either assay to detect prostate cancer metastasis at a rate far superior to any clinical staging modalities currently being used. Although more studies would be needed for better understanding, the data suggest that it is currently possible to utilize PSM mRNA-based RT-PCR for the assessment of metastatic risks, clinical staging, and evaluation of responses to therapies in patients with prostate cancer.

Like every new technology being introduced to clinical medicine, clinical acceptance of this new modality has to be validated. Studies must be done to ascertain statistical relationships between test results and disease processes as well as to establish guidelines for clinical interpretation of test results. Comparison of this molecular modality with current clinical modalities must be done on a large sample size with long-term follow-up of these patients. Perhaps the most significant issue that must be addressed for a clinically reliable RT-PCR-based assay, however, is the development of a standard internal control. Many laboratories are currently using the mRNA produced from the human prostate cancer cell line LNCaP as an internal control for their assays. The amount of mRNA production in LNCaP cells, however, has been shown to vary extensively depending on passage number of cells and growth conditions such as the amount and lot of serum used [4]. Preparations of standards and interpretation of detection sensitivity of these assays have also differed between laboratories. It should be noted that many investigators used a calculated ratio of one prostate cancer cell per number of nonmarker-expressing cells rather than the actual number of detectable cells. Consistency in reporting as well as standardization is necessary before introduction of this assay into the clinical setting.

Future research

Investigators started out with a seemly simply task: to develop an assay at a molecular level to detect circulating prostate cancer cells in the peripheral blood, with the 'magic number' for detection limit being two cancer cells per milliliter of blood. As the investigations unfold, however, we find that, although we do need to technically improve the detection sensitivity of the assay, the 'magic number' may not be a true reference due to the variables in the actual disease process observed in previous studies. It must also be emphasized that we do not know what the presence of circulating cancer cells signifies. It is unknown whether circulating cancer cells have true metastatic potential or whether they simply represent sloughed tumor cells destined to die. It will take much more work investigating the hemodynamics and evolution of circulating cancer cells in relationship to the expression of specific tumor makers to determine how a positive test for circulating cancer cells truly relates to a patient's clinical disease course.

Several intriguing observations arise from previous investigations: 1) the uneven distribution of circulating cells, 2) disproportional test results between stages, and 3) differential expression of antigens, such as PSM and PSA. Although some explanations can be found from previous studies in other disciplines, we must do further research to completely understand these phenomena. Future research should include both in vivo and in vitro longitudinal studies to follow up the dynamics and evolution of circulating cells. It would be interesting to develop animal models to observe progression of metastasis by RT-PCR and to isolate prostate cancer cells from patients with different disease states to study their molecular and phenotypic changes. Studies involving collection of samples at different time points and at different sites of circulation in relation to different stages may help us better understand how tumor cells are distributed and the mode of collection needed to yield the most desirable information. These studies will offer more clinical understanding of RT-PCR assay results. Finally, the differential expression of PSM and PSA in circulating prostate cancer cells has also motivated investigators to look for and define more tumor markers with a hope that a panel of RT-PCR-based markers may become available to determine to what stage the disease has progressed [4].

References

1. Mukamel E, Hanna J, deKernion JB (1987). Pitfalls in preoperative staging in prostate cancer. Urology 30:318–323.
2. Epstein JI, Pizov G, Walsh PC (1993). Correlation of pathologic findings with progression after radical retropubic prostatectomy. Cancer 71:3583–3593.
3. McNeal JE, Vilers AA, Redwine EA, Freiha FS, Stamey TS (1990). Capsular penetration in prostate cancer: significance for natural history and treatment. Am J Surg Pathol 14:240–247.
4. Heston WDW (1995). Detection of hematogenous dissemination of prostate cancer by

RT-PCR with primers specific for prostate-specific membrane antigen. Clin Chem 41:1687–1688.

5. Fidler IJ, Hart IR (1982). Biological diversity in metastatic neoplasms — origins and implications. Science 217:998–1001.
6. Liotta LA, Kleinerman J, Saidel GM (1974). Quantitative relationship of intravascular tumor cells, tumor vessels and pulmonary metastases following tumor implantation. Cancer Res 34:997–1003.
7. Schirrmacher V (1985). Cancer metastasis: experimental approaches, theoretical concepts, and impacts for treatment strategies. Adv Cancer Res 43:1–73.
8. Mullis KB, Faloona F (1987). Specific synthesis of DNA in vitro via a polymerase catalyzed chain reaction method. Enzymology 155:335–350.
9. Saiki RK, Scharf S, Faloona F, Mullis KB, Horn GT, Erlich HA, Arnhein N (1985). Enzymatic amplification of ß-globin genomic sequences and restriction site analysis for diagnosis of sickle cell anemia. Science 230:1350–1354.
10. Saik RK, Gelfand DH, Stoffel S, Scat S, Higuchi R, Horn GT (1988). Primer-directed enzymatic amplification of DNA with a thermostable DNA polymerase. Science 239:487–491.
11. Hart C, Schochetman G, Spira T, Lifson A, Moore J, Sninsky J (1988). Direct detection of HIV RNA expression in seropositive subjects. Lancet ii:596–599.
12. Sambrook J, Fritsh EF, Maniatis T (eds) (1989). Molecular Cloning: A Laboratory Manual. Cold Spring Harbor Laboratory Press: Plainview, New York.
13. Qui SD, Young CY, Bilhartz DL (1990). In situ hybridization of prostate-specific antigen mRNA in human prostate. J Urol 144:1550–1556.
14. Warembourg M, Tranchant O, Atger M, Milgrom E (1986). Uteroglobin messenger ribonucleic acid: localization in rabbit uterus and lung by in situ hybridization. Endocrinology 119:1632–1640.
15. Yamada M, Wasserman R, Lange B, Reichard BA, Womer RB, Rovera G (1990). Minimal residual disease in childhood B-lineage lymphoblastic leukemia: persistence of leukemic cells during the first 18 months of treatment. N Engl J Med 232:448–455.
16. Yokota S, Hansen-Hagge TE, Ludwig WD, Reiter A, Raghavachar A, Kleinhauer E, Bartram CR (1991). Use of polymerase chain reactions to monitor minimal residual disease in acute lymphoblastic leukemia patients. Blood 77:331–339.
17. Miyomura M, Tanimoto Y, Morishima K, Horibe K, Yamamoto M, Akatsuka Y, Kodera S, Kojima K, Matsuyama K, Hirabayashi N, Yazaki M, Imai K, Onozawa Y, Kanamaru A, Mizutani S, Saito H (1992). Detection of Philadelphia chromsome-positive acute lymphoblastic leukemia by polymerase chain reaction: possible eradication of minimal residual disease by bone marrow transplantation. Blood 79:1366–1370.
18. Smith B, Selby P, Southgate J, Pittman K, Bradley C, Blair CE (1991). Detection of melanoma cells in peripheral blood by means of reverse transcriptase and polymerase chain reaction. Lancet 338:1227–1229.
19. Mattano LA, Moss TJ, Eerson SG (1992). Sensitive detection of rare circulating neuroblastoma cells by the reverse transcriptase-polymerase chain reaction. Cancer Res 52:4701–4705.
20. Deguchi T, Doi T, Ehara H, Ito S, Takahashi Y, Nishino Y, Fujihiro S, Kawamura T, Komeda H, Horie M, Kaji H, Shimokawa K, Tanaka T, Kawada Y (1993). Detection of micrometastatic prostate cancer cells in lymph nodes by reverse transcriptase-polymerase chain reaction. Cancer Res 53:5350–5354.
21. Oesterling JE (1991). Prostate-specific antigen: a critical assessment of the most useful tumor marker for adenocarcinoma of the prostate. J Urol 145:907–923.
22. Giai M, Yu H, Roagna R, Ponzone R, Katsaros D, Levesque MA, Diamandis EP (1995). Prostate-specific antigen in serum of women with breast cancer. Br J Cancer 72:728–731.
23. Israeli RS, Powell CT, Fair WR, Heston WDW (1993). Molecular cloning of a complementary DNA encoding a prostate-specific membrane antigen. Cancer Res 53:227–230.
24. Israeli RS, Powell CT, Corr JG, Fair WR, Heston WDW (1994). Expression of the prostate-specific membrane antigen. Cancer Res 54:1807–1811.

25. Moreno JG, Croce CM, Fischer R, Monne M, Vihko P, Mulholland SG, Gomella LG (1992). Detection of hematogenous micrometastasis in patients with prostate cancer. Cancer Res 52:6110–6112.
26. Katz AE, Olsson CA, Raffo AJ, Cama C, Perlman H, Seaman E, O'Toole KM, McMahon D, Benson MC, Buttyan R (1994). Molecular staging of prostate cancer with the use of an enhanced reverse transcriptase-PCR assay. Urology 43:765–775.
27. Seiden MV, Kantoff PW, Krithivas K, Propert K, Bryant M, Halton E, Gaynes L, Kaplan I, Bubley G, Dewolf W, Sklar J (1994). Detection of circulating tumor cells in men with localized prostate cancer. J Clin Oncol 12:2634–2639.
28. Ghossein RA, Scher, HI, Gerald WL, Kelly WK, Curley T, Amsterdan A, Zhang ZF, Rosai J (1995). Detection of circulating tumor cells in patients with localized and metastatic carcinoma: clinical implications. J Clin Oncol 13:1195–1200.
29. Jaakkola S, Vornanen T, Leinonen J, Rannikko S, Stenman UH (1995). Detection of prostate cells in peripheral blood: correlation with serum concentrations of prostate-specific antigen. Clin Chem 41:182–186.
30. Hamdy FC, Lawry J, Anderson JB, Parsons MA, Rees RC, Williams JL (1992). Circulating prostate specific antigen-positive cells correlate with metastatic cancer. Br J Urol 69:392–396.
31. Wood DP, Bank ER, Humphreys S, McRoberts JW, Rangnekar VM (1994). Identification of bone marrow micrometastases in patients with prostate cancer. Cancer 74:2533–2540.
32. Henttu P, Shutsung L, Vihko P (1992). Androgens up-regulate the human prostate-specific antigen messenger ribonucleic acid (mRNA) in the LNCaP cell line. Endocrinology 130:766–772.
33. Israeli RS, Miller WH, Su SL, Powell CT, Fair WR, Samadi DS, Huryk RF, DeBlasio A, Edwards ET, Wise GJ, Heston WDW (1994). Sensitive nested reverse transcription polymerase chain reaction detection of circulating prostate tumor cells: comparison of prostate-specific membrane antigen and prostate-specific antigen-based assays. Cancer Res 54: 6306–6310.
34. Israeli RS, Miller WH, Su SL, Samadi DS, Powell CT, Heston WDW, Wise GJ, Fair WR (1995). Sensitive detection of prostate hematogenous tumor cell dissemination using prostate-specific antigen and prostate specific membrane antigen-derived primers in the polymerase chain reaction. J Urol 153:573–577.
35. Loric S, Dumas F, Eschwege P, Blanchet P, Benoit G, Jardin A, Lacour B (1995). Enhanced detection of hematogenous circulating prostatic cells in patients with prostate adenocarcinoma by using nested reverse transcription polymerase chain reaction assay based on prostate-specific membrane antigen. Clin Chem 41:1698–1704.

5. Succesful separation between benign prostatic hyperplasia and prostate cancer by measurement of free and complexed PSA

Hans Lilja and Ulf-Håkan Stenman

Biosynthesis and enzyme activity of PSA

Prostate-specific antigen (PSA) is a serine protease belonging to the human glandular kallikrein gene family [1–3]. The expression of PSA is mainly androgen dependent, and the detection of very high expression levels is restricted to the prostate tissue, but extraprostatic production at much lower levels has been demonstrated in several other tissues such as normal and malignant breast epithelium, endometrium, and bulbourethral glands [4–10]. PSA is synthesized by the columnar epithelium in the glandular ducts and acini of the prostate, but not by any other cells in prostate tissue. It is secreted at high concentrations (0.2–5 mg/mL) into seminal fluid [4–6,11]. PSA is synthesized as an inactive precursor [2,3,12]. Like other glandular kallikreins, the PSA-precursor is processed stepwise by release of a leader peptide followed by liberation of an activation peptide that results in conversion of the zymogen into enzymatically active PSA [12]. This process may occur in parallel with the secretory release from the prostate epithelium and most probably occurs prior to the ejaculatory mixing of secretions from the prostate, seminal vesicles, and epididymis, since PSA is active in ejaculates collected from subjects with defective seminal vesicles and deferent ducts [1]. The protease(s) responsible for processing of the PSA precursor have not been identified. The mature 237-amino-acid form of PSA is a single-chain serine protease with extensive structural similarity to the glandular kallikreins [1,12–14]. However, the substrate specificity is uniquely different from that of the trypsin-like glandular kallikreins and resembles that of chymotrypsin, since PSA catalyzes the hydrolysis of peptide bonds' carboxy-terminal to residues of tyrosine and leucine [15–17]. Synthetic peptide substrates for chymotrypsin can be used to measure PSA activity, but they are hydrolyzed much less efficiently by PSA than by chymotrypsin and are therefore both nonspecific and insensitive in detecting PSA activity [16].

PSA in seminal fluid

About 70% of PSA in seminal fluid occurs in enzymatically active single-chain form [1,16]. The remaining 30% lacks enzyme activity either due to internal

Pienta, K.J., (ed.), DIAGNOSIS AND TREATMENT OF GENITOURINARY MALIGNANCIES.

peptide-bond cleavages at positions Lys_{145}–Lys_{146} and/or Lys_{182}–Ser_{183} [16,18] or due to complex formation with extracellular protease inhibitors [19]. Five differently charged forms of PSA can be separated by ion-exchange chromatography. Two forms, called isoenzymes A and B, are enzymatically active, whereas the other forms, isoenzymes C, D, and E, are internally cleaved at various positions and display little or no enzyme activity. The difference in charge of the A and B isoenzymes is probably attributed to a variation in number of sialic acids occurring at terminal positions in the single Asn-linked carbohydrate side chain in PSA [18]. PSA liquefies the gel forming after ejaculation by cleaving the major gel-forming proteins, namely, semenogelin I (SgI) and II (SgII), into multiple soluble fragments of SgI and SgII [1,16,17]. Less than 5% of PSA in seminal fluid occurs as a complex with protein C inhibitor (PCI), a 55-kDa seminal-vesicle-derived serine protease inhibitor occurring at levels corresponding to about 10% that of PSA [19].

Human glandular kallikein (hGK-1 or hK2)

The gene for human kallikrein 2 (hK2) displays a high degree of homology with the PSA gene, and both genes are androgen regulated and mainly expressed in the prostate [2,3,10,20–23]. The level of the hK2 mRNA in the prostate is 10%–50% of that of PSA mRNA [10,22,23], but the concentrations of hK2 antigen in prostate tissue or seminal fluid have not been determined. Due to extensive structural identity between PSA and hK2 (≈80%) [12–14,21], they have been predicted to share many antigenic determinants. The expression of hK2 by recombinant techniques has been used to solve this question, since the hK2 protein has not yet been isolated from prostate tissue or seminal fluid [24]. The recombinant forms of hK2 and PSA share remarkably few antigenic epitopes; in fact, only 5 of 18 monoclonal antibodies against PSA cross-reacted with hK2 [24]. These data have now been used to design a time-resolved fluorometric immunoassay for sensitive and specific measurement of hK2 in serum [25].

Reaction of PSA with extracellular protease inhibitors

When enzymatically PSA is added to serum in vitro, it is inactivated by complex formation with alpha-1-antichymotrypsin (ACT) and alpha-2-macroglobulin (AMG) [16]. These are major liver-derived protease inhibitors occurring at 10^4–10^5-fold molar excess to PSA in serum. However, local ACT production has also been demonstrated by immunocytochemistry and in situ hybridization techniques in both normal and malignant prostate tissue [26,27], but the levels of locally produced ACT may be low, since the abundance of ACT mRNA is suggested to be about 1% of that of the mRNA for PSA [28]. In the PSA–AMG complex, no PSA epitopes are exposed, and conventional immunoassays fail to recognize PSA in this complex [16,29]. After denaturation with SDS, PSA in the complex is exposed [16]. In the PSA–ACT complex, several independent PSA epitopes are available [30]. Only one major PSA epitope appears to be completely lost during complex formation with ACT [29,30]. The rate of complex formation with AMG in vitro is much more rapid than that of ACT [31]. Therefore, much of the PSA reaching circulation may be metabolized by complexation with AMG [31].

Molecular forms of PSA in the blood

Most of the immunodetected PSA in the blood circulation — about 50% to 95% — exists in complex with ACT [29,32]. A minute fraction, typically 1% to 3% of total PSA, occurs in complex with alpha-1-antitrypsin [32]. The free, approximately 30-kDa noncomplexed form of PSA represents 5% to 50% of total PSA [29,32]. Most of the free PSA in serum is probably inactive because active PSA in serum is unlikely to remain free, due to the large molar excess of protease inhibitors. However, it must be emphasized that the concentration of the PSA–AMG complex is presently unknown, since it is not detected by conventional immunoassays [29].

Occurrence of abnormally elevated serum concentrations of PSA

The serum levels of PSA in men over 50 years of age are normally below 4 ng/mL [33], but the levels increase with age. The majority of patients with prostate cancer have elevated serum PSA levels, probably due to breakdown of the barriers that prevent PSA from escaping into the extracellular fluids and further into circulation. However, elevated serum levels of PSA may also be caused by benign conditions, such as bacterial prostatitis, urinary retention, and benign prostatic hyperplasia (BPH) [33]. Approximately 25% of all men with a histopathologic diagnosis of BPH have serum PSA levels above 4.0 ng/mL, but a PSA level below 4.0 ng/mL does not preclude the existence of clinically significant CAP, since approximately 20% of CAP patients diagnosed by biopsy have been reported with PSA levels less than 4.0 ng/mL at the time of diagnosis. This limits the clinical sensitivity of PSA testing for the detection of CAP [33].

Improved cancer specificity by measurement of free and complexed PSA in serum

In 1991, specific measurement of PSA complexed to ACT in serum was first reproted to improve the specificity for detection of cancer [32]. The assay used polyclonal antisera against PSA and ACT to demonstrate that the proportion of PSA–ACT to total PSA in serum is higher in men with CAP than in those with BPH [32]. These results were confirmed in an independent study using three separate time-resolved immunofluorometric assays for free PSA, PSA–ACT, and total PSA (both free and complexed forms of PSA) [34]. This investigation showed not only that the proportion of PSA–ACT to total PSA is higher but also that the proportion of free PSA to total PSA is lower in CAP than in BPH ($p < 0.0001$) [34]. The median proportion of the free PSA to total PSA (PSA–F/PSA–T) in CAP was 0.18 compared to 0.28 in BPH patients ($p < 0.0001$). The difference was significant also at PSA concentrations in serum less than 10 ng/mL and showed that measurements of the proportion of both PSA–ACT to total PSA and free PSA to total PSA could improve the specific discrimination of CAP from BPH in the PSA concentration range, which is clinically important for detection of early CAP [34]. Similar results have now been published by several groups using independently developed methods [35–43].

The immunoassays for measurement of each molecular form of PSA in serum have been further refined by the generation of extensive panels of monoclonal antibodies and by optimizing the design of the assay protocols [30]. The nonspecific interference in the PSA-C assay, most probably caused by granulocyte-derived cathepsin G complexed to ACT, is efficiently reduced by the addition of heparin to the assay buffer [30]. The proportion of PSA–ACT to total PSA [35] or free and total PSA [42] can be measured simultaneously by assaying the two forms with two different fluorescent labels and time-resolved immunofluorometry. About half the false-positive results were eliminated when the proportion of PSA–ACT to total PSA was measured rather than the concentration of total PSA in serum [35]. Receiver operation characteristic (ROC) curve analysis has shown that the area under the ROC curve (AUC = 0.81) for a dual-label assay of free to total PSA was significantly higher ($p < 0.01$) than that for total PSA in serum (AUC = 0.63) in men with total PSA concentrations in serum ranging from 1 to 20 ng/mL [42]. At sensitivity levels of 60% to 90%, the proportion of free to total PSA increased specificity by more than 20% compared to analysis of total PSA concentration in serum [42]. The improved performance of dual label methods may at least partly be due to elimination of the effect of pipetting errors arising from doing the determinations in the same vial. It also makes the determination more economical and less time consuming by eliminating the work load added by an additional assay of the free or complexed form of PSA.

The results obtained by direct immunoassays have been confirmed by Stamey et al., who separated free and complexed PSA by gel filtration before analysis by immunoassays detecting total PSA [44]. The proportion of complexed PSA to total PSA in serum is substantially higher (range 88%–98%) in CAP than in 10 BPH patients (range 73%–84%) [44]. In patients with PSA concentrations between 2 and 40 ng/mL, a proportion of free to total PSA in serum below 0.15 differentiated CAP from BPH [37].

Most studies on the various forms of PSA have concerned selected patient materials. In a study on unselected archival samples, the use of the proportion of PSA–ACT to total PSA (PSA-C/PSA-T) was found to reduce the false-positive results by about 50% [43]. Recent studies confirm that measurement of the proportion of free PSA in serum also can increase specificity in a screening population [38]. In men with elevated serum PSA, 39% of the prostate biopsies could be eliminated while still detecting 93% of the cancers using either a suspicious rectal examination or percent-free PSA $\leq$18 as biopsy criteria [38]. Several other investigators have recently confirmed the utility of determinations of free PSA and total PSA [39–41]. Taken together, these results suggest that measurement of the ratio of the various forms of PSA in serum can be used to considerably reduce the number of confirmatory tests required in a screening setting such as that performed in the U.S. However, this needs to be confirmed in a true screening study with fresh samples.

Metabolism of free and complexed PSA in serum

Three separate assays have been used to study the turnover rates of each molecular form of PSA in serum after radical retropubic prostatectomy in patients with localized CAP [45]. Free PSA has a very rapid clearance rate (half-life in the serum of $\approx$1.5 hours), which is consistent with elimination by glomerular filtration through the kidneys. The much longer half-life of PSA–ACT ($\approx$3.0 days) is consistent with its approximately 90-kDa size that prevents clearance by glomerular filtration. The half-time of total PSA in serum [45] was consistent with that reported by Stamey et al. (2.2 days), and Oesterling et al. (3.2 days) [46,47]. Recently, van Straalen et al. reported a biphasic disappearance pattern of PSA from plasma with a half-time of 1.6 hours for the α-phase and 4.6 days for the β-phase [48]. These correspond to the clearance rates of free and complexed PSA, respectively [45].

Age-dependent changes of free and complexed PSA in serum

The serum concentrations of each molecular form of PSA, namely, PSA-F, PSA-C, and PSA-T, have been determined in a randomly selected group of 422 healthy men aged 40 to 79 years in whom prostate cancer was excluded by biopsy [49]. The concentrations of each form increased with age; therefore, separate reference ranges were determined. Interestingly, the reference range for the proportion of free PSA to total PSA in serum was not age dependent. The lower reference limit based on fifth percentile was 0.15 in all age groups. The corresponding upper reference limit for PSA-C/PSA-T was less than 0.70 and that for PSA-F/PSA-C was greater than 0.25 with no dependence on age [49].

Mechanisms causing differences in the proportions of the various forms of PSA in serum

The occurrence of PSA–ACT complexes as a major proportion of the total serum PSA suggest that much of the PSA escaping from the prostate into extracellular fluids may be catalytically active, thus being able to form PSA–ACT complexes. The proportion of PSA–ACT complex present in the general blood circulation is probably influenced by many local factors such as the posttranslational processing of PSA, access of ACT and competing complex ligands such as AMG and PCI. The kinetics of the generation of complexes with different complex ligands has been investigated [16,19,31]. It has been shown that enzymatically active PSA readily forms complexes with both ACT and AMG in vitro, but preferentially with the latter [16,31]. However, the internally cleaved, two- or multichain forms of PSA still react with AMG but not with ACT, though the reaction rate with AMG of the internally cleaved forms is much slower than that of the fully active forms [31]. A possible explanation for the higher proportion of PSA–ACT to total PSA in CAP could be that a larger proportion of the PSA released from prostate cancer consists of enzymatically active forms of PSA [50].

Another potential explanation is local production of both ACT and PSA in normal and malignant prostate tissue. Specific immunostaining with different monoclonal and polyclonal antibodies against ACT and in situ hybridization with oligonucleotide probes have shown that cells producing both ACT and PSA were abundant in most prostate cancers, particularly in well-differentiated ones [26,27]. It is not unlikely that the local production of ACT and PSA by prostate tumor cells could provide conditions optimal for the formation of PSA–ACT complexes, which later enter the general blood circulation. By contrast, the reported lack of ACT production in BPH nodules may facilitate the release of free PSA into circulation [26,27].

Preanalytical factors

Most studies on free and complexed PSA have been performed on samples that have been stored refrigerated, frozen at −20°C or at −70°C for various periods of time. Thus, results obtained by the analysis of stored samples may not be directly comparable to those obtained with fresh samples. Furthermore, very little data are currently available on the short-term stability of the different PSA forms in serum samples or on the stability in anticoagulated blood plasma samples. However, under optimized storage conditions, purified PSA from seminal fluid and PSA–ACT complexes formed in vitro are stable for several weeks [30]. Storage of serum containing PSA, especially at elevated temperatures, causes loss of total PSA immunoreactivity by few changes in PSA–ACT [35]. This finding is probably explained by slow complex formation between free PSA and AMG causing loss of total and free PSA [31]. This effect may strongly affect the proportion of free to total but also complexed to total PSA. Prolonged storage of serum at −20°C has been shown to reduce the concentration of PSA, especially that of PSA–ACT [43]. This finding could be explained by slow hydrolysis of PSA–ACT. The released PSA would then lose immunoreactivity by complex formation with AMG. If methods for assay of free, complexed, and total PSA are used for screening, it is important that the effects of preanalytical factors have been elucidated. In particular, the ratio of free to total may be strongly dependent on storage time [50].

References

1. Lilja H (1985). A kallikrein-like serine protease in prostatic fluid cleaves the predominant seminal vesicle protein. J Clin Invest 76:1899–1903.
2. Riegman PH, Vlietstra RJ, van der Korput J, Pomijn J, Trapman J (1989). Characterization of the prostate-specific antigen gene: a novel human kallikrein-like gene. Biochem Biophys Res Commun 159:95–102.
3. Lundwall Å (1989). Characterization of the gene for prostate-specific antigen, a human glandular kallikrein. Biochem Biophys Res Commun 161:1151–115.
4. Nadji M, Tabei SZ, Castro A, Chu TM, Murphy GP, Wang MC, Morales AR (1981). Prostate-specific antigen: an immunohistologic marker for prostatic neoplasms. Cancer 48:1229–1232.
5. Papsidero LD, Kuriyama M, Wang MC, Horoszewicz J, Leong SS, Valenzuela L, Murphy GP, Chu TM (1981). Prostate antigen: a marker for human prostate epithelial cells. J Natl Cancer Inst 66:37–42.
6. Ford TF, Butcher DN, Masters JRW, Constance Parkinson M (1985). Immunocytochemical localisation of prostate-specific antigen: specificity and application to clinical practice. Br J Urol 57:50–55.
7. Kamoshida S, Tsutsumi Y (1990). Extraprostatic localization of prostatic acid phosphatase and prostate-specific antigen: distribution in cloacogenic glandular epithelium and sex-dependent expression in human anal gland. Hum Pathol 21:1108–1111.
8. Frazier HA, Humphrey PA, Burchette JL, Paulson DF (1992). Immunoreactive prostatic specific antigen in male periurethral glands. J Urol 147:246–248.
9. Yu H, Diamandis EP, Monne M, Crocc C (1995). Oral contraceptive-induced expression of prostate specific antigen in the female breast. J Biol Chem 270:6615–6618.
10. Henttu P, Lukkarinen O, Vihko P (1990). Expression of the gene coding for human prostate-specific antigen and related hGK-1 in benign and malignant tumors of the human prostate. Int J Cancer 45:654–660.
11. Ahlgren G, Rannevik G, Lilja H (1995). Impaired secretory function of the prostate in men with oligo-astenozoospermia. J Androl 16:491–498.
12. Lundwall Å, Lilja H (1987). Molecular cloning of human prostate specific antigen cDNA. FEBS Lett 214:317–322.
13. Schaller J, Akiyama K, Tsuda R, Hara M, Marti T, Rickli E (1987). Isolation, characterization and amino-acid sequence of gamma-seminoprotein, a glycoprotein from human seminal plasma. Eur J Biochem 170:111–120.
14. Watt K, Lee P-J, M'Timkulu T, Chan W-P, Loor R (1986). Human prostate-specific antigen: structural and functional similarity with serine proteases. Proc Natl Acad Sci USA 83:3166–3170.
15. Akiyama K, Nakamura T, Iwanaga S, Hara M (1987). The chymotrypsin-like activity of human prostate-specific antigen, g- seminoprotein. FEBS Lett 225:168–172.
16. Christensson A, Laurell C-B, Lilja H (1990). Enzymatic activity of prostate-specific antigen and its reactions with extracellular serine proteinase inhibitors. Eur J Biochem 194:755–763.

17. Lilja H, Abrahamsson P-A, Lundwall Å (1989). Semenogelin, the predominant protein in human semen. J Biol Chem 264:1894–1900.
18. Zhang W-M, Leinonen J, Kalkkinen N, Dowell B, Stenman U-H (1995). Purification and characterization of different molecular forms of prostate specific antigen in human seminal fluid. Clin Chem 41:1567–1573.
19. Christensson A, Lilja H (1994). Complex formation between protein C inhibitor and prostate-specific antigen in vitro and in human semen. Eur J Biochem 220:45–53.
20. Riegman PH, Vlietstra RJ, Klaassen P, van der Korput J, Geurts van Kessel A, Romijn J, Trapman J (1989). The prostate-specific antigen gene and the human glandular kallikrein-1 gene are tandemly located on chromosome 19. FEBS Lett 247:123–126.
21. Schedlich LJ, Bennetts B, Morris BJ (1987). Primary structure of a human glandular kallikrein gene. DNA 6:429–437.
22. Chapdelaine P, Paradis G, Tremblay RR, Dubé JY (1988). High level of expression in the prostate of a human glandular kallikrein mRNA related to prostate-specific antigen. FEBS Lett 236:205–208.
23. Young CY-F, Andrews PE, Montgomery BT, Tindall DJ (1992). Tissue-specific and hormonal regulation of human prostate-specific glandular kallikrein. Biochemistry 31:818–824.
24. Lövgren J, Piironen T, Övermo C, Dowell B, Karp M, Pettersson K, Lilja H, Lundwall Å (1995). Production of recombinant PSA and hK2 and analysis of their immunologic cross-reactivity. Biochem Biophys Res Commun 213:888–895.
25. Piironen T, Lövgren J, Karp M, Eerola R, Lundwall Å, Dowell B, Lövgren T, Lilja H, Pettersson K (in press). A novel immunofluorometric assay for the sensitive and specific measurement of human prostatic glandular kallikrein (hK2) in serum. Clin Chem.
26. Bjartell A, Björk T, Matikainen MT, Abrahamsson PA, diSant' Agnese A, Lilja H (1993). Production of alpha-1-antichymotrypsin by PSA-containing cells of the human prostate epithelium. Urology 42:502–510.
27. Björk T, Bjartell A, Abrahamsson PA, Hulkko S, diSant' Agnese A, Lilja H (1994). Alphal-antichymotrypsin production in PSA producing cells is common in prostate cancer but rare in benign prostatic hyperplasia. Urology 43:427–434.
28. Gershagen S, Schoen S, Cockett ATK, Abrahamsson P-A, Lilja H (1994). Characterization of the prostatic production of α_1-antichymotrypsin and its implications on the regulation of prostate-specific antigen. J Urol 151(Suppl.): 366A(abstract 553).
29. Lilja H, Christensson A, Dahlén U, Matikainen MT, Nilsson O, Pettersson K, Lövgren T (1991). Prostate-specific antigen in human serum occurs predominantly in complex with α_1-antichymotrypsin. Clin Chem 37:1618–1625.
30. Pettersson K, Piironen T, Seppälä M, Liukkonen L, Christensson A, Matikainen M-T, Suonpää M, Lövgren T, Lilja H (1995). Free and complexed prostate-specific antigen (PSA): in vitro stability, epitope map, and development of immunofluorometric assays for specific and sensitive detection of free PSA and PSA-α_1-antichymotrypsin complex. Clin Chem 41:1480–1488.
31. Leinonen J, Zhang W-M, Stenman U-H (1996). Complex formation between PSA isoenzymes and protease inhibitors. J Urol 155:1099–1103.
32. Stenman UH, Leinonen J, Alfthan H, Ranniko S, Tuhkanen K, Alfthan O (1991). A complex between prostate-specific antigen and α_1-antichymotrypsin is the major form of prostate-specific antigen in serum of patients with prostatic cancer: assay of the complex improves clinical sensitivity for cancer. Cancer Res 51:222–226.
33. Oesterling JE (1991). Prostate-specific antigen: a critical assessment of the most useful tumor marker for adenocarcinoma of the prostate. J Urol 145:907–923.
34. Christensson A, Björk T, Nilsson O, Dahlén U, Matikainen MT, Cockett ATK, Abrahamsson PA, Lilja H (1993). Serum prostate-specific antigen complexed to α_1-antichymotrypsin as an indicator of prostate cancer. J Urol 150:100–105.
35. Leinonen J, Lövgren T, Vornanen T, Stenman UH (1993). Double-label time-resolved immunofluorometric assay of prostate-specific antigen and of its complex with a1-antichymotrypsin. Clin Chem 39:2098–2103.

36. Lilja H, Björk T, Abrahamsson PA, Stenman UH, Shaw N, Dowell B, Oesterling JE, Pettersson K, Piironen T, Lövgren T (1994). Improved separation between normals, benign prostatic hyperplasia (BPH) and carcinoma of the prostate (CAP) by measuring free (F), complexed (C) and total (T) concentrations of prostate specific antigen (PSA). J Urol 151:400A.
37. Prestigiacomo A, Stamey TA, Lilja H, Pettersson K, Wolfert B (1995). Comparison of patients with benign prostatic hyperplasia and prostate cancer by measuring non-complexed 'free' prostate-specific antigen (PSA): the 'best case' scenario. J Urol 153:462A.
38. Catalona WJ, Smith DA, Wolfert B, Wang TJ, Rittenhouse HG, Ratliff TL (1995). Increased specificity of PSA screening through measurment of percent free PSA in serum. J Urol 153:312A.
39. Bangma CH, Kranse R, Blijenberg BG, Schröder FH (1995). The new delfia prostate specific antigen (PSA) assays of free and total PSA: results of the first comparative evaluation. J Urol 153:294A.
40. Partin AW, Kelly CA, Subong ENP, Walsh PC, Chan DW (1995). Measurements of the ratio of free PSA to total PSA improves prostate cancer detection for men with total PSA levels between 4.0 and 10.0 ng/mL. J Urol 153:295A.
41. Wang TJ, Hill T, Norton K, Sokoloff R, Frankenne F, Rittenhouse HG, Wolfert RL (1995). Specific immunoassays for free PSA and its clinical relevance. J Urol 153:295A.
42. Mitrunen K, Pettersson K, Piironen T, Björk T, Lilja H, Lövgren T (1995). Dual-label one-step immunoassay for simultaneous measurement of free and total prostate specific antigen concentrations and ratios in serum. Clin Chem 41:1115–1120.
43. Stenman U-H, Hakama M, Knekt P, Aromaa A, Teppo L, Leinonen J (1994). Serum concentrations of prostate specific antigen and its complex with α_1-antichymotrypsin before diagnosis of prostate cancer. Lancet 344:1594–1598.
44. Stamey TA, Chen Z, Prestigiacomo A (1994). Serum prostate-specific antigen binding alpha-1-antichymotrypsin: influence of cancer volume, location and therapeutic selection of resistant clones. J Urol 152:1510–1514.
45. Björk T, Abrahamsson PA, Lilja H, Pettersson K, Cockett ATK (1995). Rates of clearance of free and complexed forms of PSA in serum after radical prostatectomy and transurethral microwave therapy. J Urol 153:294A.
46. Stamey TA, Yang N, Hay AR, McNeal JE, Freiha FS, Redwine E (1987). Prostate-specific antigen as a serum marker for adenocarcinoma of the prostate. N Engl J Med 317:909–916.
47. Oesterling JE, Chan DW, Epstein JI, Kimball AW Jr, Bruzek DJ, Rock RC, Brendler CB, Walsh PC (1988). Prostate specific antigen in the preoperative and postoperative evaluation of localized prostatic cancer treated with radical prostatectomy. J Urol 139:766–772.
48. Van Straalen JP, Bossens MMF, de Reijke TM, Sanders GTB (1994). Biological half-life of prostate-specific antigen after radical prostatectomy. Eur J Clin Chem Biochem 32:53–55.
49. Oesterling JE, Jacobsen SJ, Klee GG, Pettersson K, Piironen T, Abrahamsson PA, Stenman UH, Dowell B, Lövgren T, Lilja H (1995). Free, complexed and total serum prostate specific antigen: the establishment of appropriate reference ranges for their concentrations and ratios. J Urol 154:1090–1095.
50. Stenman U-H, Leinonen J, Zhang W-M (in press). Problems of PSA determinations. Eur J Clin Chem Clin Biochem.

Surgical and Radiation Advances

6. Retroperitoneal lymphadenectomy in staging and treatment of clinical stage I and II nonseminomatous testis cancer (NSGCT): the development of nerve-sparing techniques

J.P. Donohue

Two decades ago, the extended bilateral suprahilar retroperitoneal lymphadenectomy was described using special exposure techniques via the midline abdominal approach [1]. This wide template of dissection (figure 6-1) encompassed all the known sites of lymphatic drainage within the retroperitoneum. The rationale behind this somewhat extensive procedure was that it provided the best guarantee of removing all microscopic deposits of infradiaphragmatic metastatic disease in an era when relapse was often fatal owing to poor chemotherapy rescue. Results from that period justified this intensive surgical approach in nonseminomas; the lower relapse rate combined with improved survival was marginally better than prophylactic irradiation programs, the only other alternative treatment available at that time.

Since the mid-1960s, we have performed just over 2000 retroperitoneal lymph node dissection (RPLND) operations at the Indiana University Medical Center. It is against this background of experience that we have gradually but consistently modified our surgical techniques. The initial impetus for modifying the type of operation we performed came from an improvement in our understanding of the specific sites of nodal metastases from testis cancer. Thus, the wide field of dissection in the suprahilar operation could be scaled down without jeopardizing its potential for accurate staging or therapeutic benefit if nodes were involved. The other reason for wishing to modify our operative approach was that surgical morbidity became a significant factor to be taken into consideration when effective chemotherapy became available for nonseminomatous testis cancer [2]. In particular, patients and surgeons alike focused on the loss of ejaculatory function as the principal area of concern because it invariably followed the standard bilateral lymphadenectomy [3]. In this chapter, we will trace the historical development of RPLND, including the downscaling of resection templates and the subsequent development of nerve-sparing techniques. The technique of nerve-sparing modified RPLND is then described in the manner that we perform these operations today. The role of primary retroperitoneal lymphadenectomy and the choice between surgery or surveillance as the most appropriate management option in clinical stage I NSGCT is not within the scope of this chapter.

Pienta, K.J., (ed.), DIAGNOSIS AND TREATMENT OF GENITOURINARY MALIGNANCIES.

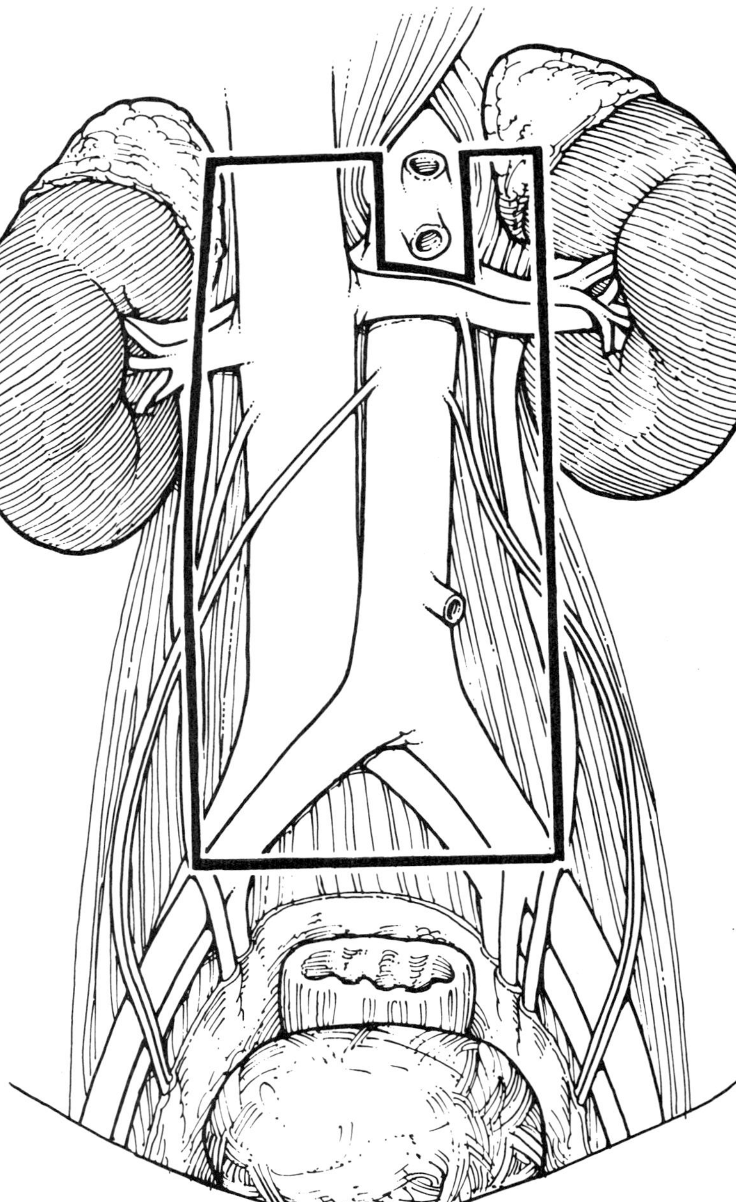

Figure 6-1. Template for bilateral RPLND with bilateral suprarenal hilar extension. Following studies of positive nodal distribution, this template was downscaled to a modified right and a modified left template, shown in figures 6-2A and 6-2B.

Sequential modifications in operative techniques

Our first modification to the traditional operation of bilateral suprahilar RPLND was omission of the suprahilar component of dissection. This reduction in the surgical template was considered appropriate when studies showed that the suprahilar lymph nodes were not a primary zone of metastatic spread in testis cancer unless there was gross involvement of the lower (infrahilar) para-aortic nodes [4]. The safety of omitting a routine suprahilar dissection was confirmed by subsequent surgical series [5,6]. In addition to the efficacy of the bilateral infrahilar approach, the operation gained popularity because it was technically less demanding than its predecessor and operative time was also reduced.

Considering the time period involved, the bilateral infrahilar RPLND was a safe and effective tool in the urologist's armamentarium against low-stage cancer of the testis. The previous training for performing suprahilar dissections was not in vain, and it became invaluable when operating for bulky disease in the postchemotherapy setting. However, the principal drawback of the bilateral infrahilar operation related to its morbidity, especially the loss of ejaculatory function, which occurred in all cases [7]. This direct complication of surgery became of increasing importance when new developments in radiology and serum markers made it possible to evaluate disease stage more accurately using noninvasive methods. Also, the dawning of the era of chemotherapy with the introduction of cisplatin made it possible to rescue patients with relapse reliably. With this new emphasis on the morbidity of treatment, there was growing pressure to reject primary surgery in favor of surveillance in early-stage nonseminomas, and this approach was adopted in several countries including the U.K. and Scandanavia [8,9]. Meanwhile, surgical centers that were committed to RPLND further downscaled the boundaries of dissection in an effort to preserve postoperative ejaculation [6,10]. Resulting modified unilateral templates (figures 6-2a and 6-2b) were based on prior knowledge of the zones of metastatic spread and a general recognition that the critical region in preserving ejaculation was the para-aortic tissues below the level of the inferior mesenteric artery [11–13]. This region contains the lumbar sympathetic chain and the postganglionic fibers from the ganglia L2 to L4 (figure 6-3). Studies of male sexual dysfunction following RPLND pointed to the injury of the sympathetic nerves as the key to this problem, and further dissection work, both at Indiana University and elsewhere, elucidated the course of the sympathetic postganglionic nerves [12,14,15]. Traveling in the para-aortic tissues, these fibers decussate to form the so-called hypogastric plexus. The terminal nerve truns from the plexus pass inferiorly to terminate in the ejaculatory apparatus of the seminal vesicles and ampullary portion of the vas.

These modified unilateral templates preserving sympathetic fibers were associated with greater preservation of ejaculation in the range of 60% to 80%. This reduction in surgical morbidity has led to the adoption of unilateral modified RPLND by most surgical centers treating cancer of the testis. The

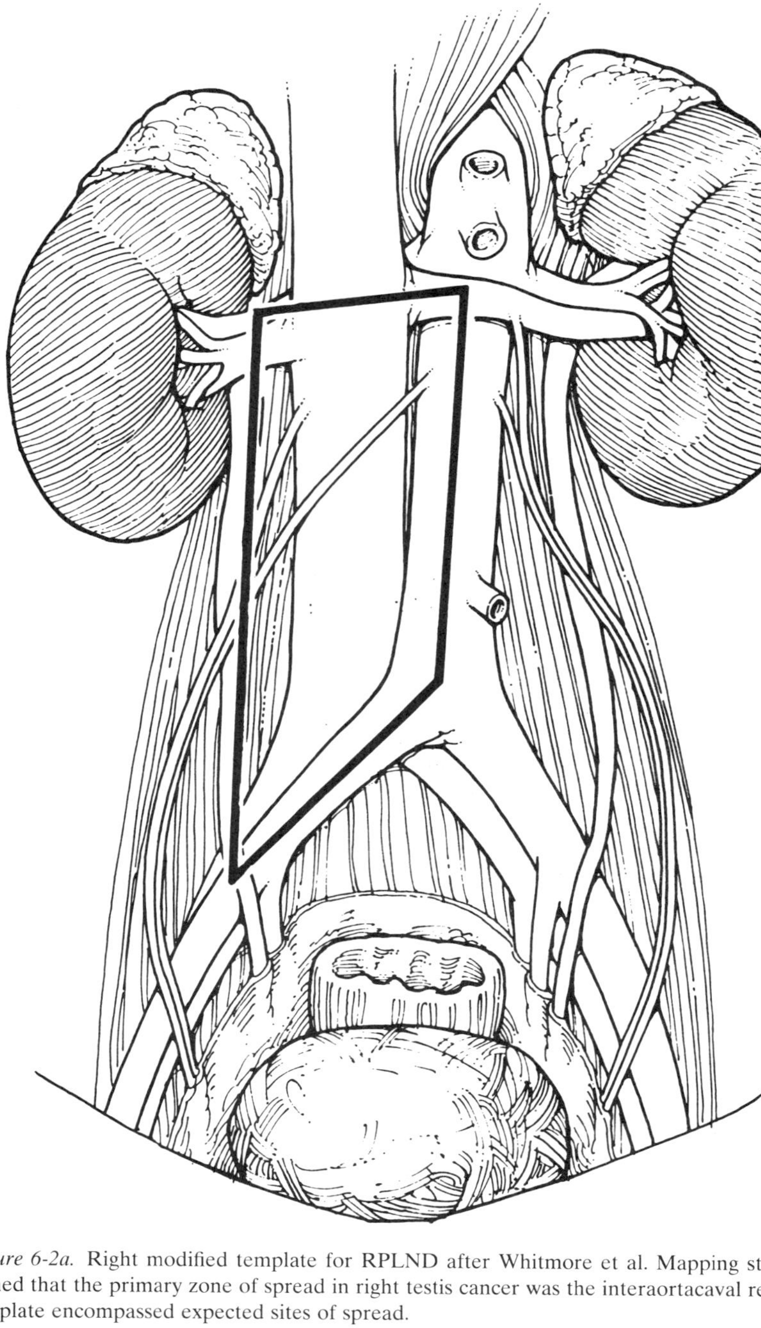

Figure 6-2a. Right modified template for RPLND after Whitmore et al. Mapping studies confirmed that the primary zone of spread in right testis cancer was the interaortacaval region. This template encompassed expected sites of spread.

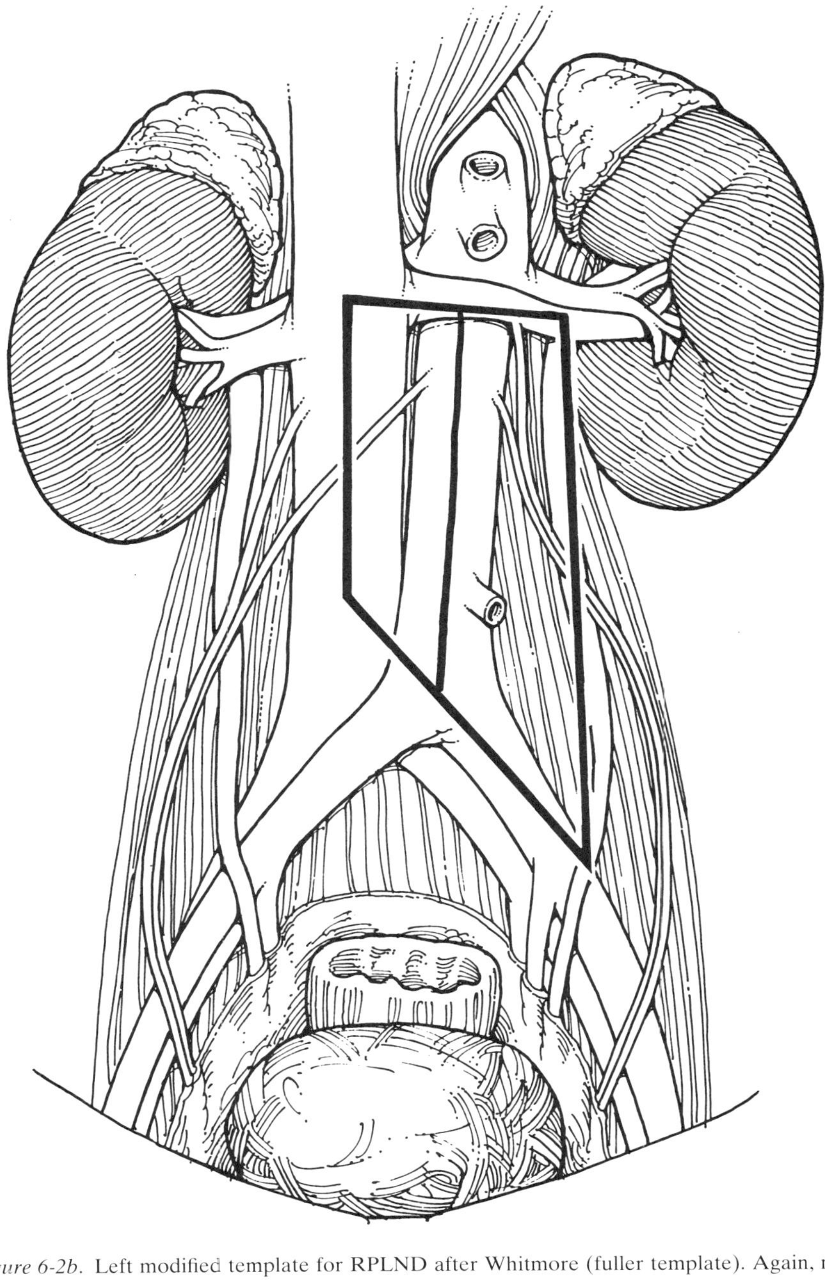

Figure 6-2b. Left modified template for RPLND after Whitmore (fuller template). Again, mapping studies showed that the primary zone of spread with left-sided primary was left para-aortic. Therefore, Whitmore's larger template was further subdivided to be restricted to the left para-aortic zone only.

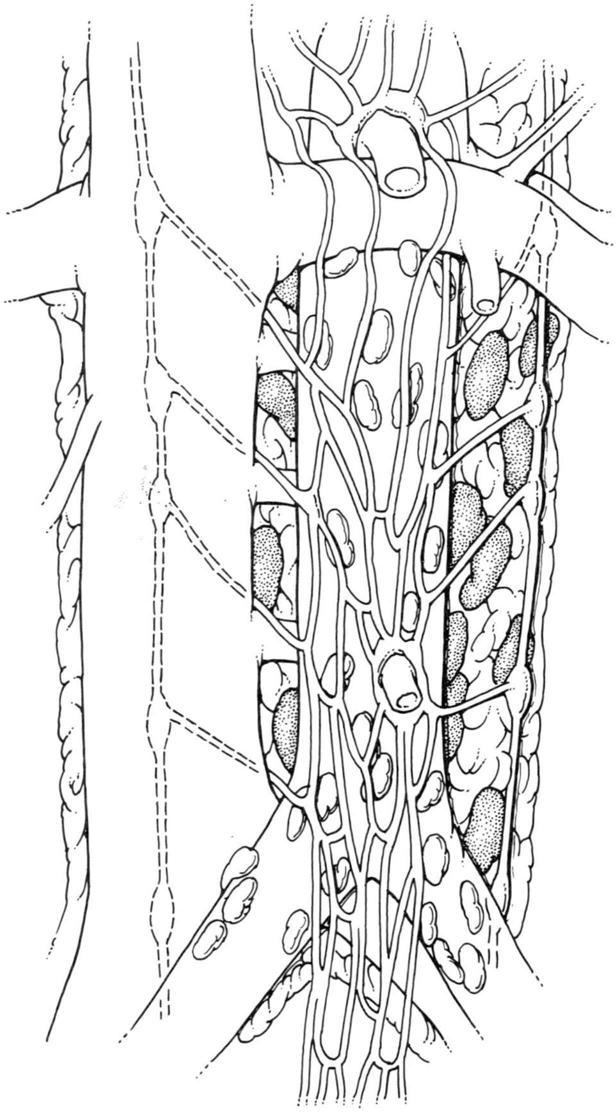

Figure 6-3. A schematic diagram of the lumbar sympathetic nervous system and its relation to the great vessels. Postganglionic fibers on the right side pass under the vena cava and emerge pre-aortic at the hypogastric plexus. From the left side, postganglionic fibers rise directly up pre-aortic, joining the hypogastric plexus below the inferior mesenteric artery, which then passes cauded into the pelvis.

benefits of a modified unilateral approach in combining a complete cancer operation with perhaps a better than even chance of ejaculatory preservation was a significant development in the management of early-stage disease, particularly in view of the increasing number of relapse rates reported by centers using surveillance only [8,9].

The modified template significantly reduced surgical morbidity, but it was felt that a more proactive role for the surgeon was indicated because the means of preserving the nerves in the modified unilateral operation simply relied on their exclusion from the dissected template. The results indicate that in about half of cases, the nerves can be damaged using the modified template. Therefore, as long ago as 1978, we began our first efforts to identify prospectively sympathetic fibers in the course of RPLND. It was our belief that if dissection of the sympathetic fibers was done before lymphadenectomy, then preservation of ejaculation might be preserved in virtually all RPLND patients. In carefully selected patients with low risk of recurrent disease, we gradually introduced a nerve-sparing modification when performing a modified unilateral procedure. By 1984 we were convinced that some patients could have their postganglionic fibers identified and preserved during the course of an effective staging lymphadenectomy [15]. The intermingling of sympathetic fibers with the lymphatic tissues is such that their preservation can be tedious and add significantly to operation time. However, as the results show in a later section, we find that a nerve-sparing procedure is not only feasible but also removes the only remaining morbidity of primary RPLND.

The surgical technique of nerve-sparing modified retroperitoneal lymph node dissection

As described earlier, the templates for resection are different for right- and left-sided testis tumors. Therefore, our operative approach varies according to the side of initial testis primary.

Nerve-sparing modified retroperitoneal lymph node dissection for right-sided tumors (technique)

The retroperitoneum is exposed by incising the root of the small bowel from the cecum to the ligament of Treitz. The small bowel mesentery is separated from the anterior aspect of Gerota's fascia, giving access to the great vessels. The gonadal veins are clearly visible. This exposure is maintained by the use of laparotomy pads and a large ring retractor.

Sometimes the terminal nerve trunks of the sympathetic hypogastric plexus are visible in the preaortic area near the origin of the right iliac artery, but in most patients these delicate strands are obscured by fat. Therefore, it is usually simplest to begin dissecting in the traditional manner at the level of the renal vein. The lymphatics on the anterior aspect of the left renal vein are divided, and this dissection is carried medially and thence in a caudal direction to the crossing of the external iliac artery. Dissecting in the anterior midline of the cava (12 o'clock) avoids damaging the nerve roots where they emerge medially from underneath the cava toward the aorta (figure 6-4). This anterior division of the lymphatics over the great vessels is called *the anterior split*. The subsequent dissection of this package off the great vessels medially and laterally is called the *roll* technique — hence, the term *split and roll*. Using this technique, one can readily identify the nerve roots of L1, 2, and 3 in the packet of tissue that is rolled medially off the cava. A plastic vessel loop is placed around each nerve branch to make it more obvious and to permit gentle traction during subsequent dissection. Once the roots of L1, 2, and 3 are taped, it is a simple matter to dissect distally and connect with the decussation of fibers that form the distal trunks of the hypogastric plexus as they pass anterior to the iliac vessels and down into the pelvis. In the course of this dissection, the anterior set of interaortocaval lymph nodes can be resected off the nerve roots that lie posteriorly. The more substantial and difficult portion of the dissection follows, and this involves mobilization of the remaining interaortocaval lymph nodes, which lie posterior to the nerve roots. These posterior interaortocaval nodes lie in a sulcus bounded by the nerve roots laterally, the anterior spinous ligaments and lumbar vessels posteriorly, and the aorta medially. This package is delivered by sharp and blunt dissection from the overlying nerve roots, which are gently elevated in the vessel loops. This part of the dissection can be most tedious if the prepared nerve roots are to be preserved. Major lymphatics

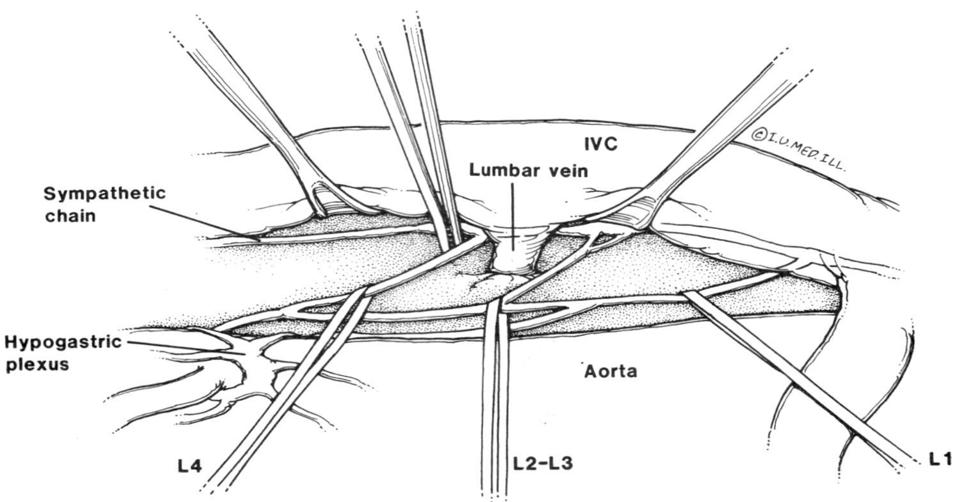

Figure 6-4. The right post ganglionic fibers of L1 thru L4 rise from the right sympathetic trunk dorsal to the cava. They emerge into the interaortocaval and pre-aortic area, where they commingle with splanchnic fibers in larger trunks. Prior to lymphadenectomy, these are prospectively identified and isolated in vessels loops as shown.

are secured by clips, especially distally and those against the posterior body wall. The cephalad limit of the dissection is the right renal artery. The L2 to L4 nerve roots lie inferior to the renal artery, but care must be taken when squaring out at the apex of the dissection so as not to catch the L1 nerve root as it passes to its ganglion just above and posterior to the renal artery. Ultimately, the interaortocaval lymph node package is drawn out from under the nerve roots. Usually the specimen is removed en bloc, but sometimes this is difficult and nodal tissue must be removed in segments so as to preserve the nerves. There is a significant amount of nodal tissue between the aorta and nerve trunks along the posterior body, wall and it may be necessary to divide the lumbar vessels during the course of removing these nodes. The right para-aortic sulcus is now clear, and one can see the anterior spinous ligaments, aorta, and nerve roots cleanly dissected.

The right-sided modified dissection is virtually complete, having removed the interaortocaval node group. The name *interaortocaval* distinguishes these nodes from those on the opposite side of the vena cava (the right paracaval group). Nodes in this latter group are rarely involved in primary testis tumors and are not of paramount importance when doing a nerve-sparing operation. However, they are easily stripped off the vena cava and the posterior body wall as a separate package. Again, care is taken to preserve the sympathetic chain and the branches of the genitofemoral and ilioinguinal nerve distally.

The interaortocaval node group (right para-aortic) is the central core of the modified template for right-sided tumors. The distal trunks below the inferior mesenteric artery and the contralateral L1 to L3 nerve roots are unlikely to be injured in such modified dissections if the zone of resection is limited to these interaortocaval parameters already mentioned. Therefore, even without ipsilateral nerve-sparing, most patients should be able to ejaculate when given a unilateral RPLND on this modified template.

Following dissection, the retroperitoneum is inspected and lymphatic leaks are clipped. The root of the small bowel is reapproximated with chromic catgut, and the abdomen is closed without external drainage.

Nerve-sparing retroperitoneal lymph node dissection for left-sided primary tumors (technique)

As previously explained, the template for resection is different in left-sided primary tumors, and we use an alternative method for exposing the retroperitoneum whereby the root of the small bowel is left intact. Instead, the left colon is elevated by dividing the left mesocolon from the level of the sigmoid up to and including the lienocolic ligament. The mesentery of the colon is separated from the underlying Gerota's fascia, revealing the gonadal vein and great vessels. Retraction is set and the gonadal vein, which traverses the field, is divided where it enters the left renal vein. This exposes the underlying ureter, which forms the lateral boundary of the dissection template.

The initial step in a left-sided nerve-sparing technique is exposure of the lumbar sympathetic chain by dissecting posterolateral to the aorta. The L1 to L3 nerve roots are easily identified as they course medial vein and inferior, decussating with contralateral sympathetic branches and splanchnic sympathetic fibers that course anterior to the aorta (figure 6-5). Occasionally the nerve roots are apparent initially when exposing the retroperitoneum. If so, they can be taped and dissected with the sympathetic chain, and the ganglia can then be identified by dissecting along the nerve roots themselves. In either case, with the sympathetic chain and nerve roots identified, the anterior set of nodes is easily dissected off them. These nodes are few in number compared to the posterior group, which is isolated from the overlying nerve roots using the same technique as described for right-sided primaries (figure 6-6). The nerve roots are dissected to permit their elevation off the nodal package lying in the sulcus bounded by the aorta medially, the spinous ligaments posteriorly, and the nerve roots themselves, which course ventrally over them. A combination of blunt and sharp dissection is useful. Again, it is critical not to inadvertently incorporate the nerve roots in the lymph node specimen when squaring off the package superiorly. Also, care should be taken to elevate the left renal vein and divide any lumber vessels that drain into it to optimize exposure at the cephalad margin of the node package.

The left renal artery is the upper limit of dissection, and the L1 to L3 nerve roots and the sympathetic chain course below this level. The node package can be dissected off the aorta with relative safety by keeping tension on the nerve roots in their plastic loops. The origin of the spermatic artery is divided and separated from the node package. As on the right, the interaortocaval nodes are drawn out from under the nerve roots while the lymphatic connections are clipped as they are encountered. Once this has been accomplished, the nerve-sparing left-sided template is complete, and the mesentery of the colon is reapproximated prior to closure.

The results of nerve-sparing modified retroperitoneal lymph node dissection

Several years ago, a review of 1180 RPLND operations performed at Indiana University Medical Center over the past 25 years found that 140 patients have had primary RPLND using the nerve-sparing technique just described. At that time, 73 patients had a median follow-up of 24 months [15]. Fifty-nine patients were pathological stage I, while the remaining 14 patients were found to have positive nodes by surgical/pathologic staging. Four patients had relapsed, of whom two cases had elevated serum markers only and another case developed chest metastases. These three cases received chemotherapy and are now disease free. Another patient who was shown to be stage IIB by RPLND and who refused adjuvant chemotherapy developed both chest and abdominal metastases. He received combination chemotherapy and underwent a subsequent postchemotherapy resection of a residual suprahilar abdominal mass,

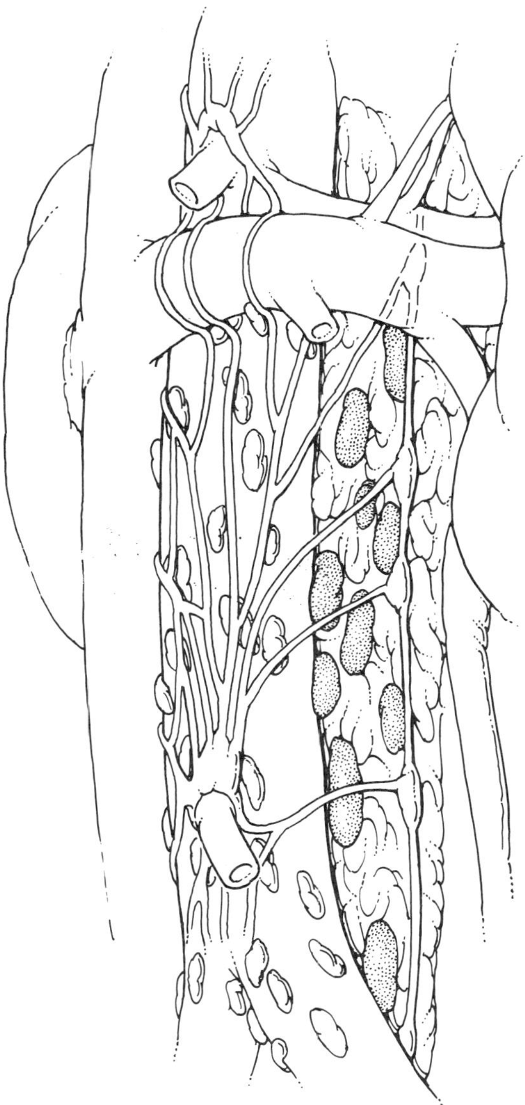

Figure 6-5. The left postganglionic sympathetic fibers are rising from L1 thru L4 ganglia of the sympathetic chain dorsal and left of the aorta, joining the pre-aortic decussation of nerve trunks (called a hypogastric plexus) just like their right-sided counterparts.

which was found to be scare and necrosis. None of the 59 patients with pathological stage I disease had relapse; this implied that modified RPLND did not miss any patient with positive nodes.

Seventy-two patients retained normal ejaculatory function after nerve-sparing RPLND [15]. One single exception was time limited and resumed

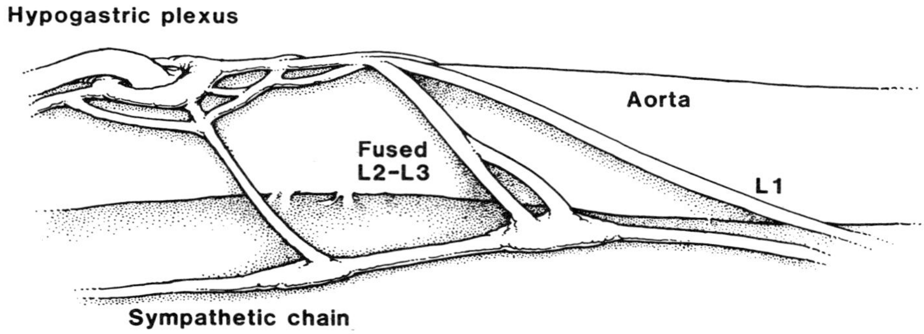

Figure 6-6. The left-sided nerve-sparing technique requires isolation of the postganglionic fibers arising from the sympathetic chain and merging in the pre-aortic area near the inferior mesenteric artery. Occasionally, the ganglia of L2 and L3 may be fused.

normal function several months later. In 1993, this group treated with NS-RPLND with more than two-year follow-up numbered 167 [16].

Also, an additional ten patients underwent nerve-sparing RPLND in the postchemotherapy setting. All had low-volume disease (stage IIA, IIB) and normal serology preoperatively. No case suffered local or distal relapse, while all these patients maintained normal ejaculatory function.

The contribution of nerve-sparing modified retroperitoneal lymph node dissection

The traditional aim of cancer surgery has been to achieve radical removal of the primary tumor with its regional zone of lymphatic drainage. As such, radical surgery offers the best chance of preventing a local recurrence and, if nodes are positive, then hopefully treatment has been early enough to prevent further, more distal relapse. However, this approach has long been known to produce considerable functional morbidity, and in urological oncology today more emphasis is therefore put on combining good quality of life with the established concept of total tumor clearance.

Clearly, the ideal with reference to patients with clinical stage I cancer of the testis is to identify those who in fact have microscopic nodal disease so they can be treated expediently. Currently, the most accurate way to achieve this aim is by RPLND. The procedure can be therapeutic for those found to be stage II and accurately directs further management. The combination of modern nerve-sparing techniques with a modified unilateral template means that this procedure can be performed without any long-term morbidity.

To conclude, it is perfectly reasonable to adopt nerve-sparing RPLND as appropriate management in early-stage cancer of the testis, considering the current state of the art in clinical staging. Similarly, the results with nerve-sparing RPLND in the postchemotherapy setting are most encouraging; it is in this latter group that the nerve-sparing procedure may well have the greatest future potential.

Our experience at Indiana University with clinical stage A and B testis cancer has been recently reported in some detail [10,16,17].

Cost-benefit and risk-benefit assessment of RPLND is now possible by virtue of this detailed analysis [17–20]. This can be of practical value to physicians and patients alike as options of management are considered (tables 6-1 and 6-2; figures 6-7 and 6-8).

Table 6-1. Risk-benefit analysis of primary therapy (for clinical stage B NSGCT testis cancer)

	1° RPLND surgery	1° chemotherapy
Failure rate (need for 2 Rx)	1/3	1/3
Death rate	2%	4%
Late relapses (>2 yrs)	0–1%	3–5%
Long-term toxicity	1–10% (anejaculation)	40–55% (infertility)
Overtreatment (clinical staging error)	20%	Unreported est. 20%

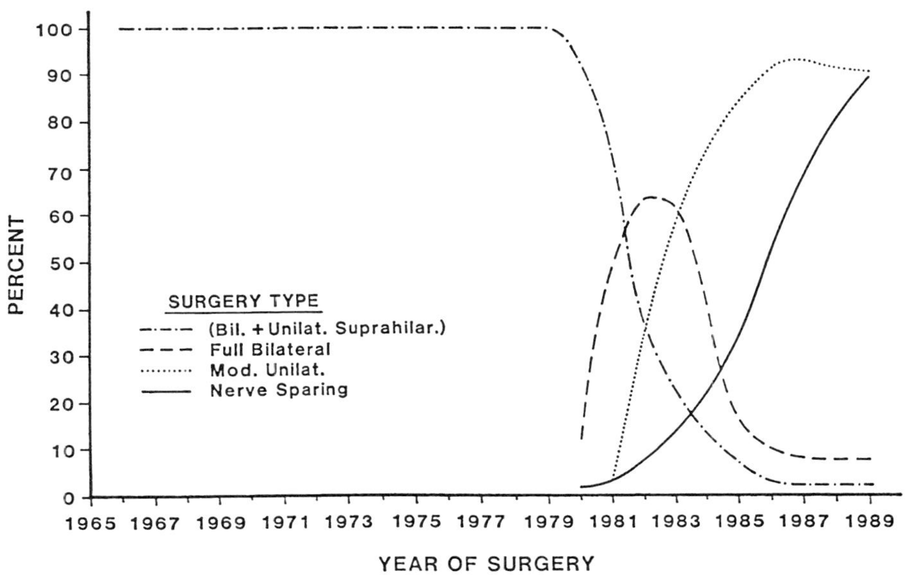

Figure 6-7. Schematic representation of the utilization of four different types of RPLND at Indiana University over a 25-year period. Bilateral and unilateral suprahilar techniques were replaced in the late 1970s with infrahilar techniques, such as bilateral infrahilar, modified unilateral, and finally prospective nerve-sparing techniques done on a modified unilateral template. In the early 1980s, modified unilateral templates combined with nerve-sparing techniques became the standard approach for RPLND for clinical stage A disease.

Table 6-2. Comparison of primary therapy for clinical stage B NSGCT

	Primary RPLND	Primary chemotherapy
Curative (as monotherapy)	2/3	2/3
Failure rate as monotherapy	1/3 (10–49%)	1/3 (20–40%)
Overall survival incl. 2° therapy	98%	96%
Late relapses	<1%	>3%
Long-term toxicity	0–10%	Unreported est. 10–30%

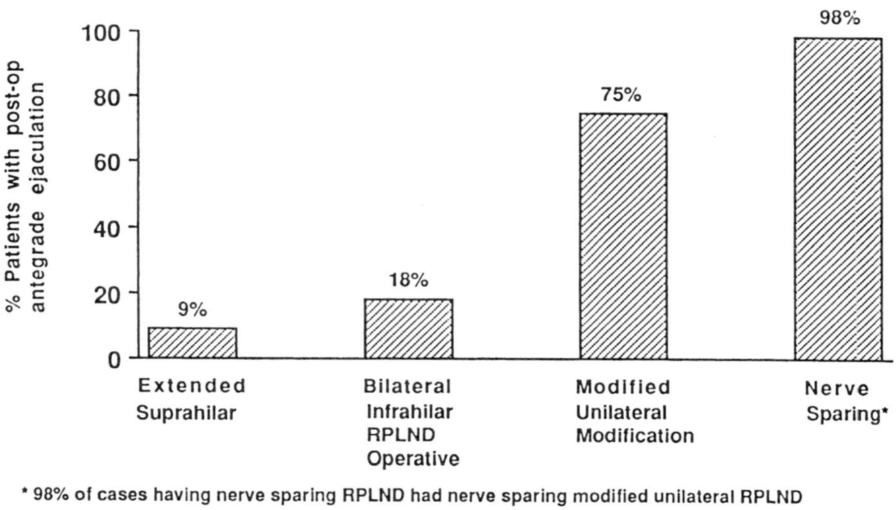

Figure 6-8. A bar graph indicates the progressive improvement in normal postoperative antegrade ejaculation with modified templates and nerve-sparing technique as opposed to former techniques without nerve sparing.

References

1. Donohue JP (1977). Retroperitoneal lymphadenectomy: the anterior approach including bilateral suprarenal-hilar dissection. Urol Clin N Am 4:509–521.
2. Einhorn LH, Donohue JP (1977). Improved chemotherapy in disseminated testicular cancer. J Urol 117:65–69.
3. Donohue JP, Rowland RG (1981). Complications of retroperitoneal lymphadenectomy. J Urol 125:338.
4. Ray B, Hajdu SI, Whitmore WF (1974). Distribution of retroperitoneal lymph node metastases in testicular germinal tumors. Cancer 33:340–348.
5. Donohue JP, Zachary JM, Maynard SD (1992). Distribution of nodal metastases in nonseminomatous testicular cancer. J Urol 128:315–320.

6. Pizzocaro G, Salvioni R, Zononi F (1985). Unilateral lymphadenectomy in intraoperative stage I nonseminomatous germinal testis cancer. J Urol 134:485–489.
7. Narayan P, Lange P, Fraley EE (1982). Ejaculation and fertility after extended retroperitoneal lymph node dissection for testicular cancer. World J Urol 127:685–688.
8. Hoskin P, Dilly S, Easton D, et al. (1986). Prognostic factors in stage I nonseminomatous germ cell testicular tumors managed by orchiectomy and surveillance: implications for adjuvant chemotherapy. J Clin Oncol 4:1031–1036.
9. Freedman LS, Jones WG, Peckham MJ, et al. (1987). Histopathology in the prediction of relapse of patients with stage I testicular teratoma treated by orchidectomy alone. Lancet ••:294–297.
10. Donohue JP, Thornhill JA, Foster RS, Rowland RG, Bihrle R (1993). Retroperitoneal lymphadenectomy for clinical stage A testis cancer (1965 to 1989): modifications of technique and impact on ejaculation. J Urol 149:237–243.
11. Jewett MA, et al. (1988). Retroperitoneal lymphadenectomy for testicular tumor with nerve-sparing for ejaculation. J Urol 139:1220–1224.
12. Lange PH, Chang WY, Fraley EE (1987). Fertility issues in the therapy of nonseminomatous testicular tumors. Urol Clin N Am 14:731–745.
13. Richie JP, Garnick MB (1987). Modified retroperitoneal lymphadenectomy for patients with clinical stage I testicular tumor. J Urol 137:212A.
14. Colleselli K, Poisel S, Schachtner W, Bartsch G (1990). Anatomic study and operative approach to nerve-sparing bilateral retroperitoneal lymphadenectomy. J Urol 144:293–298.
15. Donohue JP, Foster RS, Geier G, et al. (1988, 1990). Preservation of ejaculation following nerve-sparing retroperitoneal lymphadenectomy (RPLND). J Urol 139:206A; 144:287–292.
16. Donohue JP, Thornhill JA, Foster RS, Rowland RG, Bihrle R (1993). Primary retroperitoneal lymph node dissection in clinical stage A nonseminomatous germ cell testis cancer. Br J Urol 71:326–335.
17. Donohue JP, Thornhill JA, Foster RS, Bihrle R, Rowland RG, Einhorn LH (1995). The role of retroperitoneal lymphadenectomy in clinical stage B testis cancer: the Indiana University experience (1965–1989). J Urol 153:85–89.
18. Donohue JP, Rowland RG, Bihrle R (1988). Transabdominal retroperitoneal lymph node dissection in diagnosis and management of genitourinary cancer. In *Genitourinary Cancer* (eds. D.G. Skinner & G. Lieskowsky), W.B. Saunders: Philadelphia, Ch. 55, pp. 802–816.
19. Baniel J, Foster RS, Rowland RG, Bihrle R, Donohue JP (1994). Complications of primary retroperitoneal lymph node dissection. J Urol 152:424–427.
20. Donohue JP, Thornhill JA, Foster RS, Rowland RG, Bihrle R (1994). Stage I nonseminomatous germ cell testicular cancer: management options and risk-benefit considerations. World J Urol 12:170–177.

7. Current therapy for invasive bladder cancer

James E. Montie

Bladder cancer commonly presents difficult treatment decisions for both the patient and the urologist. Most bladder cancers are histologically well differentiated, without invasion into the wall of the bladder (Ta), and can be successfully managed endoscopically; however, 20% to 30% of cancers demonstrate at some time invasion into the bladder wall, making conservative management unlikely to be successful. Progressive invasion of the cancer into the lamina propria (T1) or muscularis propria (T2, T3) increases the potential for incomplete transurethral resection and the risk for development of metastases. The decision to abandon endoscopic management and go on to removal of the bladder places a heavy burden on the urologist's shoulders. Removal of the bladder early in the course of the disease might improve survival results, but a certain number of patients would lose their bladder when the loss might not have been absolutely necessary. Inaccurate staging methods, variability inherent in the biology of the cancer, inconsistency in pathologic interpretation of depth of invasion, and patient lifestyle considerations make the 'tightrope' that both the patient and physician must walk between bladder preservation and bladder removal particularly difficult. Cystectomy provides excellent local control for all but the largest cancers, but undeniably has a profound impact on urinary and sexual function of the patient. Improvements in methods of urinary diversion using an orthotopic neobladder to the urethra may provide maintenance of near normal bladder function for many patients, but the new bladder will not be as good as the original one. Thus, the presence of a potentially lethal bladder cancer forces a pivotal decision about a treatment strategy of bladder preservation versus bladder reconstruction. The following review will summarize current views on the options of surgical or combined therapies for invasive bladder cancers.

Bladder preservation

Transurethral resection

Transurethral resection (TUR) has been the mainstay of bladder cancer management for most of this century. Papillary cancers confined to the inner

Pienta, K.J., (ed.), DIAGNOSIS AND TREATMENT OF GENITOURINARY MALIGNANCIES.

surface epithelium of the bladder are amenable to resection, with morbidity limited to a low risk for bleeding or bladder perforation. Once a bladder cancer invades the lamina propria of the bladder wall, complete resection is less certain, analogous to pulling a weed with uncertainty about removal of all the roots. The larger the cancer and deeper the penetration, the less likely it is that the resection will eliminate the cancer. Nonetheless, some cancers that are invasive (T1, T2) can be completely resected; TUR used as the sole therapy in selected cases provides five-year survival rates of approximately 50% [1,2]. However, the patient selection required to ensure the suitability of TUR as the sole therapy may provide even better survival if a more aggressive treatment is used. If a TUR is going to be successful, the site of the cancer in the bladder must be re-resected on several occasions to be sure that no residual disease is present; intravesical treatment (such as Bacillus Calmette Guerin, BCG) provides additional therapy to diminish the formation of new tumors.

Partial cystectomy

Removal of a portion of the bladder for an invasive cancer is attractive because it allows excision of the full thickness of the bladder wall and surrounding perivesical fat yet preserves bladder function. Partial cystectomy in selected cases yields results potentially comparable to total cystectomy [3]. However, the number of patients suitable for a partial cystectomy is unfortunately quite small, comprising only 5% of individuals with invasive cancer. To obtain good results with partial cystectomy, the tumor needs to be a single lesion in space and time (solitary and the initial tumor) and in a location in the bladder amenable to partial cystectomy with a margin of normal mucosa, muscle, and surrounding tissue without compromising bladder capacity or function. Few tumors meet these requirements; poor patient selection can cause a disastrous result that requires a later total cystectomy or renders the patient incurable secondary to an extravesical pelvic recurrence. An ill-advised partial cystectomy, all too often done with older age as the primary indication, may not only fail to eliminate the cancer but also doom salvage therapies to failure. Clinical trials at Memorial Sloan-Kettering Cancer Center and in Europe used initial systemic chemotherapy combined with partial cystectomy, but there is general agreement that this approach is of uncertain benefit and remains investigational [4,5].

External radiation therapy

The introduction of cobalt 60 irradiation in the 1950s led to many reports of its use in invasive bladder cancer. Subsequently, urologists in the United States viewed radiation therapy (R.T.) results as inferior to those obtained with cystectomy, with or without preoperative R.T. However, in some countries, external R.T. — now with improved delivery using a linear accelerator and better treatment planning — remains a commonly used treatment [6–8].

Treatment failures require a salvage cystectomy. Complete elimination of the invasive cancer and freedom from new tumors in the bladder happens in only 20% to 30% of patients. Patient selection is also important for R.T.; a complete TUR prior to R.T. and the absence of hydronephrosis yield better results. Although salvage cystectomy is feasible without a documented increase in perioperative mortality, most surgeons are less likely to use an orthotopic bladder replacement and feel that a pelvic complication after R.T. is more difficult to manage.

Systemic chemotherapy plus radiation therapy

In the 1980s, effective systemic chemotherapy for bladder cancer became available [9]. Complete response rates occurred in 15% to 30% of patients with established metastatic disease, primarily in soft tissue sites such as nodal or pulmonary metastases. These encouraging results using both the MVAC (methotrexate, vinblastine, adriamycin, cisplatin) and CMV (cisplatin, methotrexate, vinblastine) regimens also included favorable responses in the primary tumor in the bladder. Thus, it was logical to hope that either primary chemotherapy by itself or combined with external R.T. might provide elimination of the cancer and preserve bladder function [10]. Although some promising preliminary data exist, there remains a distressingly high failute rate based on incomplete destruction of the existing cancer and the development of new tumors in the bladder during follow-up [10–14]. Durable elimination of local bladder cancer while maintaining a functional bladder occurs in approximately 20% to 40% of cases [11–14]. Some of the recurrences in the bladder after chemotherapy and R.T. are noninvasive and potentially amenable to intravesical treatment, and these have been viewed as minimally threatening to the patient. Recurrent tumors in a patient whose cancer has already demonstrated an invasive and thus potentially lethal phenotype cannot be regarded lightly; long-term results of the best agent, BCG, demonstrate late failures, and considerable caution is needed in following such patients [15]. Patient selection to include patients who had a complete TUR, pure transitional cell tumors, no carcinoma in situ (CIS), and no hydronephrosis may improve results to an approximately 50% durable response [11,14,16]. However, these results are disappointing and reflect an increasing realization that the effectiveness of systemic chemotherapy for bladder cancer still leaves a great deal to be desired [9,17,18]. A personal view is that patients should be apprised of the availability of bladder preservation strategies but that control of the cancer in the pelvis with this approach is substantially inferior to cystectomy.

Bladder reconstruction

Once the bladder is removed, a method must be available for drainage and, if possible, storage of urine. Any form of urinary diversion requires that the patient be kept dry and free from renal deterioration or infection. Categories of diversion are listed in table 7-1. From 1950 to the early 1990s, the predominant method of diversion was the ileal conduit; although this requires an external appliance, it works well with few complications and a tolerable alteration in lifestyle and body image for most patients when combined with good enterostomal therapy support. However, diversion options eliminating the need for an external appliance became more feasible and attractive beginning in the early 1980s. Initial studies focused on continent cutaneous diversion that required intermittent self-catheterization of the reservoir; the marginal gain in lifestyle and the complexity of the surgical procedures precluded widespread acceptance [19,20]. More recently, orthotopic neobladders gained increased popularity in both men and women because of restoration of a near-normal voiding pattern through the urethra [21]. A successful procedure provides an enormous advantage to the patient's body image and potential to return to normal activities. Early concerns about neobladders centered on the risk for urethral recurrence and incontinence.

The often diffuse, mucosal transitional cell carcinoma (TCC) in situ can extend into the prostatic urethra and subsequently the more distal urethra. Historically, approximately 10% of men after cystectomy developed a urethral recurrence, and fear of this precluded orthotopic diversion. However, it is now clear that the presence of TCC in the prostatic urethra identifies patients at a higher risk for urethral TCC; conversely, patients without prostatic TCC are at a low risk for urethral disease and thus are good candidates for diversion to the urethra [22]. The status of the prostatic urethra can be evaluated preoperatively and intraoperatively, allowing the decision to be made about orthotopic diversion [23]. Urethral recurrences occur in 2% to 3% of men using these selection criteria [24–26]. Similarly, the risk for urethral recurrences also discouraged orthotopic diversion in women. Recent experience suggesting the absence of cancer in the bladder neck predicts a low risk for urethral recurrence in women and thus allows consideration for orthotopic diversion [27,28]. As many as 75% of men and women may be candidates for neobladders using these criteria.

Incontinence is the second major concern associated with orthotopic diversion. Experience with orthotopic diversion began in the 1950s with the use of tubular bowel segments to function as the reservoir. Because tubular bowel

Table 7-1. Common methods of urinary diversion

1. Cutaneous, incontinent (e.g.: ileal conduit)
   — requires external appliance
2. Cutaneous, continent (e.g.: Koch pouch, Indiana pouch)
   — requires intermittent self-catheterization
3. Orthotopic neobladder (e.g.: Koch ileal reservoir, Studer, Hautmann)
   — allows voiding per urethra

segments had relatively high intraluminal pressures and period contractions, continence was poor. In the 1980s, it became clear that de-tubularization of the bowel decreased the pressure in the reservoir, abolished phasic contractions, and improved compliance, allowing for substantially better storage performance. When the improved reservoirs were used for orthotopic diversion, continence became much better [21,24–28]. Currently, daytime continence is expected in more than 95% of patients; nocturnal incontinence remains more common and is a consequence of lowered urethral resistance during sleep. Reservoir function continues to improve 1, 2, and 3 years after surgery and appears durable. Patients over 70 years of age tend to have more nocturnal incontinence, presumably secondary to attenuated tone in the pelvic musculature [25]. In men, the entire prostate is removed with the bladder, using surgical techniques developed for radical prostatectomy, with preservation of the external urinary sphincter. In women, the urethra is divided at the junction with the bladder neck, avoiding any dissection of the genitourinary diaphragm [29]. In women particularly, concern about incontinence delayed trials until the last 2 to 3 years. As experience accumulates, it appears that continence in women will be at least as good and probably better than that seen in men. Urinary retention is a potential risk in both men and women and can be a late development as a consequence of decompensation of the reservoir; retention is then managed with clean, intermittent self-catheterization [30].

Late metabolic complications after incorporation of longer bowel segments into the urinary tract are a possibility. Of particular concern is a late vitamin B-12 deficiency due to removal of the terminal ileum from the gastrointestinal tract to fashion the urinary reservoir. Clinically evident vitamin B-12 deficiency is rare, but long-term follow up is limited, and it could become a serious problem in some patients. Neurologic damage, potentially irreversible, may be the first sign of the deficiency, so a high index of suspicion is needed [31,32].

An enormous literature is available on various methods of reservoir construction, and over 40 variations have been described. Reservoirs have been named after people, cities, states, and universities. Several principles have emerged from this large experience. Bowel segments need to be de-tubularized to abolish contractions, must be reconstructed to assume a spherical shape with adequate capacity, and must have good compliance to enlarge with a low intraluminal pressure. Multiple bowel configurations meet these requirements, and there is no universally accepted reservoir considered superior to the rest. It would appear that four orthotopic reservoirs occupy general acceptance with comparable results [24–26,33].

Three variations on ileal reservoirs are widely used. Koch and colleagues described a U-shaped, de-tubularized ileal reservoir that has been popularized by Skinner and associates; a unique feature of this technique is an afferent nipple valve to prevent ureteral reflux [24]. Studer et al. adopted a similar configuration of the bowel but used an afferent ileal segment for the ureteral anastomoses without specific attempts to prevent ureteral reflux [26]. No substantial differences in outcome of the upper tracts are apparent. Hautmann et al. use a W-configured ileal reservoir that has theoretically the best volume/pressure characteristics [25]. Lastly, an ileocolonic segment provides an immediate large capacity with good results [33].

Perspective

It is a personal belief that a major contributing factor to the current poor results obtained for invasive bladder cancer is delay in applying definitive, aggressive therapy to potentially lethal cancers. Cancers demonstrating any invasion may be undertreated due to patient and physician reluctance to intervene with a cystectomy or even to initiate definitive therapy with chemotherapy and R.T. Improvements in the delivery of cystectomy with an operative mortality rate anticipated of 1% to 2% and in the adjustment after cystectomy with orthotopic neobladders should translate into earlier use and better results [34]. Also, it is important to continue research in bladder preservation strategies because the potential exists to maintain the best quality of life in this way. However, currently available combinations of chemotherapy and R.T. provide disappointing long-term results. As new, effective systemic agents are identified, clinical trials with bladder preservation as a primary goal should be initiated.

References

1. Herr HW (1992). Transurethral resection in regionally advanced bladder cancer. Urol Clin N Am 19:695–700.
2. Solsona E, Iborra I, Ricos JV, Monros JL, Dumont R (1992). Feasibility of transurethral resection for muscle-infiltrating carcinoma of the bladder: prospective study. J Urol 147:1513–1515.
3. Sweeney P, Kursh ED, Resnick MI (1992). Partial cystectomy. Urol Clin N Am 19:701–711.
4. Fair WR (1992). Organ conservation in deeply invasive bladder tumors: a valid approach? World J Urol 10:8–10.
5. Sternberg CN (1992). Organ conservation in T2–3 bladder cancer: the role of transurethral resection, partial cystectomy, and primary and adjuvant chemotherapy. World J Urol 10:2–7.
6. Mameghan H, Fisher R (1989). Invasive bladder cancer, prognostic factors and results of radiotherapy with and without cystectomy. Br J Urol 63:251–258.
7. Fossa SD, Woehre H, Aass N, Jacobsen AB, Olsen DR, Ous S (1993). Bladder cancer definitive radiation therapy of muscle-invasive bladder cancer: a retrospective analysis of 317 patients. Cancer 72:3036–3043.
8. Gospodarowicz MK, Quilty PM, Scalliet P, Tsujii H, Fossa SD, Horenblas S, Isaka S, Prout GR, Shipley WU, Wijnmaalen AJ, Crawford ED, Jones WG, Kawai T (1995). The place of radiation therapy as definitive treatment of bladder cancer. Int J Urol 2:41–48.
9. Levine EG, Raghavan D (1993). MVAC for bladder cancer: time to move forward again. J Clin Urol 11:387–389.
10. Sternberg CN, Pansadoro V, Lauretti S, Platania A, Giannarelli D, Rossetti A, De Carli P, Arena MG, Cancrini A (1995). Neoadjuvant M-VAC (Methotrexate, Vinblastine, Adriamycin, and Cisplatin) chemotherapy and bladder preservation for muscle-infiltrating transitional cell carcinoma of the bladder. Urol Oncol 1:127–133.

11. Kaufman DS, Shipley WU, Griffin PP, Heney NM, Althausen AF, Efird JT (1993). Selective bladder preservation by combination treatment of invasive bladder cancer. N Engl J Med 329:1377–1382.
12. Tester W, Porter A, Asbell S, Coughlin C, Heaney J, Krall J, Martz K, Venner P, Hammond E (1993). Combined modality program with possible organ preservation for invasive bladder carcinoma: results of RTOG protocol 85-12. Int J Radiat Oncol Biol Phys 25:783–790.
13. Housset M, Maulard C, Chretien Y, Dufour B, Delanian S, Huart J, Colardelle F, Brunel P, Baillet F (1993). Combined radiation and chemotherapy for invasive transitional-cell carcinoma of the bladder: a prospective study. J Clin Oncol 11:2150–2157.
14. Given RW, Parsons JT, McCarley D, Wajsman Z (1995). Bladder-sparing multimodality treatment of muscle-invasive bladder cancer: a five-year follow-up. Urology 46:499–505.
15. Herr HW, Wartinger DD, Fair WR, Oettgen HF (1992). Bacillus Calmette-Guerin therapy for superficial bladder cancer: a 10-year followup. J Urol 147:1020–1023.
16. Logothetis CJ (1991). Organ preservation in bladder carcinoma: a matter of selection. J Clin Oncol 9:1525–1526.
17. Scher HI, Norton L (1992). Chemotherapy for urothelial tract malignancies: breaking the deadlock. Semin Surg Oncol 8:316–341.
18. Roth BJ, Bajorin DF (1995). Advanced bladder cancer: the need to identify new agents in the post-M-VAC (Methotrexate, Vinblastine, Doxorubicin and Cisplatin) world. J Urol 153:894–900.
19. Skinner DG, Lieskovsky G, Boyd S (1989). Continent urinary diversion. J Urol 14:1323–1327.
20. Wilson TG, Moreno JG, Weinberg A, Ahlering TE (1994). Late complications of the modified Indiana pouch. J Urol 151:331–334.
21. Martins FE, Bennett CJ, Skinner DG (1995). Options in replacement cystoplasty following radical cystectomy: high hopes for successful reality. J Urol 153:1363–1372.
22. Wood DP Jr, Montie JE, Pontes JE, Medendorp SV, Levin HS (1989). Transitional cell carcinoma of the prostate in cystoprostatectomy specimens removed for bladder cancer. J Urol 141:346–349.
23. Wood DP Jr, Montie JE, Pontes JE, Levin HS (1989). Identification of transitional cell carcinoma of the prostate in bladder cancer patients: a prospective study. J Urol 141:83–85.
24. Skinner DG, Boyd SD, Lieskovsky G, Bennett C, Hopwood B (1991). Lower urinary tract reconstruction following cystectomy: experience and results in 126 patients using the kock ileal reservoir with bilateral ureteroileal urethrostomy. J Urol 146:756–760.
25. Hautmann RE, Miller K, Steiner U, Wenderoth U (1993). The ileal neobladder: 6 years of experience with more than 200 patients. J Urol 150:40–45.
26. Studer UE, Danuser H, Merz VW, Springer JP, Zingg EJ (1995). Experience in 100 patients with an ileal low pressure bladder substitute combined with an afferent tubular isoperistaltic segment. J Urol 154:49–56.
27. Stein JP, Stenzl A, Esrig D, Freeman JA, Boyd SD, Lieskovsky G, Cote RJ, Bennett C, Colleselli K, Draxl H, Janetschek G, Poisel S, Bartsch G, Skinner DG (1994). Lower urinary tract reconstruction following cystectomy in women using the kock ileal reservoir with bilateral ureteroileal urethrostomy: initial clinical experience. J Urol 152:1404–1408.
28. Cancrini A, De Carli P, Fattahi H, Pompeo V, Cantiani R, Von Heland M (1995). Orthotopic ileal neobladder in female patients after radical cystectomy: 2-year experience. J Urol 153:956–958.
29. Montie JE (1995). Orthotopic bladder replacement in women. In Urinary Diversion, Webster GD, Goldwasser B (ed), Isis Medical Media: Oxford.
30. Keetch DW, Klutke CG, Catalona WJ (1992). Late decompensation of neobladder. J Urol 148:806–810.
31. Steiner MS, Morton RA, Marshall FF (1993). Vitamin B12 deficiency in patients with ileocolic neobladders. J Urol 149:255–257.
32. Matsui U, Topoll B, Miller K, Hautmann RE (1993). Metabolic long-term follow-up of the ileal neobladder. Eur Urol 24:197–200.

33. Goldwasser B (1995). The colonic orthotopic bladder. Urology 45:190–192.
34. Montie JE, Pavone-Macaluso M, Tazaki H, Albrecht W, Bono A, Karthaus P, Miyanaga N, Ueda T, von Eschenbach A (1995). What are the risks of cystectomy and the advances in perioperative care? Int J Urol 2:89–104.

8. Beyond the nerve-sparing radical prostatectomy

Robert C. Smith, Gary D. Steinberg, and Charles B. Brendler

Radical prostatectomy remains the most effective long-term treatment for patients with localized adenocarcinoma of the prostate. In the past it did not gain widespread popularity because many urologists believed the operation was technically difficult and was associated with significant intraoperative hemorrhage and postoperative impotence and incontinence. Over the past 15 years, an anatomical approach to radical retropubic prostatectomy has been developed that has greatly reduced the morbidity and mortality of the procedure. Delineation of the anatomy of the dorsal vein complex in 1979 by Reiner and Walsh enabled the procedure to be performed in a relatively bloodless field [1]. In 1982, Walsh and Donker described the anatomic course of the pelvic nerve plexus that provides innervation to the corpora cavernosa [2] and determined that impotence after radical prostatectomy was caused by injury to this plexus during dissection of the prostate. With the knowledge of the anatomy of the neurovascular bundles to the prostate and corpora carvernosa of the penis, the urologic surgeon may either spare the bundles or excise them when a wider margin is required to remove all of the tumor. Increased emphasis on the preservation of the striated urethral sphincter with an accurate sutured vesicourethral anastamosis that includes mucosal coaptation has led to a reduction in postoperative incontinence and bladder neck contracture [3]. This anatomic approach to radical prostatectomy has led to decreased blood loss and incontinence and has allowed many men to regain erectile potency. Thus, radical prostatectomy has become more acceptable to both patients and physicians.

There has been an extraordinary increase in the incidence of prostate cancer in the United States (60% from 1990 to 1993), and the incidence continues to rise [4]. This is in part due to increasing use of the PSA blood test as a screening tool by primary care physicians [5]. This increase in incidence coupled with the perception that radical prostatectomy is a superior form of treatment for localized prostate cancer has led to an annual sixfold increase in the number of radical prostatectomies performed from 1987 to 1992 [6]. Olsson et al. predict that approximately 52% of patients newly diagnosed with prostate cancer will be treated with radical prostatectomy [7].

Pienta, K.J., (ed.), DIAGNOSIS AND TREATMENT OF GENITOURINARY MALIGNANCIES.

Early detection

Presently, there is no curative therapy for patients with metastatic prostate cancer; therefore, efforts have focused on aggressive screening to detect the disease while it is still organ confined and potentially curable. Widespread use of serum PSA and transrectal ultrasound (TRUS) to screen for prostate cancer has resulted in earlier detection of tumors, many of which are nonpalpable (T1c). The biologic significance of these tumors is uncertain, and some of these may be clinically insignificant. It is estimated that screening may identify up to 10 million men with prostate cancer; however, it is estimated that only approximately 900,000 men would die of their cancer if left untreated [8]. Unfortunately, it is not possible to differentiate tumors that will progress from those that will not. Clinically useful markers for predicting the clinical course of the disease are being studied by various investigators. True progress, however, will not be made until delineation of the cellular and molecular pathways of metastatic progression are identified.

The clinical and pathological characteristics of nonpalpable prostate cancers identified with PSA screening have recently been reported in several studies [9–12] (table 8-1). Incidental prostate cancers detected at the time of cystoprostatectomy have a mean tumor volume of 0.04cc, 78% are less than 0.5cc, and 87% are organ confined [13]. In contrast, T1c prostate cancers are approximately 50 times larger and generally more extensive. Oesterling et al. reported on 208 patients with T1c prostate cancer treated with radical prostatectomy [9]. Only 53% of the patients had organ-confined cancer (11% with less than 0.5cc of tumor), 34% had positive surgical margins, 9% had seminal vesicle invasion, and 3% had pelvic lymph node metastases. Humphrey and Catalona reported on 53 men undergoing radical prostatectomy for stage T1c prostate cancer [10]. In this series, only 19% of these tumors were less than 0.5cc, 43% demonstrated extracapsular extension and/or positive surgical margins, and only 8% of tumors were Gleason score 2–4. Epstein et al. reported on 157 stage T1c prostate cancer patients treated with radical prostatectomy [11]. Only 51% of the patients had organ-confined prostate cancer (26% less than 0.5cc of tumor), 34% had extensive extracapsular extension, 17% had positive surgical margins, 6% had seminal

Table 8-1. Pathologic characteristics of clinical stage T1c tumors at radical prostatectomy

Study	No. Pts.	OC	+SM	+SV or +LN	Min. tumor (<0.5cc)
Oesterling et al. [9]	208	53%	34%	12%	11%
Humphrey et al. [10]	53	57%	43%[a]		19%
Epstein et al. [11]	157	51%	17%	10%	26%
Scaletscky et al. [12]	142	68%	26%	7%	35%[b]

[a] ECP and/or positive surgical margins.
[b] Less than 1.0ml.

vesicle invasion, and 4% had positive pelvic lymph nodes. Thus, the majority of stage T1c prostate cancers appear to be clinically significant tumors.

Epstein et al. also examined multiple preoperative clinical and pathological parameters in an attempt to identify patients with insignificant tumors who might be considered for conservative therapy. Criteria used to identify patients with insignificant tumors (tumor volume less than 0.2 cc) were a PSA density less than 0.1 ng/cc, no Gleason grade 4 or 5 tumor on needle biopsy, less than three positive biopsy cores, and less than 50% involvement of any single biopsy core. Using these criteria, 19 of 26 insignificant tumors were correctly identified.

In another study, Epstein et al. reported on 153 radical prostatectomy specimens removed for nonpalpable prostate cancer [14]. They evaluated 720 individual tumor foci in these 153 specimens. There was a weak correlation ($r = 0.254$) between tumor grade and volume. Of 106 peripheral tumors containing any Gleason pattern 4 or 5, 45% were less than 1.0 cc in volume, and overall 9% of the prostates contained tumor foci that were predomiantly Gleason pattern 4 or 5 and measured 1 cc or less. Therefore, prostate cancer does not only dedifferentiate as it grows, but can be high grade early in its course. Thus, patients followed conservatively should undergo widespread needle sampling of the prostate to enhance detection of foci of high-grade disease in the prostate.

Cancer control

Paulson recently presented his 20-year experience with radical perineal prostatectomy for clinically localized prostate cancer [15]. The cancer-specific survival at 13.5 years was 90% for patients with organ- and specimen-confined tumors, but only 60% for patients with margin-positive disease (table 8-2). Of 222 patients with margin-positive disease, 66 underwent immediate adjuvant radiation therapy (within six months of surgery). Early postoperative adjuvant radiation therapy did not appear to enhance survival over those patients that did not receive such therapy. In addition, the survival of patients with margin-positive, node-negative disease and patients with node-positive disease was similar. Thus, margin-positive disease appears to represent systemic disease that is incurable by local measures.

Prostate-cancer-specific survival at ten years for patients with localized prostate cancer treated by radical prostatectomy has been reported by several groups [16–19]. Partin et al. recently presented the ten-year experience at Johns Hopkins with anatomic radical prostatectomy [16]. This study included 955 men, average age of 59.4 ± 6.4 years, with clinical stage T1–2 prostate cancer with a mean follow-up of 53 months. Patients in this series had an actuarial likelihood of cancer-specific survival at ten years of 93%. Similar results were found by Zincke et al., who reported their data by clinical stage

Table 8-2. Actuarial likelihood of cause-specific survival at 10 and 13.5 years for patients with localized prostate cancer treated with radical prostatectomy

Study	Actuarial timepoint	Stage/grade	Prostate cancer-specific survival
Paulson [15]	13.5 years	Organ- and specimen-confined	90%
		margin positive	60%
Partin et al. [16]	10 years	cT1-2	93%
Stein et al. [17]	10 years	cT1-3	91%
Trapasso et al. [18]	10 years	cT1-T2N0	94%
Zincke et al. [19]	10 years	cT1	95%
		cT2a	90%
		cT2b,c	88%
		Gleason ≤ 3	95%
		Gleason 4–6	90%
		Gleason ≥ 7	82%

and grade [19]. Not surprisingly, the actuarial ten-year cancer-specific survival was highest for patients with cT1 tumors (95%), and lower for cT2a (90%) and for cT2b,c (88%) tumors. When analyzed by grade, the highest ten-year survival was found for Gleason scores of 3 or less (95%), and lower for Gleason scores between 4 and 6 (90%) and for Gleason scores of 7 or more (82%).

Disease-free survival from prostate cancer can now be assessed more accurately because of the widespread availability of the PSA blood test. Several groups have reported the actuarial likelihood of remaining PSA free at 5 and 10 years following radical prostatectomy for clinically localized prostate cancer [15–20] (table 8-3). Partin et al. recently reported in their series that the actuarial likelihood of disease recurrence as measured by a detectable PSA increased with pathologic stage and Gleason score [16]. The ten-year actuarial likelihood of freedom from PSA relapse was 85% for men with organ-confined disease, 82% with focal capsular penetration, 54% with established capsular penetration and Gleason score less than 7, 42% with established capsular penetration and Gleason score 7 or greater, and 43% with seminal vesicle involvement. Therefore, in men with high-grade tumor (Gleason score 7 or greater) and capsular penetration or seminal vesicle involvement, cure is less likely. No patient with lymph node metastases had an undetectable serum PSA at ten years. In patients treated with adjuvant radiation therapy to the prostatic bed for a detectable PSA, only 10% had a reduction in PSA to the undetectable range that was sustained at least two years.

Zincke et al. reported the 25-year experience with over 3000 patients undergoing radical prostatectomy for clinically localized prostate cancer at the Mayo Clinic and identified prognostic and treatment variables [19]. Twenty-six percent of the patients received adjuvant therapy (19% received hormonal therapy, 5% received radiation therapy, and 1% received radiation and hormonal therapy). The overall 10- and 15-year undetectable PSA rates were 52

Table 8-3. Actuarial likelihood of remaining free of disease recurrence at 5 and 10 years as determined by PSA relapse in patients with clinically localized prostate cancer treated with radical prostatectomy

			Likelihood of remaining PSA free	
Study	No. pts.	Stage/grade	5 years	10 years
Paulson[a] [15]	613	Organ confined	85%	72%
		Specimen confined	50%	40%
		Margin positive	42%	37%
Partin et al. [16]	894	Organ confined	97%	85%
		Focal capsular penetration	90%	82%
		Established capsular penetration Gleason < 7	88%	54%
		Established capsular penetration Gleason ≥ 7	68%	42%
		Seminal vesicle involvement	47%	43%
		Lymph node involvement	15%	0%
Trapasso et al. [18]	601	Organ confined	92%	
		Capsular penetration	74%	
		Positive sem. ves.	56%	
Zincke et al. [19]	3170	cT1		70%
		cT2a		56%
		cT2b,c		47%
		Gleason grade ≤ 3		71%
		Gleason grade 4–6		53%
		Gleason grade ≥ 7		35%
Catalona et al. [20]	925	pT1 or pT2	94%	
		pT3a	84%	
		pT3b	60%	
		N1	56%	

[a] Numbers were approximated from a Kaplan–Meier curve in which the data were originally presented.

± 1.4% and 40 ± 1.9%, respectively. The crude 10- and 15-year survival rates are comparable to the expected survival rate for age-matched patients in Minnesota. Patients with cT1 tumors had the highest likelihood of remaining PSA free at ten years (70%), with lower disease-free survival from cT2a (56%) and cT2b,c (47%) tumors. Gleason score and pathological stage were prognostic factors; however, adjuvant therapy did not significantly affect recurrence or survival.

Catalona and Smith reported five-year tumor recurrence rates in 925 men with localized prostate cancer treated with anatomical radical retropubic prostatectomy with a mean follow-up of 28 months [20]. They assessed the effect of clinical stage and preoperative serum PSA on surgical outcome. The overall five-year probability of recurrence was 22%, with recurrence being related to both the PSA level and clinical stage. The five-year probability of recurrence was 7% for men with a preoperative PSA of 4.1–9.9 ng/ml and 29% for a preoperative PSA of 10 ng/ml or greater. At five years, 97% of nonpalpable tumors were free of biochemical progression as opposed to 74% of men who had palpable disease. Thus, preoperative PSA and clinical stage are important predictors of surgical outcome. However, these patients will need additional follow-up to assess long-term survival.

Recent pathologic studies have demonstrated a 40% to 63% incidence of extensive capsular perforation (ECP) in clinical stage T2 prostate cancer [21–24]. Rosen et al. found that 87% of ECP occurs in the region of the neurovascular bundles and that 57% of the positive surgical margins occur in this region [24]. Wide excision of the neurovascular bundle(s) ipsilateral to a nodule or an area of induration has been found to reduce the incidence of positive surgical margins [25]. Extended follow-up of patients that have undergone wide excision demonstrates that the probability of having an undetectable PSA at five years is 47% in patients with negative surgical margins versus 6% in patients with positive surgical margins. This new knowledge suggests that nerve-sparing prostatectomy should not be performed on the side of palpable induration and perhaps not at all for apical tumors.

Ohori et al. reported in a study of 500 patients with a mean follow-up of 36 months that patients with a Gleason score of 7 or greater had a higher cancer progression rate when treated with radical prostatectomy than patients with a Gleason score less than 7 [26]. The nonprogression rate at five years was 92 ± 4% for patients with a Gleason score less than 7 and 55 ± 12% for patients with a Gleason score of 7 or greater. Tumor volume and extracapsular disease increased significantly with increasing grade, with only 30% of high-grade tumors being organ confined. However, progression in tumors confined to the prostate did not appear to be influenced by grade, since 85% of patients with both low- and high-grade, organ-confined prostate cancer had no evidence of progression at five years. Furthermore, Partin et al. reported the clinical outcome of 72 men with Gleason scores of 8–10 on needle biopsy and clinically localized disease [27]. Nine patients (13%) did not undergo radical prostatectomy because of positive lymph nodes on frozen section. Of the 63 men who underwent radical prostatectomy, 32% had positive pelvic lymph nodes. All patients were followed for at least 24 months. The actuarial likelihood of having an undetectable PSA at five years was 43% for men with negative lymph nodes and 45% for men with specimen-confined disease. Thus, radical prostatectomy may cure some patients with poorly differentiated tumor.

The treatment of clinical stage T3 prostate cancer with radical prostatectomy remains controversial. While radiotherapy is the most frequently used modality in the treatment of patients with locally advanced disease, it is least effective when applied to large volume disease [28]. It is therefore not surprising that postirradiation biopsies in patients with T3 disease have been found to be positive in as many as 74% of patients [28,29]. In addition, the inability to obtain local tumor control appears to increase the rate of distant metastasis in patients treated with radioactive iodine seed implantation as compared to those in whom local tumor control is obtained [30]. While surgical extirpation of prostate cancer offers the best likelihood of local control, many have viewed it as a poor treatment modality because of early studies that reported poor ten-year survival rates [31,32]. However, van den Ouden et al. recently found that 38% of patients who underwent radical retropubic prostatectomy after a negative staging lymphadenectomy for clinical T3 disease were free of disease, with a mean follow-up of 43 months [33]. Both grade and serum PSA level were found to be important prognostic variables in assessing those at high risk for progression. van den Ouden et al. found that the subset of patients with high-grade disease or a PSA greater than 20 ng/ml had less than a 10% probability of remaining free of progression. These variables in addition to nodal status may allow for identification of those patients most likely to benefit from surgery.

Lerner et al. recently reported on 812 patients with clinical stage T3 tumors treated with radical prostatectomy [34]. These tumors all had disease limited to the immediate periprostatic tissue and seminal vesicles, with no extension to the pelvic side walls or involvement of the bladder base or trigone and no evidence of distant metastases. Mean follow-up was 4.5 years, with 60% of patients receiving adjuvant therapy (radiotherapy in 7%, androgen ablation in 43%, and both in 10%). Actuarial cancer-specific survival, freedom from PSA relapse, and freedom from local recurrence were 69%, 30%, and 71%, respectively, at 15 years. This compares favorably to the 26% to 33% cancer-specific survival at 15 years obtained with radiotherapy [28,35]. The effect of androgen ablation therapy appeared to have a significant impact on progression-free survival but not on cause-specific survival.

Careful patient selection is likely to be the important factor in determining which patients with clinical stage T3 disease might benefit from radical prostatectomy. It appears that patients with less extensive local disease, negative lymph nodes, well or moderately differentiated histology, and a serum PSA of less than 20 ng/ml have the best chance of benefiting from surgery. The role of adjuvant therapy in these patients remains unproven. Furthermore, several studies have demonstrated that between 17% and 30% of patients with clinical stage T3 tumors are overstaged and have pathologic T2 tumors that can potentially be cured by surgery alone [33,34,36].

The role of radical prostatectomy in the management of stage D1 prostate cancer is also controversial. Although cure is unlikely, some men survive for long periods of time clinically free of metastatic disease. In a series of 113 men that underwent radical prostatectomy for clinical stage T1 or T2 disease who were found to have pathologic stage D1 prostate cancer, prognosis was dependent on Gleason score [37]. None of the patients received adjuvant hormonal therapy until metastatic disease developed. No patient with positive lymph nodes had an undetectable PSA at three years. In patients with positive nodes and a Gleason score less than 8, the likelihood of distant metastases was 18% and 41% at 5 and 10 years, respectively, whereas 85% of men with a Gleason score of 8–10 had distant metastases by five years. Therefore, urologists who believe that patients with stage D1 disease benefit from local control of their tumor with radical prostatectomy need not perform frozen sections at the time of surgery if the preoperative prostate biopsy revealed a Gleason score of 7 or less. However, a meticulous search for positive nodes should be performed in patients with a Gleason score of 8 or greater to avoid a procedure that offers no benefit.

Morbidity and mortality

Andriole et al. reported a 7.4% early complication rate in 1342 radical prostatectomies performed over a five-year period [38]. Mortality and cardiovascular complications increased with patient age; however, there were only 0.2% deaths and 1.4% cardiovascular complications overall. In 2.6% of patients, thromboembolic events occurred (8 deep venous thromboses and 22 pulmonary emboli). Moreover, a recent study of the use of external sequential compression devices (SCDs) in the prevention of postoperative thromboembolic events failed to demonstrate a reduction in the rate of thromboembolic events in patients undergoing radical retropubic prostatectomy [39]. The only apparent difference noted was that SCDs delayed the onset of the thromboembolic events from 11 to 20 days postoperatively. This finding suggests that most patients suffering these complications will do so as an outpatient, and they should be instructed about signs and symptoms of these events prior to discharge.

Knowledge of the anatomy of the dorsal venous complex has led to a reduction in the amount of blood lost during radical prostatectomy. A recent study evaluated the effect of epidural anesthesia versus epidural plus general anesthesia versus general anesthesia on blood loss [40]. Mean blood loss in the epidural group (1490 ± 90 ml) was significantly less than in the combined epidural/general group (1810 ± 100 ml) or the general anesthesia alone group (1940 ± 130 ml) ($p < 0.01$). Since blood loss was similar in the groups receiving general anesthesia, either alone or when combined with epidural anesthesia, it implies that epidural anesthesia did not reduce bleeding, but, rather, that general anesthesia increased blood loss. Positive pressure ventilation used during general anesthesia has been shown to increase venous pressure, and this finding may explain the higher blood loss seen with general anesthesia.

Inadvertent rectal injury is a well-known complication of radical prostatectomy, occurring in approximately 0.5% to 1.2% of patients [41–43]. McLaren et al. at the Mayo Clinic retrospectively reviewed 2212 patients that had undergone radical retropubic prostatectomy and found 27 documented rectal injuries (1.2%) [43]. Six patients received a diverting colostomy, two immediate and four delayed; one of the four patients undergoing delayed colostomy died of sepsis. This patient had not undergone a preoperative bowel preparation. Two of the four rectourethral fistulae occurred in patients that had not received a bowel preparation. No patients received an omental interposition to fortify the repair. Borland and Walsh at Johns Hopkins administered only a single Fleets enema the evening prior to surgery in their series of

1000 nonirradiated patients undergoing radical retropubic prostatectomy [42]. Ten rectal injuries occurred (1.0%), nine of which were discovered at the time of surgery and repaired with a double-layered closure and a reinforcing pedicle of omentum over the suture line. One injury was discovered on postoperative day 2 and was repaired in the same fashion with the addition of a diverting colostomy. No patient developed a wound infection, abscess, or fistula. Thus, intraoperative recognition is essential to avoid sepsis and the requirement of a delayed colostomy. Omental interposition may aid in decreasing the incidence of rectourethral fistula.

Urinary incontinence is one of the most disabling complications of radical prostatectomy. Walsh reported on the first 593 men who underwent anatomical radical retropubic prostatectomy [44]. Only two men required artificial urethral sphincter implantation, 92% were completely dry, and 8% had stress incontinence. However, only 86% of men aged 70 years old or greater were completely dry. Most other series have reported less favorable urinary continence rates [45–50] (table 8-4). Chodak et al. studied the quality of life of patients following radical prostatectomy [51]. Patients treated by eight academic urologists returned almost 500 questionnaires. While only 4% reported wearing more than two pads per day, 37% of patients reported urinary leakage at least once a day. Urinary incontinence after radical prostatectomy is multifactorial but does not appear to be related to injury to the cavernosal nerves. Hopefully, anatomic studies of the puboprostatic ligaments and striated urethral sphincter as well as bladder neck will shed additional light on the mechanisms of postprostatectomy incontinence. In addition, postoperative intraurethral injection of collagen may help some men with mild stress incontinence after radical prostatectomy.

The restoration of sexual function, defined as the ability to achieve an erection sufficient for intercourse, after radical prostatectomy is related to age, clinical and pathological stage, and surgical technique. Sexual function was preserved in 91% of men less than 50 years old, 75% of men aged 50–60 years old, 58% of men 60–70 years old, and 25% of men 70 years or older in the Hopkins series [52]. However, others have been unable to reproduce these results [41,49,50,53–55] (table 8-5). Geary et al. reported potency rates of 35%

Table 8-4. Urinary continence after radical prostatectomy

Study	Continent: no pads	Minor incontinence: 1–2 pads/day	Severe incontinence: 3–5 pads/day	Complete incontinence
Johns Hopkins [44]	92.0%	6.0%	2.0%	0.3%
Mayo Clinic [45]	78.8%	15.7%	4.2%	0.8%
Stanford [46]	80.1%	8.1%	6.6%	5.2%
USC [47]	88.0%	5.4%	2.5%	Not stated
Baylor [48]	86.0%	7.0%	7.0%	Not stated
ACS [49]	81.1%	11.2%	4.1%	3.6%
Wash. Univ. [50]	94.0%	Not stated	Not stated	Not stated

for men undergoing bilateral and 15% for men undergoing unilateral nerve-sparing prosatectomy [53]. They found that potency was most stongly related to the number of bundle(s) spared, preoperative frequency of intercourse, postoperative incontinence or strictures, and cancer volume. Zimmern et al. reported potency results of 46% after 'nerve sparing' radical prostatectomy [54]. Their assessment of postoperative potency included not only patient and spouse interview, but also nocturnal penile tumescence and penile Doppler blood flow after PGE-1 injection. In addition, Zimmern reported that many patients noted poor quality and unpredictable erections. In the American College of Surgeons survey, only 27.6% of patients regained potency [49]. Chodak et al., in their study of the quality of life of almost 500 patients following radical prostatectomy, found that, compared to before surgery, 53% reported having sex much less often, 52% reported never having sex after surgery, and 81% were unable to achieve an erection [51]. Despite this, 84% had little trouble adjusting after surgery, and 86% reported overall satisfaction with surgery. These findings are consistent with those of Litwin et al., who found that, although patients treated with surgery had a greater degree of sexual dysfunction than patients treated with either radiation or observation, their ability to tolerate such problems was great [56]. Moreover, the general health-related quality of life of patients treated with surgery was no different from patients that received observation only. Thus, surgical techniques must be further refined, and additional factors important in the preservation of potency need to be identified so that the majority of men undergoing radical prostatectomy will remain potent after surgery.

Table 8-5. Recovery of sexual function after nerve-sparing radical prostatectomy

Reference	Mean age	No. pts. in study	NVB(s) spared	Potency (no.)
Quinlan et al. [52]	59	503	Bil. (291) Unil. (109)	76% (220) 56% (61)
Geary et al. [53]	64	459	Bil. (69) Unil. (203)	31.2% (22) 13.3% (27)
Zimmern et al. [54]	45–70	41	Bil. (19) Unil. (56)	46% (35) (combined)
Murphy et al. [49]	Not stated	1059	Not stated	28% (193)
Leandri et al. [41]	68	106	Bil. (106)	71% (75)
Catalona et al. [50]	64	295	Bil. (236) Unil. (59)	63% (149) 41% (24)
Drago et al. [55]	64	151	Not stated Unil. (109)	66% (100) 56% (61)
Total			Bil. (702) Unil. (371)	66% (446) 30% (112)
			Overall (2614)	35% (906)

Abbreviations: NVB(s), neurovascular bundles; Bil., bilateral; Unil., unilateral.

Neoadjuvant therapy

Recently there has been considerable interest in the use of neoadjuvant hormonal therapy to 'downstage' clinical stage B2 and C (T2c or T3) prostate cancer prior to radical prostatectomy. Oesterling et al. treated 22 patients with clinical T2c or T3 prostate cancer with hormonal deprivation prior to radical prostatectomy and compared the pathologic findings with 22 similar patients who did not receive hormonal deprivation [57]. These researchers noted no difference in pathologic stage, tumor volume, or DNA ploidy status between the two groups. Twenty of the 21 patients treated with hormonal deprivation prior to radical prostatectomy were pathological stage T3 or greater. Similarly, Plummer et al. noted that 33 of 34 patients with clinical stage T2c or T3 prostate cancer treated with hormonal deprivation prior to surgery had pathologic stage T3 disease or greater [58]. Thus, neoadjuvant hormonal therapy does not result in pathological downstaging in most patients with stage T3 disease. However, recent studies by Soloway et al. [59] and Goldenberg et al. [60] report that patients with clinical stage T1 and T2 prostate cancer treated with preoperative androgen deprivation have a lower rate of positive surgical margins than similar patients not pretreated. It is unclear, however, whether this reduction is related to improved surgical technique secondary to a somewhat smaller prostate, elimination of cells that have escaped the prostatic capsule, or hormonal therapy simply making it more difficult for the pathologist to identify extracapsular disease. It would seem unlikely that neoadjuvant hormonal therapy will sterilize extracapsular disease, and it is unknown whether the apparent reduction in positive surgical margins will translate into improved disease-free survival. Longer follow-up of these patients is necessary in order to determine if neoadjuvant hormonal therapy before radical prostatectomy will improve survival for men with clinical T1–2 prostate cancer.

Adjuvant therapy

Pathologic upstaging from clinical stage T1c and T2 to pT3 disease occurs in approximately 32%–49% and 44%–66%, respectively, of patients undergoing radical prostatectomy [9–12,16,19,32]. This finding has led to the use of adjuvant radiation therapy in an attempt to improve local control and to improve disease-free survival. Several studies have demonstrated a lower rate of local recurrence following adjuvant radiation therapy [61–63]. Gibbons et al. found that the incidence of local recurrence was lower (5%) in patients that received adjuvant radiotherapy versus a comparable group of patients that did not (30%) [61]. Using PSA as a measure of recurrence, there is a transient decrease in serum PSA in 53%–64% of men after postoperative radiation with limited follow-up [64]. Partin et al. reported only a 10% response to radiation therapy (undetectable serum PSA for greater than two years) for men with isolated elevations of PSA and a 29% response for those with documented local recurrence [16]. Eisbruch et al. noted no improvement in survival for patients with either positive margins or seminal vesicle involvement treated with adjuvant external beam radiation therapy [65]. Thus, locoregional control appears to be improved in some patients with pathologically advanced tumors; however adjuvant therapy has not been shown to decrease the development of distant metastases or improve survival. A randomized trial of adjuvant radiation therapy following radical prostatectomy is presently being conducted for patients with pathologic stage T3 prostate cancer by the South West Oncology Group (SWOG).

Use of adjuvant hormonal therapy has also been used in an attempt to increase both local control and disease-free survival in patients with T3NO and T3N1 disease. The first suggestion that radical prostatectomy combined with early endocrine therapy (EET) might be advantageous was made by Scott in 1964 [66]. He performed immediate orchiectomy in patients with grossly extracapsular disease at the time of radical perineal prostatectomy. At 15 years he found that 29% of the patients were disease free, which was superior to historical controls [67]. Other groups have reported improved local control with adjuvant hormonal therapy. There was initially great enthusiasm for adjuvant hormonal therapy in patients with T2–3N1 disease due to the findings of Zincke et al. [68]. They reported a statistically significant improvement in disease-free survival in patients who underwent radical prostatectomy and EET. However, cause-specific survival was not found to be significantly better in patients treated with EET. Studies by Myers et al. and deKernion et al. have also failed to find a significant cause-specific survival advantage to EET following radical prostatectomy [69,70].

Ploidy analysis has been used to subclassify patients with T3N1 disease. Myers et al. studied the effect of EET in patients with T3N1 disease in patients that underwent radical prostatectomy and found that those with diploid tumors had a significantly better cause-specific survival than those undergoing delayed endocrine therapy [70]. However, Winkler et al. determined that ploidy alone had a powerful impact on prognosis, with progression occurring in only 15% of patients with diploid tumors and in 75% of patients with nondiploid tumors ($p < 0.0001$), regardless of treatment with EET [71]. Furthermore, no patient with a diploid tumor died of prostate cancer with a median followup of 7.5 years. Prospective, randomized studies are needed to demonstrate whether EET improves cause specific survival in patients with T3N1 disease.

Prognostic markers

At present, the prognosis for men with prostate cancer depends on pathologic stage and Gleason score. However, additional possible prognostic markers have been studied. Lieber et al. analyzed 494 patients (pathological stages B,

C, D1) who underwent radical prostatectomy at the Mayo Clinic from 1967 to 1981 [72]. The nuclear DNA ploidy patterns were assessed from paraffin-embedded tissue. In a multivariate analysis, these researchers found that Gleason score, pathologic stage, and DNA ploidy were independently pathologic prognostic variables for progression and cause-specific survival. Within each pathological stage and Gleason-score grouping, patients with a nondiploid tumor had a 2.7-fold higher chance of disease progression or death from prostate cancer. Gleason score enhanced prognostication when added to ploidy. Carmichael et al. reported that DNA ploidy analysis was able to predict disease recurrence in patients with well- to moderately differentiated (Gleason score less than 7) clinical stage T2 prostate cancer treated with radical prostatectomy [73]. Additional pathological parameters that may help predict prognosis in the future include nuclear morphometry, metalloproteinase, bcl-2 or e-cadherin expression, and identification of metastasis suppressor genes [74–78].

Conclusions

Radical prostatectomy is the most effective therapy for prostate cancer pathologically confined to the prostate, and recent advances in surgical technique have made radical prostatectomy more widely acceptable. Further improvements in surgical technique as well as in the training of urologic surgeons will continue to decrease the morbidity and mortality of this operation. The development of clinical criteria and molecular markers to identify patients at high risk for progression may ultimately reduce the number of men that will require surgery. The success rate of adjuvant therapy in patients with advanced disease remains unsatisfactory. Current research is directed towards providing a better understanding of the molecular genetics of prostate cancer, and hopefully this will aid in the development of more effective adjuvant therapies.

References

1. Reiner WG, Walsh PC (1979). An anatomical approach to the surgical management of the dorsal vein and Santorini's plexus during radical retropubic surgery. J Urol 121:198–200.
2. Walsh PC, Donker PJ (1982). Impotence following radical prostatectomy: insight into etiology and prevention. J Urol 128:492–497.
3. Walsh PC, Partin AW, Epstein JI (1994). Cancer control and quality of life following anatomical radical retropubic prostatectomy: results at 10 years. J Urol 152:1831–1836.
4. Boring CC, Squires TS, Tong T (1993). Cancer statistics. CA 43:7–26.
5. Jacobsen SJ, Katusic SK, Bergstralh EJ, Oesterling JE, Ohrt D, Klee GG, Chute CG, Lieber MM (1995). Incidence of prostate cancer diagnosis in the eras before and after serum prostate-specific antigen testing. JAMA 274:1445–1449.
6. Lu-Yao GL, McLerran D, Wasson J, Wennberg JE (1993). An assessment of radical prostatectomy: time trends, geographic variation and outcomes. JAMA 269:2633–2636.
7. Olsson CA, Golubuff ET (1994). Detection and treatment of prostate cancer: perspective of the urologist. J Urol 152:1695–1699.

8. Scardino PT, Weaver R, Hudson MA (1992). Early detection of prostate cancer. Hum Pathol 23:211–222.
9. Oesterling JE, Suman VJ, Zinke H, Bostwick DG (1993). PSA-detected (clinical stage T1c or BO) prostate cancer; pathologically significant tumors. Urol Clin N Am 20:687–693.
10. Humphrey PA, Catalona WJ (in press). Clinical and pathological characteristics of non-palpable prostate cancers. J Urol.
11. Epstein JI, Walsh PC, Carmichael M, Brendler CB (1994). Pathologic and clinical findings to predict tumor extent of nonpalpable (stage T1c) prostate cancer. JAMA 271:369–374.
12. Scaletscky R, Koch MO, Eckstein CW, Bicknell SL, Gray GF, Smith JA (1994). Tumor volume and stage in carcinoma of the prostate detected by elevations in prostate specific antigen. J Urol 152:129–131.
13. Kabalin JN, McNeal JE, Price HM, Feiha FS, Stamey TA (1989). Unsuspected adenocarcinoma of the prostate in patients undergoing cystoprostatectomy for other causes: incidence, histology and morphometric observations. J Urol 141:1091–1094.
14. Epstein JI, Carmichael M, Partin AW, Walsh PC (1994). Small high grade adenocarcinoma of the prostate in radical prostatectomy specimens performed for nonpalpable disease: pathogenic and clinical implications. J Urol 151:1587–1592.
15. Paulson DF (1994). Impact of radical prostatectomy in the management of clinically localized disease. J Urol 152:1826–1830.
16. Partin AW, Pound CR, Clemens JQ, Epstein JI, Walsh PC (1993). Serum PSA after anatomic radical prostatectomy: The Johns Hopkins experience after 10 years. Urol Clin N Am 20:713–725.
17. Stein A, deKernion JB, Smith RB, Dorey F, Patel H (1992). Prostate specific antigen levels after radical prostatectomy in patients with organ confined and locally extensive prostate cancer. J Urol 147:942–946.
18. Trapasso JG, deKernion JB, Smith RB, Dorey F (1994). The incidence and significance of detectable levels of serum prostate specific antigen after radical prostatectomy. J Urol 152:1821–1825.
19. Zincke H, Oesterling JI, Blute ML, Bergstralh EJ, Meyers RP, Barrett DM (1994). Long-term (15 years) results after radical prostatectomy for clinically localized (stage T2c or lower) prostate cancer. J Urol 152:1850–1857.
20. Catalona WJ, Smith DS (1994). 5-year tumor recurrence rates after anatomical radical retropubic prostatectomy for prostate cancer. J Urol 152:1837–1842.
21. Catalona WJ, Bigg SW (1990). Nerve-sparing radical prostatectomy: evaluation of results of 250 patients. J Urol 143:538–544.
22. Villers A, McNeil JE, Redwine EA, Freiha FS, Stamey TA (1989). The role of perineural space invasion in the local spread of prostatic adenocarcinoma. J Urol 142:763–768.
23. Walsh PC (1988). Radical prostatectomy with reduced morbidity: an anatomic approach. NCI Monogr 7:133–137.
24. Rosen MA, Goldstone L, Lapin S, Wheeler T, Scardino PT (1992). Frequency and location of extracapsular extension and positive surgical margins in radical prostatectomy specimens. J Urol 148:331–337.
25. Smith RC, Partin AW, Epstein JI, Brendler CB (1996). Extended followup of the influence of the neurovascular bundle(s) on prognosis in men with clinically localized prostate cancer and extensive capsular perforation. J Urol 156:454–458.
26. Ohori M, Goad JR, Wheeler TM, Eastham JA, Thompson TC, Scardino PT (1994). Can radical prostatectomy alter the progression of poorly differentiated prostate cancer? J Urol 152:1843–1849.
27. Partin AW, Lee BR, Carmichael M, Walsh PC, Epstein JI (1994). Radical prostatectomy for high grade disease: a reevaluation. J Urol 151:1583–1586.
28. Bagshaw MA, Cox RS, Ray GR (1988). Status of radiation treatment of prostate cancer at Stanford University. NCI Monogr 7:47–60.
29. Scardino PT, Wheeler TM (1988). Local control of prostate cancer with radiotherapy: fre-

quency and prognostic significance of positive results of post-irradiation prostate biopsy. NCI Monogr 7:95–103.

30. Fuks Z, Leibel SA, Wallner KE, Begg CB, Fair WR, Anderson LL, Hilaris BS, Whitmore WF (1991). The effect of local control on metastatic dissemination in carcinoma of the prostate: long-term results in patients treated with ^{125}I implantation. Int J Radiat Oncol Biol Phys 21:537–547.
31. Boxer RJ, Kaufman JJ, Goodwin WE (1977). Radical prostatectomy for carcinoma of the prostate: 1951–1976. A review of 329 patients. J Urol 117:208–213.
32. Elder JS, Jewett HJ, Walsh PC (1982). Radical perineal prostatectomy for clinical stage B2 carcinoma of the prostate. J Urol 127:704–706.
33. van den Ouden D, Davidson PJT, Hop W, Schroeder FH (1994). Radical prostatectomy as a monotherapy for locally advanced (stage T3) prostate cancer. J Urol 151:646–651.
34. Lerner SE, Blute ML, Zincke H (1995). Extended experience with radical prostatectomy for clinical stage T3 prostate cancer: outcome and contemporary morbidity. J Urol 154:1447–1452.
35. Scardino PT (1989). Is radiotherapy effective for locally advanced (stage C or T3) prostate cancer? Prog Clin Biol Res 303:223–239.
36. Morgan WR, Bergstralh EK, Zincke H (1993). Long-term evaluation of radical prostatectomy as treatment for clinical stage C (T3) prostate cancer. Urology 41:113–120.
37. Sgrignoli AR, Walsh PC, Steinberg GD, Steiner MS, Epstein JI (1994). Prognostic factors in men with stage D1 prostate cancer: identification of patients less likely to have prolonged survival after radical prostatectomy. J Urol 152:1077–1081.
38. Andriole GL, Smith DS, Rao G, Goodnough L, Catalona WJ (1994). Early complications of contemporary radical retropubic prostatectomy. J Urol 152:1858–1860.
39. Cisek LJ, Walsh PC (1993). Thromboembolic complications following radical retropubic prostatectomy: influence of external sequential pneumatic compression devices. Urology 42:406–408.
40. Shir Y, Raja SN, Frank SM, Brendler CB (1995). Intraoperative blood loss during radical retropubic prostatectomy: epidural versus general anesthesia. Urology 45:993–999.
41. Leandri P, Rossignol G, Gautier J-R, Ramon J (1992). Radical retropubic prostatectomy: morbidity and quality of life. Experience with 620 consecutive cases. J Urol 147:883–887.
42. Borland RN, Walsh PC (1992). The management of rectal injury during radical retropubic prostatectomy. J Urol 147:905–907.
43. McLaren RH, Barrett DM, Zincke H (1993). Rectal injury occurring at radical retropubic prostatectomy for prostate cancer: etiology and treatment. Urology 42:401–405.
44. Walsh PC, Quinlan DM. Morton RA, Steiner MS (1990). Radical retropubic prostatectomy: improved anastamosis and urinary incontinence. Urol Clin N Am 17:679–684.
45. Blute ML, Bergstralh EJ, Zincke H (1995). Morbidity assessment of contemporary radical retropubic prostatectomy for clinicall localized prostate cancer. J Urol 151:487A.
46. Geary ES, Dendinger TE, Stamey TA (1995). Impotence, incontinence and vesical neck strictures following nerve-sparing radical prostatectomy. J Urol 151:488A.
47. Simoneau R, Grossfeld GD, Lieskovsky G, Chen S-C, Skinner DG (1995). Complications of radical retropubic prostatectomy. J Urol 151:487A.
48. Goad JR, Rogers E, Ohori M, Boone TB, Scardino PT (1995). Incontinence after radical prostatectomy in 315 patients: the outcome and risk factors. J Urol 151:488A.
49. Murphy GP, Mettlin C, Menck H, Winchester DP, Davidson A-M (1994). National patterns of prostate cancer treatment by radical prostatectomy: results of a survey by the American College of Surgeons commission on cancer. J Urol 152:1817–1819.
50. Catalona WJ, Basler JW (1993). Return of erections and urinary continence following nerve sparing radical retropubic prostatectomy. J Urol 150:905–907.
51. Chodak GC, Sinner M, Rukstalis DB, Pontes E, Montie J, Schellhammer P, Williams R, Resnick M (1995). Patient reported outcomes following radical prostatectomy performed at eight academic institutions. J Urol 153:390A.

52. Quinlan DM, Epstein JI, Carter BS, Walsh PC (1991). Sexual function following radical prostatectomy: influence of preservation of neurovascular bundles. J Urol 145:998–1003.
53. Geary ES, Dendinger TE, Freiha FS, Stamey TA (1995). Nerve sparing radical prostatectomy: a different view. J Urol 154:145–149.
54. Zimmern PE, Leach GE, Roskamp D, Kaswick J (1994). A prospective evaluation of potency following nerve sparing radical prostatectomy. J Urol 151:488A.
55. Drago JR, Badalment RA, York JP, Simon J, Riemenschneider H, Nesbitt J, Perez J (1992). Radical prostatectomy: OSU and affiliated hospitals experience 1985–1989. Urology 39:44–47.
56. Litwin MS, Hays RD, Fink A, Ganz PA, Leake B, Leach GE, Brook RH (1995). Quality-of-life outcomes in men treated for localized prostate cancer. JAMA 273:129–135.
57. Oesterling JE, Andrews PE, Suman VJ, Zincke H, Meyers RP (1993). Preoperative androgen deprivation therapy: artificial lowering of serum PSA without downstaging the tumor. J Urol 149:779–782.
58. Plummer K, Crawford ED, Dangeshari F, Andros B, Pfister S, Miller GJ (1994). Hormonal pretreatment does not affect the final pathologic stage in locally advanced prostate cancer. Urology 44:38–41.
59. Soloway MS, Sharifi R, Wajsman Z, McLeod D, Wood DP Jr, Puras-Baez A (1995). Randomized prospective study comparing radical prostatectomy alone versus radical prostatectomy preceded by androgen blockade in clinical stage B2 (T2bNxMo) prostate cancer. J Urol 154:424–428.
60. Goldenberg SL, Klotz LH, Jewett MAS, Srigley J, Barkin J, Mador D, Fradet Y, Chin JL, Paquin J-M, Laplante S (1995). Randomized controlled study of neoadjuvant reversible androgen withdrawal therapy with cyproterone acetate in the surgical management of localized prostate cancer. J Urol 153:254A.
61. Gibbons RP, Cole BS, Richardson RG, Correa RJ Jr, Brannon GE, Mason JT, Taylor WJ, Hafermann MD (1986). Adjuvant radiotherapy following radical prostatectomy: results and complications. J Urol 135:65–68.
62. Jacobson GM, Smith JA Jr, Stewart JR (1987). Postoperative radiation therapy for pathologic stage C prostate cancer. Int J Radiat Oncol Biol Phys 13:1021–1024.
63. Bahnson RR, Garnett JE, Grayhack JT (1986). Adjuvant radiation therapy in stages C and D1 prostatic adenocarcinoma: preliminary results. Urology 27:403–406.
64. Lange PH, Lightner DJ, Medini E, Reddy PK, Vessella RL (1990). The effect of radiation therapy after radical prostatectomy in patients with elevated prostate specific antigen levels. J Urol 144:927–933.
65. Eisbruch A, Perez CA, Roessler EH, Lockett MA (1994). Adjuvant irradiation after prostatectomy for carcinoma of the prostate with positive margins. Cancer 73:384–387.
66. Scott WW (1964). An evaluation of endocrine therapy plus radical perineal prostatectomy in the treatment of advanced carcinoma of the prostate. J Urol 91:97–102.
67. Scott WW, Boyd HL (1969). Combined hormonal control therapy and radical prostatectomy in the treatment of selected cases of advanced carcinoma of the prostate: a retrospective study based on 25 years of experience. J Urol 101:86–92.
68. Zincke H (1989). Extended experience with surgical treatment of stage D1 adenocarcinoma of the prostate: significant influences of immediate adjuvant hormonal therapy (orchiectomy) on outcome. Urology 33(Suppl 5):27–36.
69. deKernion JB, Neuwirth H, Stein A, et al. (1990). Prognosis of patients with stage D1 prostate carcinoma following radical prostatectomy with and without early endocrine therapy. J Urol 144:700–703.
70. Myers RP, Larson-Keller JJ, Bergstralh EJ, Zincke H, Oesterling JE, Lieber M (1992). Hormonal treatment at time of radical retropubic prostatectomy for stage D1 prostate cancer: results of long-term follow-up. J Urol 147:910–915.
71. Winkler HZ, Rainwater LM, Myers RP, Farrow GM, Therneau TM, Zincke H, Leiber MM (1988). Stage D1 prostatic adenocarcinoma: significance of nuclear DNA ploidy patterns studied by flow cytometry. Mayo Clin Proc 63:103–112.

72. Leiber MM, Murtaugh PA, Farrow GM, Myers RP, Blute ML (1995). DNA ploidy and surgically treated prostate cancer. Cancer 75:1935–1943.
73. Carmichael MJ, Veltri RW, Partin AW, Miller MC, Walsh PC, Epstein JI (1995). Deoxyribonucleic acid ploidy analysis as a predictor of recurrence following radical prostatectomy for stage T2 disease. J Urol 153:1015–1019.
74. Partin AW, Steinberg GD, Pitcock RV, Wu L, Piantadosi S, Coffey DS, Epstein J (1991). Use of nuclear morphometry, Gleason histologic scoring, clinical stage and age to predict disease free survival among patients with prostate cancer. Cancer 70:161–168.
75. Pajouh NS, Nagle RB, Breatnnack R, Finch JS, Brawer MK, Bowden GT (1991). Expression of metalloproteinase genes in human prostate cancer. J Cancer Res Clin Oncol 117:144–150.
76. McDonnell TJ, Tronscoso P, Brisbay SM, Logothetis C, Chung LWK, Hsieh J-T, Tu S-M, Campbell (1992). Expression of protooncogene bcl-2 in the prostate and its association with emergence of androgen-independent prostate cancer. Cancer Res 52:6940–6944.
77. Umbas R, Schalken JA, Aalders TW, Carter BS, Karthaus HFM, Schaafsman HE, Debruyne FMJ, Isaacs WB (1992). Expression of the cellular adhesion molecule E-cadherin is reduced or absent in high-grade prostate cancer. Cancer Res 52:5104–5109.
78. Rinker-Schaeffer CW, Hawkins AL, Ru N, Dong J-T, Stoica G, Griffin CA, Ichikawa T, Barret JC, Isaacs JT (1994). Differential suppression of mammary and prostate cancer metastasis by human chromosome 17 and 11. Cancer Res 54:6249–6256.

9. Three-dimensional conformal therapy (3D-CRT) for prostate cancer

Paul J. Chuba, Arthur T. Porter, and Jeffrey D. Forman

Three-dimensional conformal therapy (3D-CRT) is the logical outgrowth of the need of radiation oncologists to maximize the radiation dose to the tumor and to minimize the dose to the normal tissues. Only a short time ago, the methods described here were unworkable or inefficient due to constraints of the computer hardware and software required for treatment planning and imaging systems. Conformal radiotherapy may be defined as the attempt to conform the radiation dose distribution as closely as possible to the tumor. The resultant sparing of normal tissue structures may reduce complication rates and allow increased radiation dose to be delivered to the tumor. As used here, the term *therapeutic ratio* refers to the comparison of tumor control and normal-tissue complication probabilities. When these factors are optimized and lead to improved outcome, we have achieved therapeutic gain.

Particularly in the field of prostate cancer radiotherapy, progress made in improving the planning process has already borne fruit in the form of improved dosimetric and clinical results. The first application of conformal radiotherapy may be ascribed to the use of intraurethral radium in 1911 [1], which had the goal of conforming the radiation dose to the shape of the prostate. Later, in the 1930s, the poor penetration of orthovoltage irradiation led to the introduction of multiple beam angles, which may be considered the forerunner of modern 3D-CRT [2]. Megavoltage radiation using linear accelerators was used with rotational arcs at Stanford in the 1960s [3], and Perez instituted a four-field technique, sometimes with an added perineal beam [4]. Simulator-based treatment planning approximately coincided with the use of cerrobend cast blocks for beam shaping in the 1970s and 1980s. Purdy may be credited with calculation of dose in multiple two-dimensional sections in the mid-1960s, thus introducing computer dosimetry for use in conformal treatment planning [5].

In the following discussion, current concepts for 3D-CRT for prostate irradiation are outlined. Current 3D-CRT methods are illustrated, and the process of optimizing beam arrangements for maximizing target-volume definition and minimizing normal-tissue irradation is described. It will become clear that the present state of the art requires interactive effort and human evaluation of the therapeutic ratio. In the future we may expect to find the

Pienta, K.J., (ed.), DIAGNOSIS AND TREATMENT OF GENITOURINARY MALIGNANCIES.

integration of mathematical models of dose–response relationships using biologic data and biologic effective dose with computer-based treatment planning.

Features of the 3D treatment planning system

In its most elementary form, 3D-CRT consists of simulation, treatment planning, evaluation of treatment plans, and treatment delivery. The components of 3D treatment planning systems vary widely; however, the common denominator among successful systems is a user-friendly interface. The physician must be able to easily contour anatomic structures and to define the beam aperture as part of a beam's-eye view (BEV) display in real time on the computer screen. Also, the ability to quickly and easily change beam arrangements for the interactive comparison of plans cannot be underestimated. This appears to be the major limitation of many systems at present. Although 3D volume rendering and the 3D rendering of conformal dose distributions are esthetically pleasing and useful for presentation graphics, these features are not essential, since wire-loop models are adequate, and 3D rendering is not useful if it increases the processing time and expense of the system.

Ideally, the system will accept input from magnetic tape or will be hardwired to the treatment planning CT-scanner. The planning software will be called upon to input and store data describing electron and photon beam characteristics. The ability to add bolus or to use tissue compensators is also useful. The output of the BEV display [6], isodose plans, and digital reconstruction radiographs requires laser printers and (color) plotters. Some systems will require specialized equipment or software. For example, brachytherapy planning and the integration of brachytherapy and external beam treatment planning may be desired. Although mostly invisible to the physician, the calculation algorithms required for fully 3D planning are highly critical components. The validation of these algorithms can only be done by experienced medical physicists. At Wayne State University, the in-house software (named VRS-plan) uses algorithms developed by George Sherouse [7]. The ability to use 3D planning in fully conformal treatment with fast neutrons using the superconducting cyclotron at Harper Hospital has been added.

In order to introduce the versatility of the 3D system in enabling human optimization, representations of two different commonly used beam arrangements for prostate irradiation are shown in figure 9-1. In this particular view, the skin, pelvic bones, prostate, and seminal vesicles have been contoured. In both the four-field 'box' (figure 9-1a) and six-field 'crossfire' axial plans (figure 9-1b [8]) the central ray of each beam passes through the axial CT plane to intersect with the other beams at the isocenter, which is placed within the prostate. Although each beam arrangement irradiates the prostate and seminal vesicles, each has differing consequences with respect to normal-tissue dose. For the four-field box beam arrangement, it can be seen that the bladder

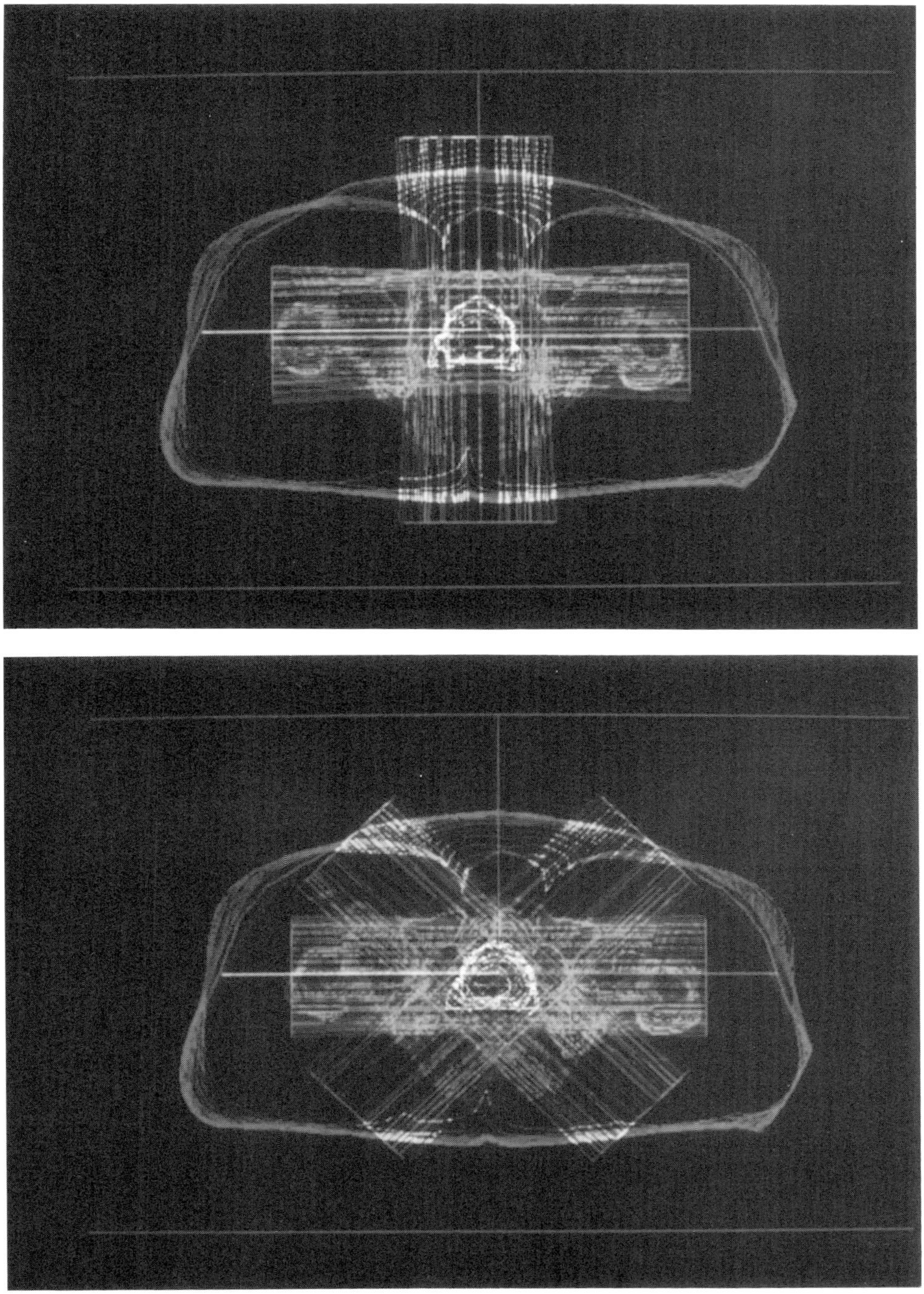

Figure 9-1. Visualization of two different external beam arrangements in the AP BEV window. Both were planned on a single data set from one patient. The four-field (**a**) and six-field 'crossfire' axial (**b**) beam arrangements are shown.

and rectum lie entirely within the AP and PA field. It should be clear that in the extreme case, delivering the entire dose by use of straight laterals would spare significantly more bladder and rectum than the four-field box, but at the expense of giving a high dose to the subcutaneous tissue and femoral heads. In the six-field technique, the AP and PA fields are replaced with opposed right and left lateral obliques. Not surprisingly, the dose to normal tissue is spread out over a larger area, and critical normal tissues may be spared. As both the four-field (figure 9-1a) and six-field (figure 9-1b) techniques are axial (in the axial CT plane) and coplanar (all central rays are in one plane), the dose calculations are facilitated. It is for this reason that the four- and six-field techniques (and others) may be used without true 3D-planning capability.

Practical simulation and treatment planning

At Wayne State University, either conventional simulation followed by CT simulation or CT simulation alone ('virtual simulation') is done. Prior to simulation, the patient is given a solution of oral contrast to drink for radiographic visualization of the small bowel. Immobilization is performed by constructing a polyurethane foam cradle around the patient's buttocks and thighs. Next, a Foley catheter is inserted into the bladder using sterile technique and 50 cc of dilute bladder contrast is introduced. Seven cc of undilute bladder contrast are used for inflating the Foley balloon. For conventional simulation, the catheter is withdrawn slightly so that the Foley balloon rests firmly against the bladder neck (thus defining the base of the prostate). For CT scanning, the balloon and catheter are removed. Note that in patients who have had a previous prostatectomy, the catheterization step is omitted. No contrast is introduced into the rectum to avoid problems with iatrogenically produced prostate motion. A second catheter is typically introduced into the penile urethra for the purpose of performing a urethrogram. A penile clamp is placed near the base of the penis and 10 cc of contrast are injected, followed by removal of the catheter. The penile clamp remains in place until completion of the CT scan. In general, catheterized patients are prescribed a short course (three days) of antibiotic prophylaxis (trimethoprim/sulfamethoxazole or ciprofloxacin).

Next, simulation radiographs are prepared. Under fluoroscopic guidance, the isocenter is placed at the center of the prostate (approximately midway between the bottom of the Foley balloon and a point approximately 1.0 cm above the apex of the urethrogram). Simulation radiographs for AP, lateral, or oblique beams are taken. Since CT simulation will follow, it is unnecessary to determine exact field sizes at this time. The isocenter is marked on patient's skin using the room lasers, and the patient is brought to the CT simulator.

For CT simulation, radio-opaque BBs are placed over the skin marks, and the patient is repositioned in the polyurethane cradle, reproducing the treatment position. Axial images are taken through the prostate and seminal vesicles with 5-mm table feed. In order to use inferior–superior oblique beam arrangements, it may be necessary to scan inferiorly to midthigh in order to provide sufficient skin contour to calculate the beam's entry. These data are then stored for use in the 3D-treatment planning computer.

A great number of our patients have now been simulated using this virtual simulation technique [7]. Virtual simulation implies dispensing with the conventional simulation and radiographs and performing only CT simulation, with resulting time and cost savings. To implement this, a method must be devised for mapping the isocenter determined by CT onto the patient's skin for marking (another requirement is the ability to generate digital reconstruction radiographs (DRRs), a computed representation of the X-ray, for comparison with port films or on-line portal images). At Wayne State University, a laser marking device has been developed for this purpose [9]. In effect, this device determines where the therapy room laser, directed at the isocenter, would intersect the patient's skin. The laser marking device may be free-standing or mounted in the gantry of the CT scanner. One must also be able to contour the target volume structure interactively, during or immediately after the scan is made. Once these capabilities are in place, the actual practice of virtual simulation is very simple. After the polyurethane cradle is made, bladder and urethral contrast is introduced, several axial CT images [10–12] through the prostate gland are obtained, and the prostate is contoured (for these images only) on the 3D treatment planning computer. The geometric center of the prostate is calculated automatically, and the AP and lateral projections of this isocenter are marked on the patient's skin by use of the laser marking device. Once the remaining CT image data are collected, the simulation is complete.

After simulation, treatment planning continues at the computer console. The prostate, seminal vesicles, bladder, rectum, small bowel, skin, and pelvic bone contours are entered. An autocontour routine may be used for contouring pelvic bone and skin (as well as bladder and small bowel in many cases). The base of the prostate is determined using interactive modification of the gray scale on the CT image [13]. The apex of the prostate may be difficult to determine on CT, and the urethrogram is useful in this regard [14–17]. The contours of the prostate and seminal vesicle are done separately; these correspond to the annotation 'gross tumor volume' in ICRU report 50 [10]. In patients treated postprostatectomy, an attempt is made to define the presurgical location of the prostate and seminal vesicles.

Next, the contoured 'anatomes' are reconstructed in three dimensions by the computer, and the beam's-eye view is displayed on the screen. At this point in time, any beam, beam angle, or couch position may be used, so that the BEV may be used to draw blocks on the screen. The calculated SSDs may be cross-checked with the measured SSDs. The shaped cast block may be manufactured conventionally; alternatively, data may be provided for multileaf collimation for any beam. DVHs and isodose plans allow evaluation of dose to the tumor and to critical normal tissue structures. Depending on whether virtual simulation or conventional plus CT simulation was done, the block design is transferred from the BEV to the simulation films, or DRRs are generated Subsequent verification may be made by comparing port films or on-line portal images to DRRs or simulation radiographs. It can be seen that filmless radiotherapy is very feasible when using virtual simulation, DRRs, and on-line portal imaging.

Optimization of beam arrangements

Just as in conventional radiotherapy treatment planning, the 3D-CRT plan requires a choice of beam energy, block design, beam modifiers, and beam arrangement. The goal is to hit the target volume while sparing normal tissue. The practical application of 3D-CRT presupposes that beam arrangements and target volumes may be idealized and facilitates the comparison of multiple plans. Also, 3D-CRT for the first time enables the use of noncoplanar dose calculations.

In figure 9-2, a four-field 'noncoplanar' beam arrangement [18,19] that we have used for prostate cancer patients is shown as a BEV and superimposed

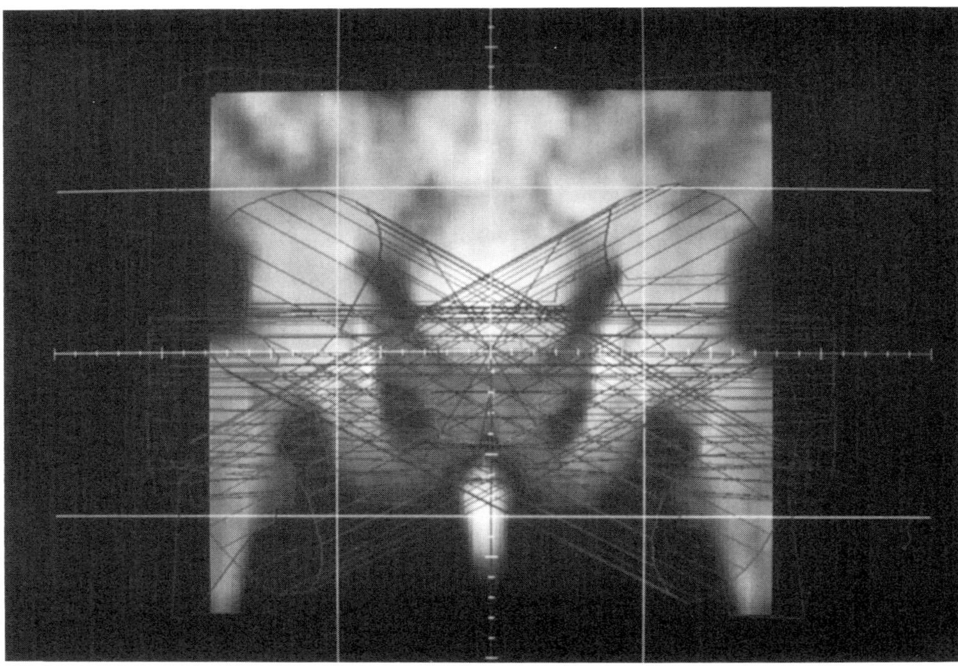

Figure 9-2. Visualization of four-field noncoplanar beam arrangement in the BEV window. Two lateral and two inferior to superior oblique beams are illustrated.

upon a DRR. The use of the BEV and DRR together allows visualization of the anatomy (pelvic bones and urethrogram) from the geometric perspective of the beam itself and facilitates shaping the beam (i.e., drawing blocks). In contrast to the four-field box and six-field crossfire obliques, in the four-field noncoplanar arrangement the AP and PA fields from the four-field 'box' have been replaced with right and left anterior–superior oblique fields (RAISO/LAISO). Note that this arrangement is both nonaxial and noncoplanar in that the central rays of the beams cannot all be found in the same plane. The entry and exit of these beams is more difficult to visualize; however, bladder and rectal sparing is maximized. The nonaxial and noncoplanar nature of this beam arrangement requires that dose calculations be performed with fully 3D computation in which beams may enter from any direction. At Wayne State University, we have for several years now typically used a four-field box technique for delivery of the first 45 Gy and the four-field noncoplanar oblique technique for the remaining boost dose (approximately 24 Gy).

Isodose plans from the four-field box (figure 9-1a), the six-field crossfire oblique (figure 9-1b), and the four-field noncoplanar (figure 9-2) beam arrangements presented above are shown superimposed on the axial CT image

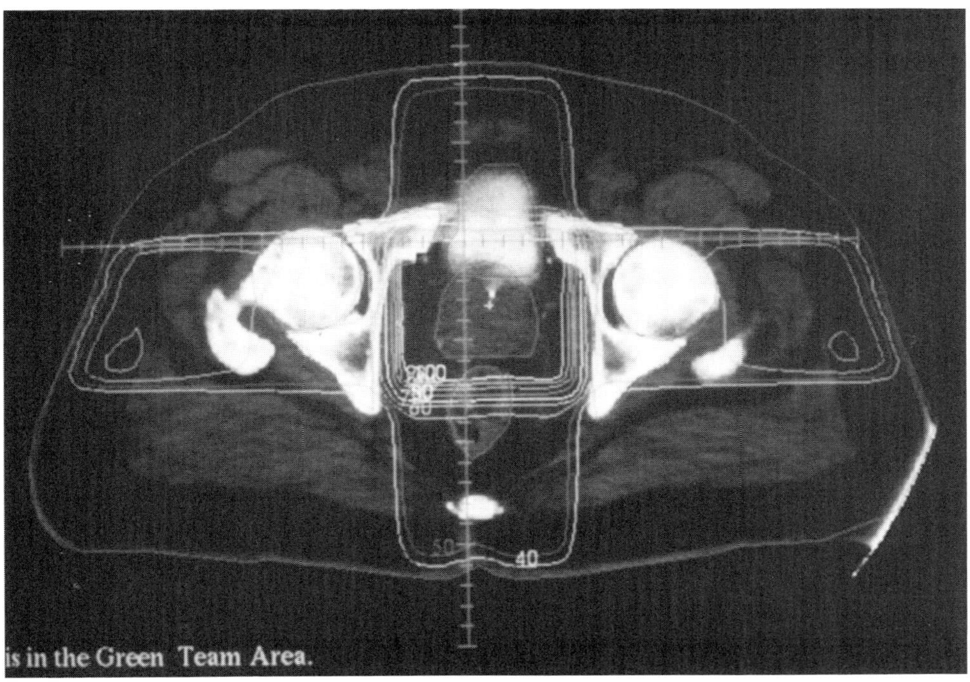

a

Figure 9-3. Dose distributions for the four-field (**a**), six-field crossfire axial (**b**), and four-field noncoplanar (**c**) beam arrangements are shown in the axial CT plane.

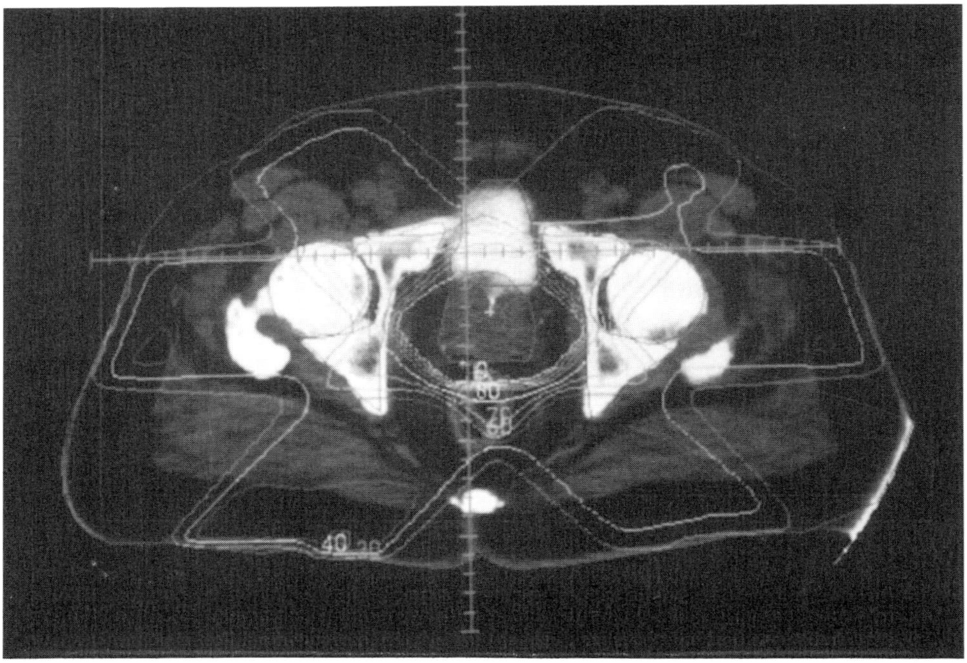

b

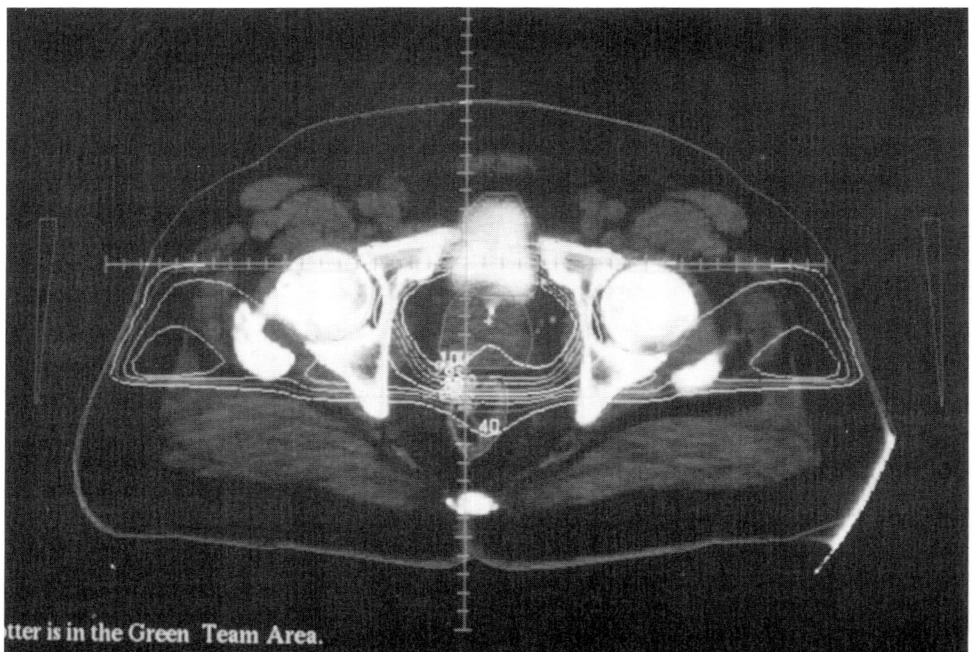

c

Figure 9-3. (*Continued*)

at the central axis in figure 9-3a–c. In each plan, the prostate is contained within the 100% isodose line. By inspection of these plans, it can be concluded that bladder and rectal sparing (at the central axis region) is greater for the six-field crossfire oblique arrangement (figure 9-3b) than for the four-field box (figure 9-3a). Similarly, bladder and rectal sparing is greater for the four-field noncoplanar beam arrangement (figure 9-3c) than for either of the other two plans.

The four-field coronal oblique plan shown in figure 9-4 is somewhat unconventional but serves to further illustrate the value of 3D-CRT in optimization of treatment planning. In this arrangement, right and left inferior oblique ports (RIO and LIO) are paired with opposed superior oblique ports (RSO and LSO). This plan has actually been used for part of the treatment in patients treated according to hyperfractionated mixed neutron-photon protocols at Wayne State University. Interestingly, the four coronal obliques have the property of sparing the femoral head, which appears to be at greater risk for complications in dose-escalation studies [20]. In figure 9-5, the dose distributions for this field arrangement are shown in the axial (figure 9-5a), coronal (figure 9-5b), and sagittal (figure 9-5c) planes. It may be seen that with the

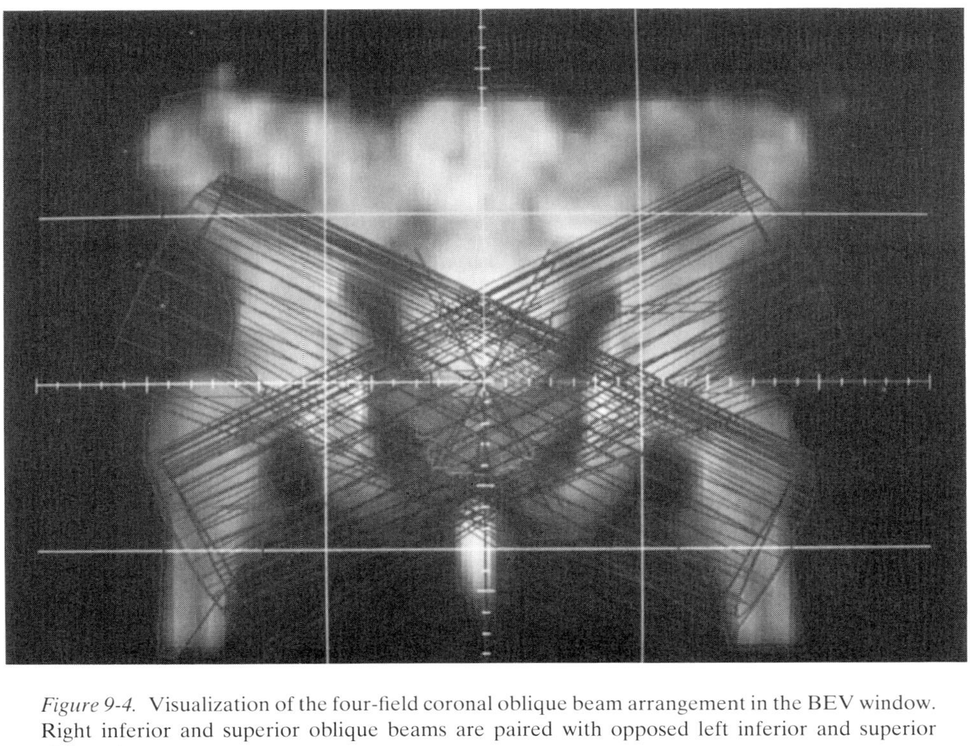

Figure 9-4. Visualization of the four-field coronal oblique beam arrangement in the BEV window. Right inferior and superior oblique beams are paired with opposed left inferior and superior oblique beams.

ability to visualize the dose distribution in three dimensions, the value of the coronal obliques in sparing the femoral head becomes obvious.

Dose volume histogram (DVH) analysis allows an unbiased evaluation for comparison of beam arrangements [20,21]. The cumulative DVH shows the percent of any 3D structure (anatome) that receives any percent of the dose. A comparison of DVHs for bladder for the four different beam arrangements we have so far discussed is shown in figure 9-6. For actual treatment planning, DVHs for rectum, for small bowel, and for the femoral head would also be prepared. Sparing of bladder tissue is greatest when using the four-field noncoplanar technique (figure 9-6), although some small percentage of the bladder is treated to nearly full dose with all four beam arrangements. A limitation of the DVH at the present time is that we cannot be certain which part of the structure contains the hot spot unless comparing side-by-side with the anatomy. Still, the DVH provides information that in the past has been completely inaccessible or extremely laborious to obtain. Naturally, the biologic significance of a part of a structure receiving a part of the dose remains to be completely defined [22].

a

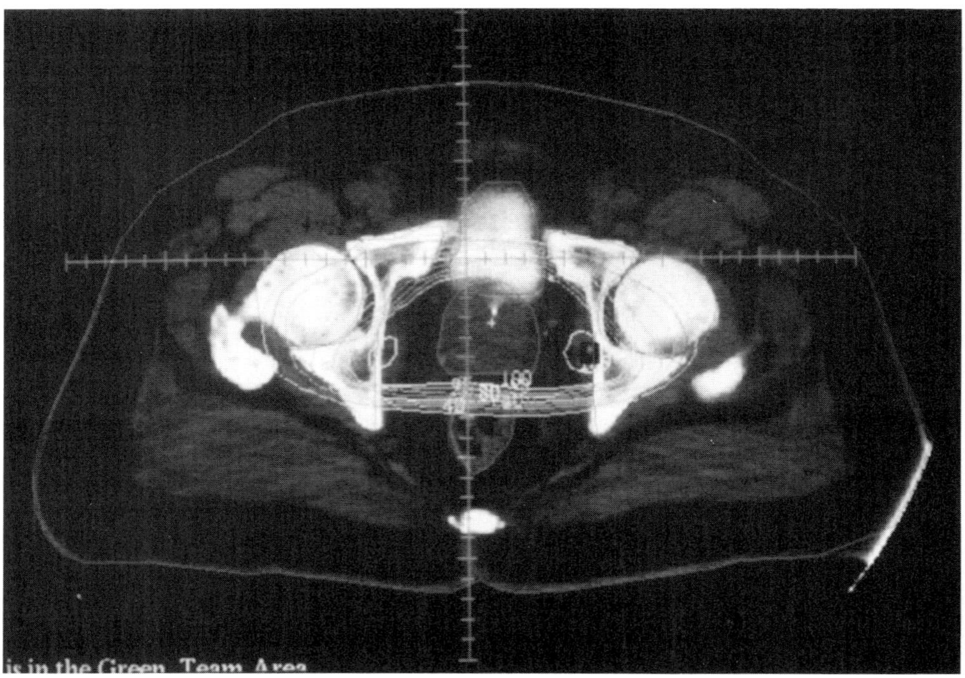

Figure 9-5. Dose distribution for the four-field coronal oblique plan is shown in three different planes. The axial (**a**), coronal (**b**), and sagittal (**c**) CT planes are shown with the isodose plans superimposed on the reconstructed CT images.

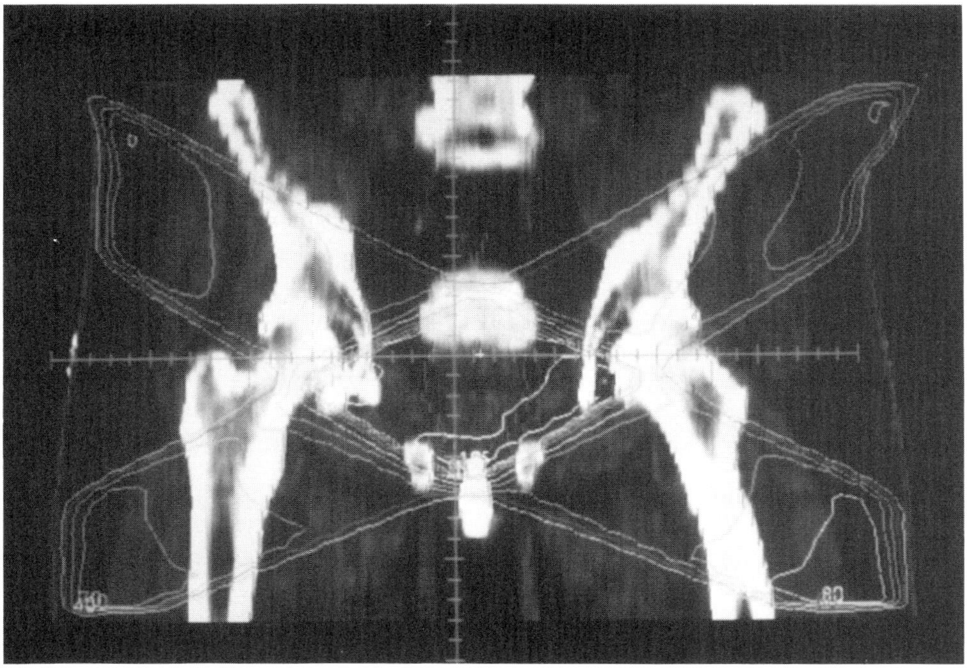

b

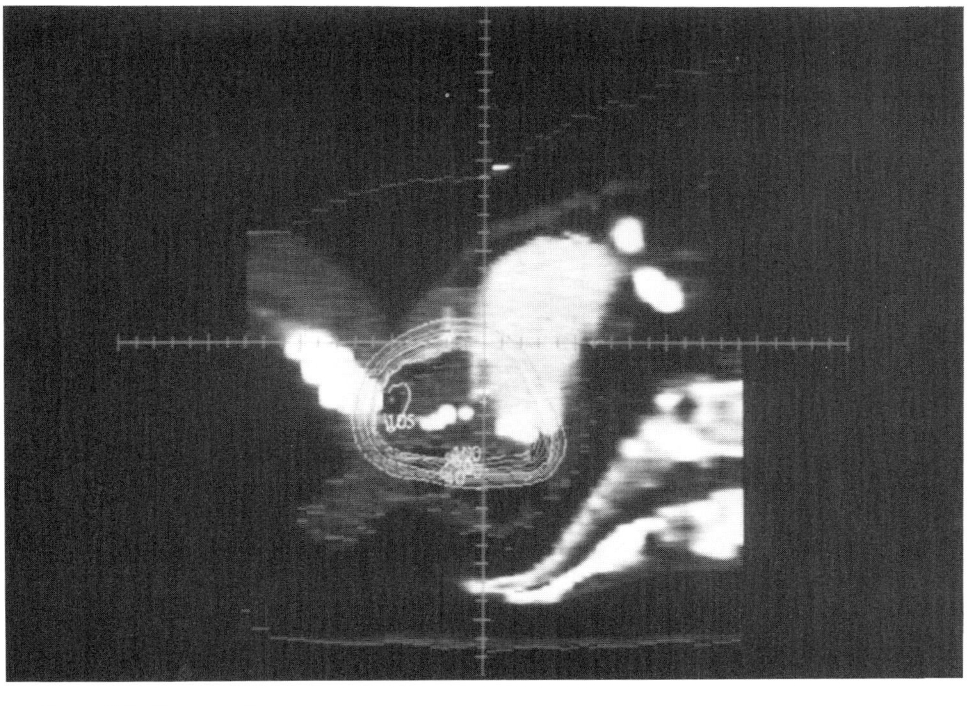

c

Figure 9-5. (*Continued*)

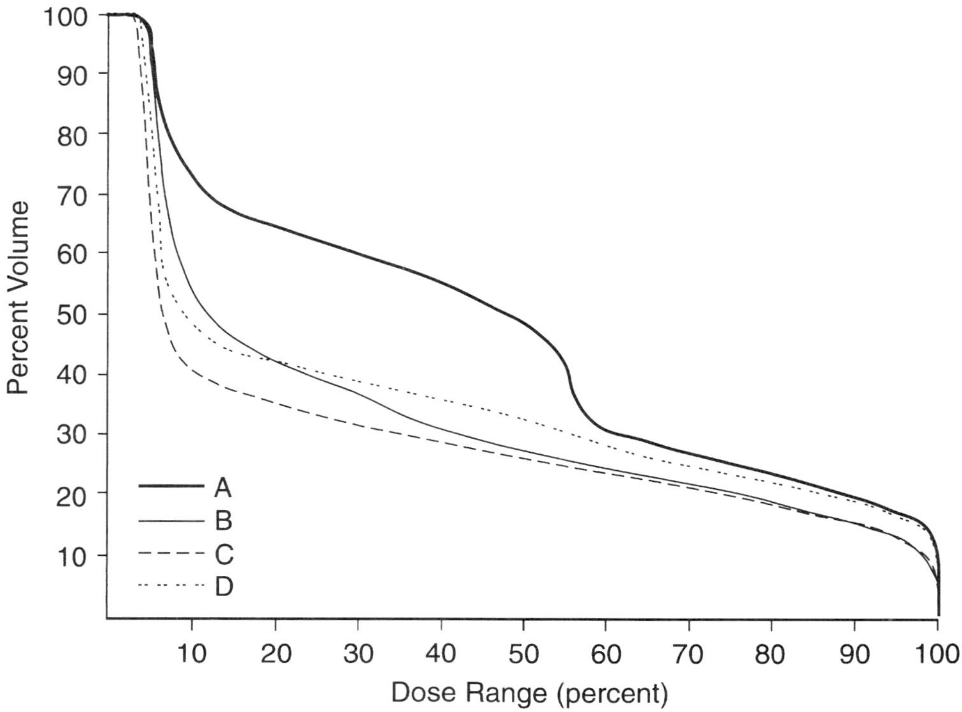

Figure 9-6. Dose–volume histogram analysis for bladder irradiation based on the four different beam arrangements: A, four-field axial; B, six-field crossfire axial; C, four-field coronal oblique; D, four-field noncoplanar.

Technical factors related to outcome

We now turn our attention to outcome parameters. Improved outcome for 3D-CRT for prostate cancer may be a result of refinement in target volume definition or of increased normal tissue sparing. In the ideal situation, these two parameters may be adjusted to allow for the safe delivery of higher radiation doses (dose escalation).

Target volume definition

Initial studies of the usefulness of 3D-CRT treatment planning for prostate cancer suggested that conventional methods yielded poor target volume definition. Ten-Haken et al. [23] compared treatment plans for shaped fixed fields in the boost treatment of stage C prostate cancer with traditional 8×8 cm bilateral arcs. Interestingly, the 8×8 cm field yielded geographic misses (20% to 35% of the target volume outside the field) in all 17 patients studied. These data are particularly interesting in view of the fact that many of the patients in the early Stanford experience were treated with even smaller fields (6×6 cm, 7×7 cm).

Other studies of target volume definition that have been facilitated by 3D-CRT include prostate motion and the usefulness of bladder and urethral contrast. Largely as a result of the use of 3D-CRT treatment planning, we have recently become aware of the motion of the prostate in three-dimensional space [24–28]. At the University of Michigan [11,23], patients were CT scanned initially with an empty bladder and an empty rectum. Next, contrast was introduced, and a second scan was done in the same treatment postion. Surprisingly, in 31 out of 50 patients studied, more than 0.5-cm movement of the prostate gland could be demonstrated. In seven patients who had local recurrence after I-125 seed implants, the movement of radio-opaque seeds could be followed on the scans, thus providing elegant visualization of prostate motion [11,23]. The dosimetric consequences of prostate motion have also been studied in detail with a view towards using optimal beam arrangements [27]. Ten patients were simulated using CT scan at Wayne State University and then rescanned weekly during treatment. Prostate volumes were found to vary by +/− 10% and seminal vesicle volumes by +/− 100% during the course of treatment [27,28]. The use of the four-field nonaxial oblique method led to the least amount of bladder and rectum irradiated [28]. Partly because of prostate motion, blocks that conform too tightly to the prostate may not give excellent dose distributions, and some investigators have used the term *ideal margins* to describe the use of nonuniform margins around the prostate [29].

With regard to the relative value of the use of retrograde urethrography at the time of simulation for prostate cancer [14–17], universal agreement is still lacking. One of the implications of BEV-based block design *could be* that the apex of the prostate would be defined based on the use of CT images. In one study, it was concluded that, although the apex of the prostate could only be identified with difficulty on CT, the identification of the base of the penis was sufficient for adequately placing the lower border [15]. Another report of 89 patients found that the use of the ischial tuberosity as the lower border of the field was unacceptable if a 2-cm margin was desired [17]. It appears that the optimal method is the use of the urethrogram. In a small percentage of cases, the use of other anatomic landmarks will either underdose the prostate or unnecessarily treat the penile urethra.

The use of bladder contrast to improve the definition of the prostate base was recently reported by Sharma et al. [13]. In all 17 patients studied, an improvement in the visualization of the base of the prostate was seen by using bladder contrast, and in 16 of 17 patients, this improvement was reflected in better dose distributions. It was this study that first showed that the interactive modification of the gray scale on axial CT images would better define the prostate volume [13].

Sparing normal tissue

A reduction in the complication rate for radical radiation therapy for prostate cancer using 3D-CRT may be shown on theoretical [30] or on clinical grounds [20]. Based on the patterns of care and other studies, a serious late complication rate of less than 3% may be expected with conventional radiotherapy [31], standard fractionation, and doses of up to 70 Gy.

It is not difficult to show that an increased amount of normal tissue may be treated with conventional therapy compared with 3D-CRT. In the University of Michigan study, up to five times as much normal tissue was treated with traditional open beams as with shaped fixed 3D-CRT fields [23]. When the National Cancer Institute evaluated the usefulness of 3D-CRT in 46 prostate cancer cases, all eight institutions that were studied scored lower for normal-tissue complications when using 3D-CRT. In order to predict how the sparing of normal tissue may impact on the reduction of complications, mathematical modeling of data derived from dose–volume histograms has also been done [22]. The probabilities calculated for normal-tissue complication rates, once clinically validated, may in the future allow the tailoring of dose distributions with normal tissue tolerance in mind.

Comparison of normal tissue complication probabilities for different beam arrangements using 3D data from DVHs was done by Mesina et al. [18]. The use of the nonaxial four-field beam arrangement for boost treatment was shown to result in improved dose–volume relationships for bladder and rectum when compared with the four-field box technique. Until relatively recently, however, it has remained unclear whether this theoretical improvement in the DVH would translate into reduced complications clinically.

Clinical data suggesting a reduced *acute* complication rate for prostate radiotherapy were presented by Soffen et al. [31], who attributed this reduced rate to a 14% decrease in the volume of bladder and a 14% decrease in the volume of rectum irradiated.

A statistically significant advantage for more conformal treatment (i.e., a four-field nonaxial boost technique) in reducing the *late* complication rate has now been shown in two papers. Sandler et al. [32,33] studied the relationships between morbidity and dose with various beam arrangements in a non-randomized study. In 721 patients planned with 3D-CRT, morbidity could be correlated with dose by using a Cox proportional hazards model. With a median follow-up of 22 months, 82 patients had grade 1 or 2 complications, 12 had grade 3, and 2 had grade 4, using the RTOG scale. The four-field axial (figure 9-1a), six-field crossfire axial (figure 9-1b), and four-field noncoplanar oblique (figure 9-2) beam arrangements were all represented. Importantly, the four-field noncoplanar boost arrangement exhibited the *lowest* relative risk [33].

Ben-Josef et al. compared the four-field axial conformal treatment with four-field noncoplanar boost in 106 patients treated at Wayne State University [Edgar Ben-Josef, personal communication]. Although this study was also nonrandomized, patients were evenly distributed between the two groups. There were no grade 3 or 4 morbidities in either group. The incidence of *late* grade 1 or 2 morbidity was decreased in patients treated with a four-field noncoplanar boost. This study is currently being extended to include more patients in an attempt to use a logistic model to correlate dose–volume histogram data for the bladder and rectum with the incidence of complications.

Dose escalation and therapeutic gain

Better target-volume definition and a reduction in the normal-tissue complication rate may allow for increased local control and survival in prostate cancer, especially if dose escalation can be achieved. Dose–escalation studies [34–36] are based on the presumption that local control and survival may be impacted by increased radiation dose to the prostate and that normal tissue complications may be limited to acceptable levels by conformal treatment planning.

Over 250 patients have been treated at Wayne State University as part of five separate dose-escalation studies for prostate cancer [37–43]. Data from these studies have begun to mature, and the reader is referred to the original articles for a detailed analysis [37,40,41]. In one study, conformal techniques have been combined with hyperfractionated radiation to deliver doses of up to 83 Gy. Four studies have combined neutron radiation with photon radiation using the superconducting cyclotron at Harper Hospital in Detroit [44–46]. The neutron dose distributions have been roughly comparable to those of photons [35]. These studies have demonstrated that conformal neutron radiation is very well tolerated with no greater morbidity than conventional photon radiotherapy. Furthermore, the histologic and biochemical local control has so far been remarkable. For example, over 95% biochemical local control has been shown for the first 150 patients treated for early-stage prostate cancer with these techniques. Longer follow-up will be necessary to assess the durability of these responses.

Investigators at the Memorial Sloan Kettering Cancer Center have reported on the interim results of their phase I dose escalation study with 3D-CRT in 123 patients [34]. Four-, six-, and eight-field beam arrangements were represented. Forty-nine patients had tumor doses of 64.8 to 66.6 Gy, 46 patients had tumor doses of 70.2 Gy, and 28 had 75.6 Gy. Only 32% required medication (grade 2), and one patient died with a grade 4 complication. At MSKCC patients are treated prone with thermoplastic casts for immobilization and with bladder and rectum empty. Based on this work, their current dose level is 81 Gy at 1.8 Gy/d.

The Radiation Therapy Oncology Group has recently begun a phase I/II dose-escalation study using 3D-CRT. Patients will be stratified into one of three groups. Group I includes T1b–c, T2a–b, GS < 7, and PSA4–15. Group II patients may have the same T stages but present with GS > 6 or a PSA $>$ 15. T2c patients with PSA below 70 also qualify for group II. Group III includes stage T3 with PSA less than 70. The objectives of this study are to establish the maximum dose tolerated by the patients using 3D-CRT, to quantify the normal tissue complication probability, and to evaluate local control.

Conclusion

Largely because of advances in informatics and imaging technologies, 3D-CRT is rapidly proliferating in radiation oncology facilities around the world. The ability to visualize noncoplanar beam arrangements and to accurately estimate the dose distribution in nonaxial planes is highly attractive for the radiotherapy of prostate cancer. Oncologists must become conversant with the language and theory of 3D-CRT to participate effectively in dosimetric planning and target volume definition. The radiation physicist, dosimetrist, and therapist will similarly face unique challenges. We have attempted to show that, based on objective and quantitative information with regard to dose delivered to tumor and normal tissue, a better measure of the probability of local control and complications may be defined. On this basis, dose-escalation studies with the eventual aim of increasing survival for prostate cancer may proceed.

Too often, in the clinical arena, promising advances may be delayed on the road to therapeutic success because of premature or improperly planned trials [47,48]. It is not enough that these new methods be regarded as superior because of obviousness; rather, 3D-CRT must offer tangible improvements in a cost-effective manner. For this reason, the trials we perform today must be done judiciously and with costs in mind. As outlined here, the clinical literature has already begun to reflect the efficacy of 3D-CRT in achieving therapeutic gain in prostate cancer.

References

1. Pasteau O, Degrais J (1913). De l'emploi du radium dans le traitement des cancers de la prostate. J D'urol Paris 4:341.
2. Smith GS, Pierson EL (1930). The value of high voltage x-ray therapy in carcinoma of the prostate. J Urol 23:331–342.
3. Bagshaw MA, Cox RS, Ray GR (1988). Status of radiation treatment of prostate cancer at Stanford University. NCI Monogr 7:47–60.
4. Perez CA, Walz BJ, Zivnuska FR, Pilepich M, Prasad K, Bauer W (1980). Irradiation of carcinoma of the prostate localized to the pelvis: analysis of tumor response and prognosis. Int J Radiat Oncol Biol Phys 6:555–563.
5. Simpson JR, Purdy JA, Manolis JM, Pilepich MV, Burman C, Forman J, Fuks Z, Cheng E, Chu J, Matthews J, Mahan R, Sol n L, Tepper J, Urie M (1991). Three-dimensional treatment planning considerations for prostate cancer. Int J Radiat Oncol Phys 21:243–252.
6. Low NN, Vijaykumar S, Rosenberg I, Rubin S, Virudachalam R, Spelbring DR, Chen GTY (1990). Beam's eye view based prostate treatment planning: is it useful? Int J Radiat Oncol Biol Phys 19:759–768.

7. Sherouse GW, Borland JD, Reynolds K, McMurry HJL, Mitchell TP, Chaney EL (1990). Virtual simulation in the clinical setting: some practical considerations. Int J Radiat Oncol Biol Phys 19:1059–1065.
8. Pickett B, Roach III M, Horine P, Verhey L, Phillips TL (1994). Optimization of the oblique angles in the treatment of prostate cancer during six-field conformal radiotherapy. Med Dosimetr 19:237–254.
9. Ragan DP, Forman JD, He T, Mesina CF (in press). Clinical results of computed tomography-based simulation with laser patient marking. Int J Radiat Oncol Biol Phys 34.
10. ICRU Report 50. Prescribing, Recording, and Reporting Photon Beam Therapy. International commission on Radiation Units and Measurements (Bethesda, 1993).
11. Balter J, Sandler HM, Lam K, Bree RL, Lichter AS, Ten-Haken RK (1993). Measurement of prostate motion over the course of radiotherapy. Int J Radiat Oncol Biol Phys 27(Suppl 1):136.
12. Beard CJ, Kaplan ID, Coleman CN (1993). The challenge for conformal therapy for prostate cancer. Int J Radiat Oncol Biol Phys 26:705–707.
13. Sharma R, Duclos M, Chuba PJ, Forman JD (submitted). Enhancement of prostate tumor volume definition with intravesical contrast: a 3-D dosimetric evaluation. Int J Radiat Oncol Biol Phys.
14. Cox JA, Zagoria RJ, Raben M (1994). Prostate cancer: comparison of retrograde urethrography and computed tomography in radiotherapy planning. Int J Radiat Oncol Biol Phys 29:1119–1123.
15. Roach III M, Pickett B, Holland J, Zapotowski KA, Marsh DL, Tatera BS (1993). The role of the urethrogram during simulation for localized prostate cancer. Int J Radiat Oncol Biol Phys 25:299–307.
16. Sandler HM, Bree RL, McLaughlin PW, Grossman HB, Lichter AS (1993). Localization of the prostatic apex for radiation therapy using implanted markers. Int J Radiat Oncol Biol Phys 27:915–919.
17. Wilson LD, Ennis R, Percarpio B, Peschel RE (1994). Location of the prostatic apex and its relationship to the ischial tuberosities. Int J Radiat Oncol Biol Phys 29:1133–1138.
18. Mesina CF, Sharma R, Rissman LS, Geering L, He T, Forman JD (1994). Comparison of a conformal non-axial boost with a four-field boost technique in the treatment of adenocarcinoma of the prostate. Int J Radiat Oncol Biol Phys 30:427–430.
19. Marsh LH, Ten Haken RK, Sandler HM (1992). A customized non-axial external beam technique for treatment of prostate carcinomas. Med Dosimetr 17:123–127.
20. Chuba PJ, Sharma R, Yudelev M, Duclos M, Shamsa F, Giacalone S, Orton CG, Maughan RL, Forman JD (in press). Hip stiffness following mixed conformal neutron and photon radiotherapy: a dose-volume relationship. Int J Radiat Oncol Biol Phys.
21. Kessler ML, Ten Haken RK, Frass BA, McShan DL (1994). Expanding the use and effectiveness of dose–volume histograms for 3-D treatment planning I: Integration of 3-D dose-display. Int J Radiat Oncol Biol Phys 29:1125–1131.
22. Lyman JT (1985). Complication probability as assessed from dose–volume histograms. Radiat Res 104:S13–S19.
23. Ten Haken RK, Perez-Tamayo C, Tesser RJ, McShan DL, Fraass BA, Lichter AS (1989). Boost treatment of the prostate using shaped, fixed fields. Int J Radiat Oncol Biol Phys 16:193–200.
24. Beard CJ, Bussiere MR, Plunkett ME, Coleman NC, Kijewski PK (1993). Analysis of prostate and seminal vesical motion. Int J Radiat Oncol Biol Phys 27(Suppl 1):136.
25. Forman JD, Mesina CF, He T, Devi SB, Ben-Josef E, Pelizzari C, Vijaykumar S, Chen GT (1993). Evaluation of changes in the location and shape of the prostate and rectum during a seven week course of conformal radiotherapy. Int J Radiat Oncol Biol Phys 27(Suppl 1):222.
26. Melian E, Kutcher G, Leibel S, Zelefsky M, Baldwin B, Fuks Z (1993). Variation on prostate position: quantification and implications for three-dimensional conformal radiation therapy. Int J Radiat Oncol Biol Phys 27(Suppl 1):137.
27. Hadley S, Roeske JC, Forman JD, Vijaykumar S, Chen GTY (1995). The incorporation of

organ motion in the selection of optimal beam orientations for prostate irradiation. AAPM annual meeting.
28. Roeske JC, Armato SJ, Forman JD, Hadley S, Vijaykumar S, Chen GTY (1995). The dosimetric implications of organ motion during prostate irradiation. AAPM annual meeting.
29. Roach M III, Pickett B, Rosenthal SA, Verhey L, Phillips TL (1994). Defining treatment margins for six-field conformal irradiation of localized prostate cancer. Int J Radiat Oncol Biol Phys 28:267–275.
30. Schultheiss TE, Hanks GE, Hunt MA, Lee WR (1995). Incidence of and factors related to late complications in conformal and conventional radiation treatment of cancer of the prostate. Int J Radiat Oncol Biol Phys 32:643–649.
31. Soffen EM, Hanks GE, Hunt MA, Epstein BE (1992). Conformal static field radiation therapy treatment of early prostate cancer versus non-conformal techniques: a reduction in acute morbidity. Int J Radiat Oncol Biol Phys 24:485–488.
32. Sandler HM, McLaughlin PW, Ten Haken RK, Addison H, Forman JD, Lichter A (1995). Three dimensional conformal radiotherapy for the treatment of prostate cancer: low risk of chronic rectal morbidity observed in a large series of patients. Int J Radiat Oncol Biol Phys 33:797–801.
33. Sandler HM, Perez-Tamayo C, Ten Haken RK, Lichter AS (1992). Dose escalation for stage C (T3) prostate cancer. Minimal rectal toxicity observed using conformal therapy. Radiother Oncol 23:53–54.
34. Leibel SA, Heimann R, Kutcher GJ, Zelefsky MJ, Burman CM, Melian E, Orazem JP, Mohan R, LoSasso TJ, Lo Y, Wiseberg JA, Chapman DS, Ling CC, Fuks Z (1993). Three-dimensional conformal radiation therapy in locally advanced carcinoma of the prostate: preliminary results of a phase I dose-escalation study. Int J Radiat Oncol Biol Phys 28:55–65.
35. Sharma R, Warmelink C, Yudelev M, Mesina CF, Maughan RL, Forman JD (1995). Description of a 3D conformal neutron and photon therapy technique for prostate cancer. Med Dosimetr 30:45–53.
36. Shipley WU, Verhey LJ, Munzenrider JE, Suit HD, Urie MM, McManus PL, Young RH, Shipley JW, Zeitman AL, Biggs PJ, et al. (1995). Advanced prostate cancer: the results of a randomized comparative trial of high dose irradiation boosting with irradiation using photons alone. Int J Radiat Oncol Biol Phys 32:3–12.
37. Forman JD, Oppenheim T, Liu H, Montie J, Porter AT (1993). Frequency of residual neoplasm in the prostate following three-dimensional conformal radiotherapy. Prostate 23:235–243.
38. Forman JD, Kumar R, Haas G, Montie J, Porter AT, Mesina CF (1995). Neoadjuvant hormonal downsizing of localized carcinoma of the prostate: effects on the volume of normal tissue irradiated. Cancer Invest 13:8–15.
39. Forman JD, Lee Y, Roberson P, Montie JE, Zingas AP, Porter AT (1993). Advantages of computed tomography and beam's eye view display to confirm the accuracy of pelvic lymph node irradiation in carcinoma of the prostate. Radiology 186:889–892.
40. Forman JD, Warmelink C, Sharma R, Yudelev M, Porter AT, Maughan R (1995). Description and evaluation of 3-dimensional conformal neutron and photon radiotherapy for locally advanced adenocarcinoma of the prostate. Am J Clin Oncol 18:231–238.
41. Forman JD, Duclos M, Sharma R, Chuba PJ, Hart K, Yudelev M, Devi S, Court WS, Shamsa F, Littrup P, Grignon D, Porter AT, Maughan R (in press). The therapeutic ratio of conformal mixed neutron and photon irradiation in localized and locally advanced prostate cancer. Int J Radiat Oncol Biol Phys.
42. Forman JD, Shamsa F, Maughan RL, Orton CG (submitted). Improving the therapeutic ratio of radiation in locally advanced prostate cancer. Mixed neutron/photon vs. hyperfractionated photon irradiation.
43. Forman JD, Duclos M, Giacalone S, Yudelev M, Porter AT, Maughan RL (submitted). Conformal neutron and photon irradiation in localized (T1/T2N0M0) prostate cancer.
44. Maughan RL, Kruger DG, Blosser GF, Blosser HG (1994). Calculations of x-ray and neutron transmission through multirod arrays. Med Phys 22:427–433.

45. Maughan RL, Powers WE, Blosser HG (1994). A superconducting cyclotron for neutron radiation therapy. Med Phys 21:779–785.
46. Maughan RL, Powers WE, Blosser GF, Blosser EJ, Blosser HG (1995). Radiologic properties of a prototype multi-rod collimator for producing irregular fields in photon radiation therapy. Med Phys 22:31–36.
47. Porter AT, Forman JD (1994). The role of radiotherapy in the management of locally advanced prostate cancer. Current Oncol 1:5–7.
48. Porter AT, Chuba PJ, Forman JD (1995). Radical radiotherapy for early stage prostate cancer. Current Opinion Urol 5:248–252.

10. Cryosurgical ablation of the prostate: treatment alternative for localized prostate cancer

Jeffrey K. Cohen, Gina M. Rooker, Ralph J. Miller, Jr., and Lori Merlotti

In 1995, an estimated 244,000 new cases of adenocarcinoma of the prostate will be diagnosed, making it the most common malignant tumor in men [1]. Widespread screening has lead to increased detection of prostate cancer with the aid of prostate-specific antigen, transrectal ultrasound, increased media attention and a rapidly expanding elderly population.

Numerous treatment options are available including radical prostatectomy, radiation therapy, androgen deprivation therapy, or expectant management. Despite this variety of treatment options, there exist several specific circumstances where these patients are without respectable alternatives. It is specifically for these circumstances that investigators reexamined cryosurgical techniques for treatment of this disease. Furthermore, the reality is that no single option will be acceptable for every stage, grade, and clinical presentation. To highlight these specific patient groups, one must critically examine the standard forms of therapy of prostate cancer.

Radical prostatectomy remains the choice for localized prostate cancer [2,3]. Long-term complications of impotence and incontinence have improved dramatically in the younger patient groups [4], while older patients (>70 years old) continue to have more complications [5]. Overall, elderly patients, those with comorbidities, and patients with large-volume local disease have poorer outcomes [6,7]. Clinical evidence of localized disease significantly overestimates the number of patients with pathologically organ-confined and specimen-confined disease [3].

Retrospective reviews of patients who have undergone radiation therapy reveal that as few as 20% to 38% of patients are cured with this modality [8,9]. Several authors suggest that patients with PSA greater than 20 ng/ml will not be cured after external beam therapy. Individuals with large-volume local disease and PSA values greater than 10 ng/ml benefit only marginally in these reviews [10–14].

Androgen deprivation therapy induces disease remission but is not curative; it is, thus, an unappealing option for younger patients. Observation or expectant management may be a reasonable alternative for older patients with small, well-differentiated tumors, but again is not a good choice for the younger patient [15]. In addition, a recent report has examined cause-specific

Pienta, K.J., (ed.), DIAGNOSIS AND TREATMENT OF GENITOURINARY MALIGNANCIES.

survival in patients followed for more than ten years and treated with androgen deprivation alone. This long-term follow-up shows disease-specific mortality from prostate cancer at 63% when patients are followed for ten or more years after diagnosis [16].

These inadequacies of the current therapeutic regimens prompted a reexamination of cryotherapy for the treatment of prostate cancer. Patients who have failed radiation therapy and who may have locally confined disease have no reasonable locally extirpative therapy. Patients with locally extensive cancers must accept high risks of local treatment failure as well as the risks of complications with radical prostatectomy. The chances of totally eradicating their cancer is low with radiotherapy. Finally, with widespread screening, there is an increasing segment of the population felt to be too old to undergo definitive surgery, yet these patients demand treatment in spite of admonitions against any treatment.

Cryosurgery: historical perspective and mechanism of action

It is accepted that bringing tissues rapidly to subzero temperature will induce cell death and necrosis. Cell death is an effect of ice formation and of a spectrum of events secondary to hypothermia [17]. Hypothermia begins the cascade of injury marked by decreased intracellular energy stores and a breakdown in the physical and physiological functions of the cellular membrane. Rapid hypothermia leads to intracellular dehydration and cell shrinkage. When the temperature drops below $-4°C$, ice crystals form in the extracellular space and eventually cross the cell membrane gap junctions, leading to intracellular ice, membrane rupture, and cell death. Upon completion of the freezing process, microscopic ice crystals coalesce into sheets of ice, creating shearing forces that account for additional destruction. Any viable cells that remain are suddenly faced with a markedly hypotonic environment (from the thawing of pure water) resulting in a sudden influx of free water by osmotic forces (membrane function remains inactivated). This causes cell swelling, rupture, and death. Ultimately, the freezing process causes obstruction of the vasculature, which leads to anoxia and thrombosis. This final injury completes the cytotoxic cascade of events. Tissue absorption following cryotherapy can take up to three months and is marked initially by inflammation and removal of cellular debris and later by deposition of collagen and the creation of organized scar tissue. Histologically aberrant glands can be seen following cryosurgical ablation of the prostate (CSAP), including basal cell hyperplasia, squamous cell metaplasia, and transitional cell metaplasia [18]. Neural function recovery is dependent upon the integrity of the neural sheath and may take 6 to 12 months [19].

Cryotherapeutic techniques may hold several advantages over conventional surgery. They are less invasive, are associated with a shorter hospital stay, are well tolerated by radiated tissues, and can be applied percutaneously, all of which may lead to a decrease in morbidity.

Modern cryoablation is a modification of a method originally used in the 1960s and 1970s [20]. The original freezing process was poorly controlled and monitored via digital palpation. Urethral sloughing due to freezing was a significant morbidity, and rectourethral fistulae often resulted from transmural rectal freezing. Likewise, cutaneous fistulae were associated with a perineal approach. As a result, the treatment fell into disfavor, but ten-year survival in the series was similar to surgery and radiation [21].

The modern era of CSAP was made possible by the advent of transrectal ultrasound. Due to the ultrasonically impenetrable nature of ice crystals, sound waves reflect off the frozen/ nonfrozen interface and appear on transrectal ultrasound as an advancing hyperechoic line with a anechoic shadow behind [22]. Histologic studies confirmed a precise corelation of cell death and necrosis with this ultrasonically visualized lesion [23]. It is this characteristic imaging that allows the surgeon to aggressively yet safely freeze the prostate. Once the preliminary studies were complete [24], attention was then directed toward developing a technique to freeze the prostate that would avoid the pitfalls and shortcomings of the previous attempts. The most notable issues to address included fistulization from a perineal incision and urethral sloughing.

Fistulization is avoided with ultrasound guidance, since the growth of the iceball can be monitored and stopped upon reaching the anterior rectal wall. Stopping the treatment prematurely would leave a portion of the prostate (peripheral zone) susceptible to inadequate freezing. This issue was addressed by the development of a new liquid nitrogen delivery system. This new system (Accuprobe™, Cryomedical Sciences, Inc., Rockville, MD) provided supercooled, pressurized liquid nitrogen for the procedure, which could be delivered simultaneously through multiple thin (3 mm) probes. This new technology prevented liquid nitrogen from entering a gas phase during circulation through the probes, hence enhancing more efficient heat extraction. This greater efficiency translates into colder temperatures within the ice and a steeper drop in temperature from the periphery to the probe at the core of the iceball. With this system, a smaller margin of normal tissue need be incorporated within the iceball to assure adequate cytotoxic temperatures within the prostate than was previously possible. This system eliminated the need to freeze into the rectum to achieve cytotoxic temperatures in the peripheral zone of the prostate. Percutaneous access techniques similar to the placement of a percutaneous nephrostomy were modified to allow the placement of access ports and probes transperineally into the prostate.

Urethral sloughing is avoided by use of a catheter placed in the urethra that circulates warm saline and prevents destruction of the prostatic urothelium [25]. Viable urothelium is surrounded by necrotic prostatic parenchyma that involutes, changing to scar tissue. Morbidity in the 1960s and at present is related to the warming device. The more effectively it preserves urothelium, the less the morbidity.

With the areas of previous difficulty addressed by technical modifications, a pilot study was undertaken at Allegheny General Hospital, Medical College of Pennsylvania. Beginning in June 1990, eight procedures utilizing cryosurgical equipment designed in the 1960s were completed on patients. Each procedure was well tolerated. Follow-up biopsies of the treated areas revealed predominantly scar and necrosis [26]. These results provided the impetus to embark upon a formal study of the efficacy of CSAP for the treatment of prostate cancer. All subsequent patients were treated with the Accuprobe (CMSI, Rockville, MD), which allows more thorough and extensive freezing. The application of CSAP continues to evolve as new issues arise. Presented herein are the indications, techniques, and results from the studies at Allegheny General Hospital.

Patient selection and protocol

All patients with biopsy-proven adenocarcinoma of the prostate are eligible for consideration. They must be free of active infection, have a prostate volume less than 65 g by TRUS, and be able to grant informed consent. Our assessment includes review of the above studies as well as review of the histologic slides. Each patient is examined in order to assess a clinical stage. All patients participate in a group discussion encompassing the issues of prostate cancer management, history behind cryosurgery, procedures, complications, and results to date. CSAP is identified as being an alternative to the standards of care, namely, surgery and radiation. For the purpose of decision making, patients are advised that this procedure is to be considered investigational. All patients are entered into investigational protocols. As per the protocol (1990), preoperative assessment of nodal status is only recommended in patients with a PSA greater than ten, no previous androgen deprivation therapy (which would make the histology unreliable) and age less than 70 years old.

Postoperative surveillance consists of digital rectal examinations (DREs), PSA levels, and systematic prostatic needle biopsies. All patients are instructed to obtain a PSA level at 6 and 12 weeks, then every three months thereafter. Accompanying each three-month evaluation, DREs are performed, as well as a general survey for complications. Transrectal ultrasound guided prostate biopsies are performed at 3 and 24 months. Protocol biopsies involve a total of 11 cores (sextant samples from the prostate, the proximal seminal vesicle, and neurovascular bundle bilaterally and the site of the entrance of the ejaculatory duct into the prostate).

If any of the 11 cores contains evidence of persistent or recurrent adenocarcinoma, the patient is considered a local treatment failure. A consistently rising PSA in the face of two consecutive sets of negative prostatic biopsies is considered to have distant failure, thus initiating androgen deprivation therapy. Any patient with local failure is subsequently offered repeat treatment with CSAP or can elect radiotherapy, surgical therapy, androgen deprivation therapy, or watchful waiting.

Methods

All patients are admitted through the same-day surgical unit. Preoperative preparation consists of a Fleets™ (phospha-soda) enema for rectal debulking and oral antibiotics (ciprofloxacin 500 mg po BID for three doses and metronidazole 750 mg po on arrival to the hospital). Patients are counseled about anesthesia, and either a spinal or general anesthetic is chosen.

Once anesthetized, the patient is placed in a relaxed dorsal lithotomy position. Cystoscopy is performed, and a suprapubic tube is placed into the dome of the bladder. Upon cystoscopic examination, any bladder lesions, urethral obstructive lesions, or median lobe prostatic tissue are noted, since these may require further treatment postoperatively. The cystoscope is removed and a urethral warming catheter inserted. The catheter is perfused with saline at 40°C to maintain the viability of the urethra.

Transrectal ultrasound (TRUS) is then performed. We perform CSAP with a biplanar ultrasound probe. This is crucial to allow three-dimensional surveillance of the freezing process. Additionally, the sagittal or longitudinal scanner must be a linear piezoelectric (7 mHz) crystal. The linear array sagittal transducer provides better definition of the structures posterior to the prostate without the volume averaging and refractory artifacts commonly seen with mechanical sector scanning transducers. Routine volumetric analysis is performed using the formula (L X W X H) X 0.52. All hypoechoic areas are noted and any areas of suspected capsular penetration carefully documented.

We began utilizing color flow Doppler ultrasound (CFD) to monitor CSAP in March 1994. Graphic analysis of the vessels can distinguish arterial and venous wave forms. This information is utilized to detect areas of increased vascularity, areas that would act as heat sinks to prevent adequate freezing. We can then modify our cryoprobe placement, such that we encompass and ablate these vessels in the iceball and enhance the cytotoxic effects of the cryotherapy. Interestingly, the vascular supply to the prostate is not in the same position for each patient. Also, the blood flow to the rectum can be assessed during freezing to prevent fistula formation.

The probe access ports are then placed. Each port is placed similarly and begins with a percutaneous puncture of the perineum. With a diamond-tipped needle placed in a needle guide, transrectal ultrasound (transverse transducer) is utilized to guide the needle into the appropriate position in the prostate. A stiffened 0.038″ J-tipped guide wire is placed and the needle removed. A modified Amplatz dilator (Cook Urological, Spencer, IN) and Teflon introducer sheath are then advanced over the wire, again using ultrasound visualization. Once in position, the dilator and wire are removed. The sheath is irrigated with saline to remove air and debris (which would interfere with freezing) and improve ultrasonic visualization. All probe sites are subsequently placed.

Integral to the selection of probe sites is the normal geometry of the iceball that forms at the probe tip. The iceballs generated by the Accuprobe™ system are symmetric and reproducible. The ice begins at the probe tip (≤5 mm growth past the tip in the completed iceball) and extends up the shaft for a total length of five centimeters. The maximum radius of the iceball is two centimeters, with the final iceball being egg-shaped. In a multiple-probe arrangement, iceballs augment the performance of any adjacent probes. Any recesses between adjacent iceballs (probes) become filled as a result of this augmentation, so that the final contour is smooth (this process is referred to as ice sculpting).

The typical template involves five individually controlled probes. Two probes are placed anteriorly and three posteriorly (figure 10-1). The two anterior probes are placed between 5 and 8 mm from the anterior capsule at the midpoint between the urethra and the lateral capsule. The two posterolateral probes are placed such that the iceball growth will extend past the lateral capsule prior to reaching the rectum (the point of procedure termination). The posterolateral probes should, as well, be placed as anteriorly as possible (not

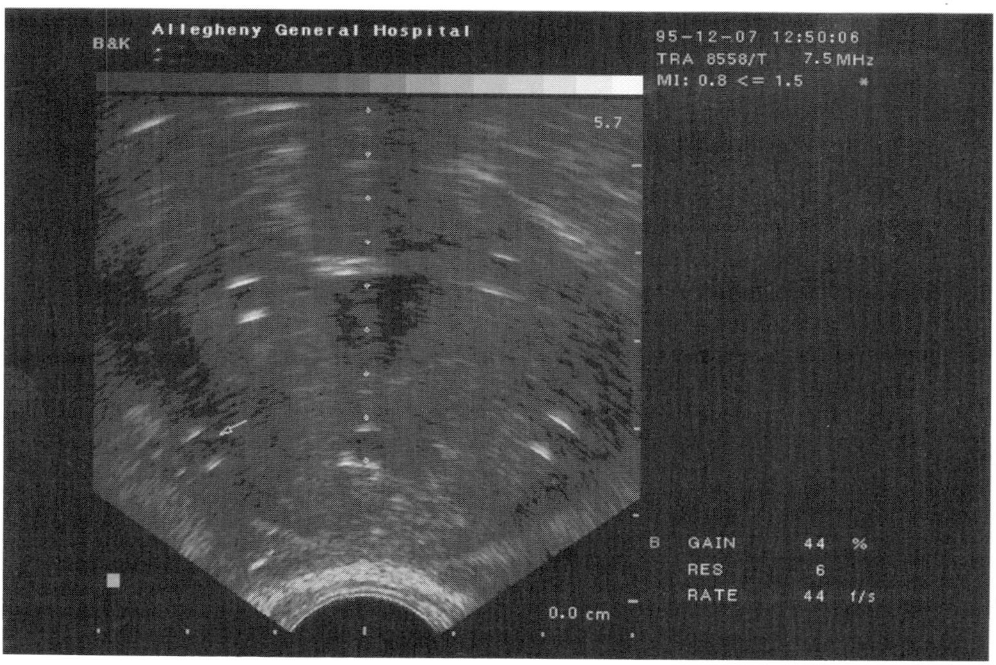

Figure 10-1. Ultrasound depiction of probe placement in the transverse plane.

beyond the 2-cm radius of the iceball) to let the iceball grow laterally to encompass the neurovascular bundles as seen by CFD and medially to augment the performance of the other probes. A fifth probe is placed in the midline posterior to the urethra. Additional access ports can be placed outside the prostate parallel to the neurovascular bundles to triangulate areas of extracapsular extension or seminal vesicle involvement.

Once all access ports are established, the cryoprobes are placed into the sheaths. The pre-slit Teflon sheaths are withdrawn and the machine is activated by circulating liquid nitrogen through the probes. This process will create a small iceball at the tip of the probe, 'sticking' the probe in place. We generally stick our probes at −70° to −100°C. The probes are suspended with rubber straps from a Bookwalter retractor ring positioned above the perineum.

Because objects close to the transducer cause acoustic interference, all manipulation, probe placement, and freezing is performed in an anterior to posterior sequence. Once all probes are stuck in place, the system is then activated to circulate pressurized, supercooled liquid nitrogen at full flow through the probes (−180° to −200°C). As the tissue temperature drops below −4°C, the tissue water changes from a liquid to a solid. This interface reflects all sound waves and is interpreted as a hyperechoic line. The lack of sound wave transmission beyond this interface is referred to as acoustic shadowing; the iceball itself is anechoic. The early freezing process is monitored in both sagittal and transverse planes to provide a three-dimensional image.

Once the advancing edge of the iceballs from the anterior probes has reached the posterior row of probes, the posterior probes are activated. The anterior probes continue to freeze until the iceballs reach the posterior prostatic capsule. This process augments the performance of the posterior probes and assures adequate margins anteriorly. Surveillance at this point is with the sagittal transducer, since it provides better delineation of the structures posterior to the prostate. A 6-cm linear-array sagittal transducer allows simultaneous visualization of the entire prostate (the ice is widest at the probe tip). The contour of the rectum does not follow a straight line. At the apex and urogenital diaphragm, the rectum is anteriorly situated compared to its location at the base. A sagittal transducer will accurately show the relationship of the iceball to the entire anterior rectal wall. As the treatment continues, there is an increase in blood flow around the prostate. The signals from the neurovascular bundles increase as the iceball approaches the rectum; in addition, portosystemic shunts through the rectum become visualized. These vascular changes are felt to be due to microvascular obstruction in the prostate. This increased peripheral flow has the potential to heat and preserve surrounding tissue. Due to this finding, we began double freezing the prostate to extinguish these signals by an encompassing iceball. The probes remain activated until the advancing edge of the iceball abuts the anterior rectal wall.

After the first freeze cycle, the prostate is then allowed to thaw (passively), after which the prostate is again refrozen (double freeze). With prostates shorter than 5 cm, the procedure is complete following the double freeze in the initial position. If the prostate length exceeds 5 cm, a pullback of the probes is necessary to adequately treat the apical and trapezoidal areas during the second freeze.

Once the freezing process is complete, the probes are thawed, then removed. Manual pressure is applied to the perineum for hemostasis, and the probe insertion sites are closed with simple sutures of 3-0 chromic. The urethral-warming catheter is left activated until the entire prostate has thawed, generally in 20 minutes. The catheter is removed, the suprapubic tube placed to straight drain, and the patient taken to the recovery room.

The usual hospital stay is one day. The following morning, the suprapubic tube is capped with a heparin lock, instructions are given, and patients are discharged to home. Postoperatively, there is generally little pain. Scrotal ecchymosis and edema (lymphedema presumably from obstructed pelvic channels) develops within 2 to 3 days and can be quite dramatic, yet invariably resolves without treatment in three weeks. Patients can resume normal activities in 1 to 2 weeks, with a return to work in a similar time frame. The suprapubic tube is removed at such time that the postvoid residuals are consistently below 100 cc. We recommend oral antibiotic coverage (ciprofloxacin) for two weeks after the procedure and for one week following suprapubic tube removal.

Results

Biopsies

Cohort 1. Through May 18, 1994, 383 patients underwent 448 procedures. The mean age of the cohort is 65.1 +/− 6.5 years (range 41–79). Mean and median follow-up are 24.3 months and 24.5 months (range 1.4–60.1). Of these patients, 359 of 383 (93.7%) have had at least one postprocedure biopsy. At the time of initial follow-up biopsy, 55 of 359 (15.3%) patients were positive for residual or recurrent carcinoma. Of those with an initial negative biopsy, 200 (65.8%) have had a subsequent biopsy and 64 of 200 (32%) are positive. Combining these two groups, overall treatment failure occurred in 119 of 359 (33.1%) of patients in this cohort. Demographics by stage, grade, and PSA are listed in tables 10-1 and 10-2 for this group. Biopsy results by stage, grade, and PSA category are listed in tables 10-3 and 10-4 for this group.

Cohort 2. From May 1994 through October 1, 1995, 158 patients underwent 168 procedures. The mean age of the cohort was 65.5 years (range 47–79). Mean and median follow-up are 8.2 months and 8.5 months (range 1.0–16.7). Of this group, 8 of 104 (7.8%) have had an initial positive biopsy and 2 of 11 (18.2%) have had a subsequent positive biopsy. Combining these groups, treatment failure occurred in 10 of 104 (9.6%) of patients. Demographics by

Table 10-1. Demographics by treatment group (cohort 1)

	N	A	B	C	D	2–4	5–7	8–10	Unkn
Virgin	235	65	93	54	23	89	130	16	0
ADT	84	17	30	20	17	21	47	14	2
XRT	23	4	5	13	1	1	12	10	0
XRT/ADT	17	1	3	7	6	1	10	4	2

Virgin, no prior local treatments; ADT, prior androgen deprivation therapy; XRT, prior external beam radiation therapy; XRT + ADT, prior external beam radiation therapy and androgen deprivation therapy; A–D, Jewitt classification; Gleason scores: 2–4, well differentiated; 5–7, moderately well differentiated; 8–10, poorly differentiated.

Table 10-2. Treatment groups by pre-op PSA (cohort 1)

	Unknown	PSA $\leq$ 4.0	PSA 4–10	PSA 10–30	PSA > 30
Virgin	2	31	116	79	16
ADT	0	7	31	29	23
XRT	0	0	6	12	6
XRT – ADT	0	0	4	9	6

Virgin, no prior local treatments; ADT, prior androgen deprivation tehrapy; XRT, prior external beam radiation therapy; XRT + ADT, prior external beam radiation therapy and androgen deprivation therapy.

Table 10-3. Biopsy results by stage and grade (cohort 1)

	N	Initial Bx (+)	(+) biopsy after (−) biopsy	Overall (+) biopsy after (−) biopsy
A1	35	3 (8.6%)	5	8 (22.9%)
A2	42	4 (9.5%)	5	9 (21.4%)
Unspec. A	10	0	3	3 (30.0%)
Overall A	87	7 (8.0%)	13	20 (23.0%)
B1	47	4 (8.5%)	10	14 (29.8%)
B2	78	13 (16.7%)	14	27 (34.6%)
Unspec. B	6	0	1	1 (16.7%)
Overall B	131	17 (13.0%)	25	42 (32.1%)
C	94	21 (22.3%)	17	38 (40.4%)
D0	32	5 (15.6%)	8	13 (40.6%)
D1	15	5 (33.3%)	1	6 (40.0%)
Overall D	47	10 (21.3%)	9	19 (40.4%)
2–4 (WD)	112	10 (8.9%)	16	26 (23.2%)
5–7 (MD)	199	34 (17.1%)	37	71 (35.7%)
8–10 (PD)	44	10 (22.7%)	11	21 (47.7%)
Unkn	4	1 (25.0%)	0	1 (25.0%)

A–D, Jewitt stage; 2–4, 5–7, 8–10, Gleason scores; WD, well differentiated; MD, moderately well differentiated; PD, poorly differentiated; (+), positive; (−), negative.

Table 10-4. Biopsy results by PSA (cohort 1)

After first procedure

PSA category	(+) at initial Bx	(+) at follow-up Bx	Total (+) Bx
Unknown	0/2	1/2 (50.0%)	1/2 (50.0%)
≤4.0 ng/ml	1/37 (2.7%)	3/20 (15.0%)	4/37 (10.8%)
4.1–10.0 ng/ml	19/152 (12.5%)	30/91 (33.0%)	49/152 (32.2%)
10.1–30.0 ng/ml	24/120 (20.0%)	22/62 (35.5%)	46/120 (38.3%)
>30.0 ng/ml	11/48 (22.9%)	8/22 (36.4%)	19/48 (39.6%)

After last procedure

PSA category	(+) at initial Bx	(+) at follow-up Bx	Total (+) Bx
≤4.0 ng/ml	1/37 (2.7%)	2/20 (10.0%)	3/37 (8.1%)
4.1–10.0 ng/ml	4/148 (2.7%)	23/88 (26.1%)	27/148 (18.2%)
10.1–30.0 ng/ml	13/116 (11.2%)	15/59 (25.4%)	28/116 (24.1%)
>30.0 ng/ml	5/45 (11.1%)	7/22 (31.8%)	12/45 (26.7%)

Table 10-5. Demographics by treatment group (cohort 2)

	N	A	B	C	D	Unkn
Virgin	99	40	29	20	6	4
ADT	34	10	9	8	6	1
XRT	16	2	3	8	2	1
XRT + ADT	9	3	4	2	0	0

Virgin, no prior local treatments; ADT, prior androgen deprivation therapy; XRT, prior external beam radiation therapy; XRT + ADT, prior external beam radiation therapy and androgen deprivation therapy.

treatment group are listed in table 10-5. Biopsy results by stage and grade are listed in table 10-6.

Radiation therapy failures

Forty patients in cohort 1 have been treated with cryosurgical ablation after previously failed external beam radiation therapy. Of that group, 23 had received radiation only (XRT), and 17 had received radiation therapy and androgen deprivation (XRT + ADT) prior to CSAP.

After one or more CSAP treatments, 40.9% of the XRT group and 41.1% of the XRT + ADT group had positive biopsies. At one year, 75.0% of XRT and 50.0% of XRT + ADT patients have a positive biopsy. At two years after treatment, 56.4% of patients treated with XRT alone have a positive biopsy, while 53.3% of those treated with XRT + ADT have a positive biopsy.

Within the XRT group at 21 or more months after treatment, mean and

Table 10-6. Biopsy results by stage and grade (cohort 2)

	N	Initial Bx (+)	(+) biopsy after (−) biopsy	Overall (+) biopsy
A1	8	0	0	0
A2	12	0	0	0
Unspec. A	21	0	1/1 (100%)	1/21 (4.8%)
Overall A	41	0	1/2 (50.0%)	1/41 (2.4%)
B1	10	0	0	0
B2	19	1/19 (5.3%)	0	1/19 (5.3%)
Unspec. B	1	0	0	0
Overall B	30	1/30 (3.3%)	0	1/30 (3.3%)
C	25	6/25 (24.0%)	0	6/25 (24.0%)
D0	6	1/6 (16.7%)	1/2 (50.0%)	2/6 (33.3%)
D1	2	0	0	0
Overall D	8	1/8 (12.5%)	1/2 (50.0%)	2/8 (25.0%)
2–4 (WD)	15	0	0	0
5–7 (MD)	78	5/78 (6.4%)	2/8 (25.0%)	7/78 (9.5%)
8–10 (PD)	13	3/13 (23.1%)	0	3/13 (23.1%)
Unkn	2	0	0	0

A–D, Jewitt stage; 2–4, 5–7, 8–10, Gleason scores; WD, well differentiated; MD, moderately well differentiated; PD, poorly differentiated; (+), positive; (−), negative.

median PSA in the group with negative biopsies was 1.6 and 1.6 ng/ml. In the positive biopsy group, mean and median PSA was 1.62 and 1.83 ng/ml.

Cohort 2 included 11 patients who were treated with CSAP after XRT failure and five patients who were treated after XRT + ADT. Median follow-up is 14 months, and at this time period, 18.2% of the XRT patients have a positive biopsy while 40.0% of the XRT + ADT group have a positive biopsy. Tables 10-7 and 10-8 include the above data.

Stage T3 patients

Ninety-four of our patients presented with stage T3 disease prior to CSAP. Review of this group reveals 54 with no prior treatments (virgin), 20 with previous androgen deprivation (ADT), 13 with previous radiation therapy (XRT), and 7 with prior radiation and androgen deprivation therapy (XRT + ADT).

Ninety-two patients have evaluable biopsy and PSA data after one or more procedures. Of this group, 25 of 92 (26.6%) have positive biopsies, including 10 of 53 (18.9%) virgin patients, 6 of 19 (31.6%) ADT patients, 6 of 13 (46.1%) XRT patients, and 3 of 7 (42.9%) patients treated with XRT + ADT.

Thirty-two patients have evaluable biopsy results at 21 months or more after treatment. Of this group, 6 of 32 (18.8%) are positive for persistent disease.

Fifty-eight patients have evaluable PSA data at 21 months or more after treatment. Mean and median PSA for those with negative biopsies is 1.27 and

Table 10-7. Biopsy results after CSAP in previously irradiated patients (cohort 1) (n = 23)

	Radiation Therapy (XRT)				XRT + ADT			
Stage	N	Initial Bx (+)	(+) Bx after (−) Bx	Total (+) Bx	N	Initial Bx (+)	(+) Bx after (−) Bx	Total (+) Bx
A	4	0	1	1 (25%)	1	0	0	0
B	5	3 (60%)	1	4 (80%)	3	1 (33.3%)	1	2 (33.3%)
C	13	4 (30.8%)	4	8 (61.5%)	7	1 (14.3%)	2	3 (42.9%)
D	1	0	0	0	6	2 (33.3%)	1	3 (75%)

A–D, Jewitt stage; XRT, prior external beam radiation therapy; XRT + ADT, prior external beam radiation therapy and androgen deprivation therapy; (+), positive; (−) negative.

Table 10-8. Biopsy results after CSAP in previously irradiated patients (cohort 2) (n = 16)

	XRT				XRT + ADT			
Stage	N	Initial Bx (+)	(+) Bx after (−) Bx	Total (+) Bx	N	Initial Bx (+)	(+) Bx after (−) Bx	Total (+) Bx
A	2	0	0	0	3	0	1 (50%)	1 (33.3%)
B	2	0	0	0	1	0	0	0
C	7	2 (28.6%)	0	2 (28.6%)	1	1 (100%)	0	1 (100%)

A–C, Jewitt stage; XRT, prior external beam radiation therapy; XRT + ADT, prior external beam radiation therapy and androgen deprivation therapy; (+), positive; (−) negative.

0.20 ng/ml, respectively, and for those with positive biopsies is 0.41 and 0.12 ng/ml, respectively. Overall, 28 of 58 (48.3%) of patients have a PSA of 0.4 ng/ml or less at 21 months or more after treatment, and 40 of 58 (69.0%) have a PSA of 1.0 ng/ml or less at the same time period.

Combination CSAP and external beam radiation

A small cohort of patients with large-volume moderately to poorly differentiated tumors has been treated with combined CSAP and external beam radiation therapy in an attempt to improve local disease control.

Thirteen patients have follow-up data and include one stage A2, three stage B1, one stage B2, six stage C, one stage D0, and one stage D1 prior to CSAP. Gleason scores prior to CSAP showed one well-differentiated tumor, five moderately differentiated tumors, and seven poorly differentiated tumors. All 13 patients who failed CSAP had positive biopsies detected at 3 to 24 months after CSAP. All subsequently underwent external beam radiation therapy and were treated with 5500 rads after CSAP failure.

Mean and median serum PSA after completion of radiation therapy are 1.35 and 0.4, respectively. Only one patient has a positive biopsy after completion of XRT, detected at three months posttreatment. The remainder are biopsy negative with stable PSA values at a mean of 14.6 months after completion of radiation therapy.

Two-year results

Cohort 1 includes 239 patients who have been followed for at least 21 months after cryoablation therapy. All patients on hormonal ablation discontinued treatment after cryotherapy. Of these 239 patients, 119 (49.8%) have undergone a subsequent set of systematic prostate needle biopsies between 21 and 36 months following treatment. One hundred and fourteen patients had received no prior local treatments (83 virgin patients and 31 androgen deprivation therapy only). Five patients had received prior external beam radiation therapy and were excluded from these statistics. Eight patients from this group initially had a positive biopsy following an earlier application of CSAP, have subsequently been retreated (using CSAP), and have been followed for a minimum of 21 months after an initial negative biopsy. Mean follow-up in this group is 32 months, with a range of 21.5 to 57.4 months. Overall, 64 of 364 patients (17.6%) had a positive biopsy after one or more treatments at some time period during follow-up.

At 21 or more months, mean and median PSA at the time of a positive biopsy in the virgin group was 1.26 and 0.88 ng/ml, respectively, and in the ADT group was 1.75 and 1.45 ng/ml, respectively. These results were in contrast to the mean and median PSA values at the time of a negative biopsy in the virgin group of 1.05 and 0.20 ng/ml, respectively, and in the ADT group of 0.83 and 0.60 ng/ml, respectively. There are 101 patients with and 62 patients without biopsies who have evaluable PSA data 21 months or more after treatment. Among all patients, 80.4% (264 of 328) and 90.2% (296 of 328) achieved a nadir PSA of 0.4 ng/ml and 1.0 ng/ml or less, respectively, in the first year after treatment. Forty-six of 101 biopsied patients (73 virgin, 28 ADT) (45.5%) and 43 of 62 nonbiopsied patients (48 virgin, 14 ADT) (69.3%) have a PSA of 0.4 ng/ml or less 21 months or more posttreatment. Overall, 89 of 163 (54.6%) had a PSA of 0.4 ng/ml or less 21 months or more after treatment. Sixty-nine of 101 biopsied patients (73 virgin, 28 ADT) (68.3%) and 53 of 62 nonbiopsied patients (42 virgin, 11 ADT) (85.5%) have a PSA of 1.0 ng/ml or less 21 months or more after treatment. Overall, 122 out of 163 patients (74.8%) have a PSA of 1.0 ng/ml or less at 21 months or more after treatment. Tables 10-9, 10-10, and 10-11 reflect these results.

Complications

Complications of therapy in the group of patients in cohort 1 were minimal. The most prevalent of these was urethral sloughing, occurring in 9.8% of patients. As a result of CSAP, 3.6% of patients have become incontinent — defined as the need for a pad six months after treatment. Six patients experi-

Table 10-9. Median PSA results over time for patients after all treatments (cohort 1)

	(+) Biopsy				(−) Biopsy			
	Pre-Tx	3 mos	12 mos	>21 mos	Pre-Tx	3 mos	12 mos	>21 mos
Virgin	9.10	0.90	1.20	0.88	7.13	0.12	0.20	0.20
ADT	11.60	0.90	1.13	1.45	11.00	0.30	0.30	0.60
XRT	10.90	0.90	1.53	2.71	12.00	0.70	0.95	1.50
XRT + ADT	36.70	2.60	0.40	1.90	18.10	0.70	0.70	0.40

Virgin, no prior local treatments; ADT, prior androgen deprivation therapy; XRT, prior external beam radiation therapy; XRT + ADT, prior external beam radiation therapy and androgen deprivation therapy.

Table 10-10. PSA levels in patients with and without biopsy at two years: virgin patients (n = 121)[a]

PSA levels	Patients biopsied	Patients not biopsied
≤0.4 ng/ml	36/73 (49.3%)	36/48 (75.0%)
≤1.0 ng/ml	51/73 (69.9%)	42/48 (87.5%)

[a] 73 patients with a PSA level and biopsy at 21 or more months after treatment; 48 patients with a PSA level and no biopsy at 21 or more months after treatment.

Table 10-11. PSA levels in patients with and without a biopsy at two years: ADT patients (n = 42)[a]

PSA levels	Patients biopsied	Patients not biopsied
≤0.4 ng/ml	10/28 (35.7%)	7/14 (50.0%)
≤1.0 ng/ml	18/28 (64.3%)	11/14 (78.6%)

[a] 28 patients with a PSA level and biopsy at 21 or more months after treatment; 14 patients with a PSA level and no biopsy at 21 or more months after treatment.

enced prolonged urinary retention and 17 have urethral stricture disease or contracture of the bladder neck that required manipulation. There were no treatment-related deaths in this cohort, and no complications presented in a delayed fashion. Table 10-12 lists all complications for this cohort.

Cohort 2 has a shorter period of follow-up, but the 33.3% incidence of significant urethral sloughing has been considerably greater than the cohort 1 group. This difference is directly attributable to the warming device, which was not available in this patient group. A warmer manufactured from stock operating-room parts was used in this patient group after removal of the original warmer from the market by the FDA. The number of patients with urethral stricture or bladder neck contracture requiring manipulation has increased as well to 11.3%. Other complications are similar to those in cohort 1 and are listed in table 10-13. There has been one treatment-related death in this cohort from emphysematous cystitis and necrotizing fasciitis in a diabetic patient.

The original urethral warming catheter was removed from the market after May 18, 1994, for further testing by the Food and Drug Administration. Despite its use in more than 300 patients, it was reclassified as a significant risk device. Review of the first 103 cases with the new urethral warming device revealed that sloughing was more common in virgin patients (26.5%) than in androgen deprivation therapy patients (12.5%) or radiation-failure patients (6.3%). Analysis of the virgin cohort reveals that the risk of sloughing is directly proportional to gland volume. Sloughing in virgin patients with gland volumes less than 20g occurred at 1.1%. As gland volume increased above 20g, sloughing occurred at a rate of 35.7%. The original warmer has been approved by the FDA and was re-released in November of 1995.

Discussion

A new era of CSAP has begun utilizing minimally invasive techniques, transrectal ultrasound, and the concept of urethral warming/protection. Cryosurgical ablation of the prostate can now be achieved with a minimum of surgical complications as compared to historic references [27]. The average hospital stay of one day is significantly less than that for radical prostatectomy, and the recuperative period as well is much shorter for those patients treated with an effective urethral warmer.

Table 10-12. Complications (n = 448) (cohort 1)

Urethrorectal fistula	2 (0.4%)	UTI	6 (1.3%)
Sloughing syndrome	44 (0.9%)	Prostatic abscess	2 (0.4%)
After Bx	21 (47.7%)	Urinary retention	6 (1.3%)
Bleeding	9 (2.0%)	Incontinence	16 (3.6%)
Urethral stricture	10 (2.2%)	After TURP	8 (50.0%)
Bladder neck contracture	7 (1.6%)	Perineal necrosis	1 (0.2%)
Prostatitis	4 (0.9%)	Sepsis	3 (0.7%)
Epididymitis	7 (1.6%)	Balanitis/phimosis	1 (0.2%)
Perineal fistula	1 (0.2%)	Perineal pain	2 (0.4%)
Scrotal swelling	1 (0.2%)	Priapism	1 (0.2%)
Numb glans penis	1 (0.2%)		

Table 10-13. Complications (n = 168) (cohort 2)

Sloughing syndrome	56 (33.3%)	UTI	2 (1.4%)
After Bx	14 (25.0%)	Urinary retention	3 (1.8%)
Bleeding	2 (1.2%)	Perineal pain	3 (1.8%)
Urethral stricture	12 (7.1%)	Epididymitis	4 (2.4%)
Bladder neck contracture	7 (4.2%)	Lymphocele	1 (0.6%)
Incontinence	20 (11.9%)	Prostatic abscess	1 (0.6%)
After TURP	12 (60.0%)	Emphysematous cystitis and necrogizing fasciitis	1 (0.6%)
Sepsis	1 (0.6%)		

Cause-specific survival is the ultimate measure of success for the treatment of clinically localized adenocarcinoma of the prostate. Therefore, the true survival rates for patients with prostate cancer undergoing cryosurgical ablation of the prostate (CSAP) will not be known for many years to come. Serial PSA following radical prostatectomy or a rising PSA following radiation therapy can antedate clinical disease progression by months to year. Following radiation therapy, a positive prostate biopsy portends a significantly increased risk of metastasis [3,11]. A rising serum PSA and positive prostate biopsy following radiotherapy can be intimately related, as reported by Kabalin et al., who documented local failure in 93% of men demonstrating a rising PSA after external beam radiotherapy [10]. Additionally, Stamey et al. reported that only 23 of 113 patients (20%) undergoing irradiation for prostatic cancer achieve cure, defined as long-term PSA levels persistently less than 1.7 ng/ml [8]. PSA and posttreatment biopsies are therefore widely accepted as outcome measures in identifying treatment failure and make it possible to compare local treatment modalities without waiting for long-term cause-specific survival data.

Problems arise, however, when drawing comparisons to most of the historical reviews, which do not use PSA as a measurable outcome. Treatment efficacy was determined by local symptomatology and clinical examination. Recent publications have critically re-examined the results following radiotherapy for clinically localized adenocarcinoma of the prostate utilizing PSA and core biopsy. Reports quantifying these short-term measures of success following radiotherapy have enabled an interim comparison against cryotherapy.

Several recent reviews have examined the effects of external beam radiation therapy on serum PSA. Kavadi et al. presented the retrospective experience from the University of Texas, M.D. Anderson Cancer Center. This cohort shared similar stage, grade, and PSA demographics with our group undergoing CSAP. This study examined the ability of both pre- and posttreatment PSA to predict treatment response. They determined that a one-year posttreatment nadir PSA value of 1.0 ng/ml or less was a significant predictor of treatment success. Nadir PSA values of 1.0 ng/ml or less correspond with a combined clinical local and distant relapse rate of 17%. For nadir PSA values above 1.0 ng/ml, the recurrence rates exceeded 70%. From this study, 43% of patients attained a nadir PSA value of 1.0 ng/ml or less following radiotherapy, while only 12% achieved an undetectable nadir PSA of 0.3 ng/ml or less.

Furthermore, evaluation of the cohort by preoperative PSA category demonstrated significantly less favorable results with increasing preoperative PSA levels. Patients with normal preoperative PSA values (less than 4.0 ng/ml) had an 83% chance of a nadir below 1.0 ng/ml. This is in contrast to preoperative PSA values between 10 and 30 ng/ml and greater than 30 ng/ml, which had only a 19.7% and 8.5% chance, respectively, of a nadir PSA below 1.0 ng/ml [14].

A recent report by Hancock et al. reviewed external beam radiation therapy data for 110 patients followed an average of 12.4 years after treatment.

Using criteria for control established by previous reports [8], they found 42 of 110 (38%) patients maintained clinical disease-free status after radiation therapy [9] (PSA $\leq$ 4.0 ng/ml, negative digital rectal exam, and absent metastases).

A more critical review of this paper confirms the findings of Kavadi et al. [14]. Specifically, 30% achieved a long-term PSA of 1.0 ng/ml or less. In more advanced clinical stages (T2b–T3), 19% of patients maintained a PSA of 1.0 ng/ml or less. There were no patients with a Gleason's score of 7 or more who had a PSA of 1.0 ng/ml or less. Unfortunately, biopsy data are not available on this cohort of patients. Clearly, the chance for cure is limited in patients with advanced stage (T2b–T3) and grade (Gleason score $\geq$7).

In a similar review, Lee et al. presented their five-year surveillance following external beam radiotherapy at the Fox Chase Cancer Center. Patient demographics again were very similar to our cohort undergoing CSAP. They evaluated biochemical no evidence of disease (bNED) status at five years (defined as a most recent PSA value of 1.5 ng/ml or less if followed for more than one year). Though bNED was directly proportional to pretreatment clinical stage (bNED for T1, T2, and T3 disease was 62%, 53%, and 34%, respectively, at five years), multivariate analysis confirmed that the pretreatment PSA value was a more significant indicator of success. Lee et al. further determined that patients with a pretreatment PSA below 15 ng/ml had a significantly greater chance of bNED than those above this level in all clinical stages. The effects were most notable in patients with 'early stage' disease (T1, T2A, T2B) [28].

Table 10-14 highlights the results of patients following CSAP with respect to a nadir PSA value of 1.0 ng/ml or less and preoperative PSA category. In both regards, CSAP is more successful than radiotherapy in attaining these goals. The results indicate that radiotherapy fails more frequently in advanced disease, as indicated by increasing PSA and increasing clinical stage. Cryotherapy, however, is more effective in these advanced presentations.

To provide a more specific reflection of local control following radiotherapy, Crook et al. reviewed their experience of routine systematic biopsies following definitive XRT for clinically localized adenocarcinoma of the prostate. This cohort was older and generally had less advanced stage and grade

Table 10-14. Comparison of XRT to CSAP in attaining a post-treatment nadir of PSA $\leq$ 1.0 ng/ml

	% attaining nadir PSA $\leq$ 1.0 ng/ml after XRT	% attaining nadir PSA $\leq$ 1.0 ng/ml after CSAP
All patients	43%	92%
Preoperative PSA 10–13 ng/ml	15%	96%
Preoperative PSA >30 ng/ml	4%	40%

cancers than in the CSAP group. Four to six random biopsies were obtained using TRUS by a radiologist at 12 months then every six months thereafter until negative. Fifty-one percent (115 of 226) of patients had histologic evidence of viable cancer on the initial 12-month biopsy. Thirty-nine of these 115 patients eventually converted to negative biopsies, leaving an overall positive biopsy rate of 34%. The authors examined positive biopsies with a proliferating cell nuclear antigen (PCNA) stain. In patients displaying delayed conversion to negative biopsy status, 67% of those examined were negative for PCNA, suggesting 'inactivated' cancer. Thus, the delayed conversion might be predicted by the absence of PCNA [13].

In comparison to CSAP, the chances that a patient will have a positive biopsy following one or numerous cryoablation procedures is 31.0% and 18.3%, respectively, for cohort 1 and 9.6% after a single treatment in cohort 2, which has a shorter follow-up period. CSAP compares favorably in both cohorts to external beam radiation therapy when comparing biopsy status after treatment.

Direct comparisons to historical series following radical prostatectomy are difficult due to the persistence of a measurable PSA following CSAP. Epstein et al. reported a 30% rate of biochemical failure for initially localized CSAP within five years after radical prostatectomy [29]. As with radical prostatectomy, a persistently rising PSA after CSAP is indicative of residual cancer, either locally or distally. However, the presence of residual necrotic, dysplastic, or hypertrophic glands within the prostate may lead to a residual detectable PSA in the absence of persistent cancer. Following CSAP in the present series (cohort 1), treatment failure for clinical stages A1–B1, as defined by either biopsy-confirmed local recurrence or rising serial PSA values in the absence of local recurrence, occurred in 16.1% (16 of 129 or 12.4% with biopsy-proven local recurrence and 23 of 133 or 20.4% with a rising PSA and negative biopsy).

Review of several reports indicate that salvage radical prostatectomy following radiation therapy failure achieves biochemical cure in 29.4% to 47% of cases [30,31]. Patients treated with CSAP for biopsy-proven recurrence after radiation therapy in the present series (cohort 1) maintain a negative biopsy following CSAP 20.2% to 75.0% of the time after one or more treatments. In addition, 25.0% to 66.6% of patients achieve a negative biopsy with CSAP in radiation failures after one or more treatments when ADT is combined with CSAP. Results for cohort 1 are listed in table 10-14.

Conclusion

Cryosurgical ablation of the prostate incorporates modern technology and the current concepts of cancer control to apply the proven destructive abilities of cryotherapy in the eradication of prostate cancer. Though long-term results are not yet available, cryosurgical ablation of the prostate is effective as measured by PSA and biopsy status at 21 to 36 months posttreatment. A total of 78.5% of patients achieved an undetectable 12-month nadir PSA, while 60.7% of patients retain an undetectable PSA level 21 months after treatment. In addition, 89.9% achieve a 12-month nadir PSA of 1.0ng/ml or less and 76.1% retain it at 21 months after treatment. The overall positive biopsy rate after one treatment is 31.0%, with a 18.3% positive biopsy rate after one or more treatments. When compared to radiation therapy, cryotherapy exceeds current treatment results, especially in more advanced presentations. Complications were minimal when using the original urethral warmer, but increased considerably during the time of its removal from the market.

These results are the work of one center with a strong commitment to evaluating and improving a technique that is highly operator dependent. Even though cause-specific survival is not yet available, the results clearly demonstrate a role for this procedure in patients who are at significant risk for pathologically nonorgan-confined prostate cancer.

References

1. Wingo PA, Tong T, Bolden S (1995). Cancer statistics, 1995. CA 45(1):8–30.
2. Gibbons RP, Correa RJ, Brannen GE, Weissman RM (1989). Total prostatectomy for clinically localized prostatic cancer: long term results. J Urol 141:564.
3. Partin AW, Pound CR, Clemens JQ, Epstein JI, Walsh PC (1993). Serum PSA after anatomic radical prostatectomy. Urol Clin N Am 20(4).
4. Quinlan DM, Epstein JI, Carter BS, Walsh PC (1991). Sexual function following radical prostatectomy: influence of preservation of neurovascular bundles. J Urol 145:998–1002.
5. Fowler FJ, Barry JJ, Lu-Yao G, Roman A, Wasson J, Wennberg JE (1993). Patient-reported complications and follow-up treatment after radical prostatectomy. Urology 42(6):622–629.
6. McNeal JE, Villers AA, Redwine EA, Freiha FS, Stamey TA (1990). Histologic differentiation, cancer volume, and pelvic lymph node metastasis in adenocarcinoma of the prostate. Cancer 66:1225.
7. Stamey TA, McNeal JE, Freiha FS, Redwine E (1988). Morphometric and clinical studies on 68 consecutive radical prostatectomies. J Urol 139:1235.
8. Stamey TA, Ferrari MK, Schmid HP (1993). The value of serial prostate specific antigen determinations 5 years after radiotherapy: steeply increasing values characterize 80% of patients. J Urol 150:1856–1859.
9. Hancock SL, Cox RS, Bagshaw MA (1995). Prostate specific antigen after radiotherapy for prostate cancer: a reevaluation of long-term biochemical control and the kinetics of recurrence in patients treated at stanford university. J Urol 154:1412–1417.
10. Kabalin JM, Hodge KK, McNeal JE, Freiha FS, Stamey TA (1989). Identification of residual cancer in the prostate following radiation therapy: role of transrectal ultrasound guided biopsy and prostate specific antigen. J Urol 143:326–331.
11. Egawa S, Wheeler TM, Greene DR, Scardino PT (1992). Detection of residual prostate cancer after radiotherapy by sonographically guided needle biopsy. Urology 34(4):358–363.
12. Freiha FS, Bagshaw MA (1984). Carcinoma of the prostate: results of post-irradiation biopsy. Prostate 5:19.
13. Crook JM, Perry GA, Robertson S, Esche BA (1995). Routine prostate biopsies following radiotherapy for prostate cancer. Urology 45(4):624–632.
14. Kavadi VS, Zagars GK, Pollack A (1994). Serum prostate-specific antigen after radiation therapy for clinically localized prostate cancer: prognostic implications. Int J Radiat Biol Phys 30(2):279–287.

15. Terris MK, McNeal JE, Stamey TA (1992). Detection of clinically significant prostate cancer by transrectal ultrasound-guided systematic biopsies. J Urol 148:829–832.
16. Aus G, Hugosson J, Norlen L (1995). Lone-term survival and mortality in prostate cancer treated with noncurative intent. J Urol 154:460–465.
17. Baust JG, Chang AH (in press). Cryosurgery: underlying mechanisms of damage and new concepts in cryosurgical instrumentation. Proc 9th World Congress of Cryosurgery, June 1995.
18. Masson D, Bidair M, Shabaik A, Wilson S, Schmidt JD (1995). Pathologic changes in prostate biopsies following cryoablation therapy (abstract). J Urol 153(4):484A.
19. Tumble TE, Whalen JT (1992). The effects of cryosurgery and cryoprotectants on peripheral nerve function. J Reconstr Microsurg 8:53–58.
20. Gondor MJ, Soanes WA, Shulman S (1966). Cryosurgical treatment of the prostate. Invest Urol 3(4):372–378.
21. Bonney WW, Fallon B, Gerber WL, Hawtrey CE, Loening SA, Narayana AS (1982). Cryosurgery in prostate cancer: survival. Urology 19:37–42.
22. Brandt B, Hibon J, LeMaire P, Lomina D, Lardennois B (1985). Ultrasonography and cryosurgery of the prostate. Cryosurgery 7.
23. Littrup PJ, Mody A, Sparschu R, Prchevski P, Montie J, Zingas AP, Grignon D (1994). Prostatic cryotherapy: ultrasonographic and pathologic correlation in the canine model. Urology 44(2):175–184.
24. Onik G, Cobb C, Cohen J, Zabkar J, Porterfield B (1988). Ultrasound characteristics of frozen prostate. Radiology 168:629–631.
25. Cohen JK, Miller RJ (1994). Thermal protection of urethra during cryosurgery of prostate. Cryobiology 31:313–316.
26. Onik GM, Cohen JK, Reyes GD, Rubinsky B, Chang Z, Baust J (1993). Transrectal ultrasound-guided percutaneous radical cryosurgical ablation of the prostate. Cancer 72(4):1291–1299.
27. Loening S, Lubaroff D (1984). Cryosurgery and immunotherapy for prostatic cancer. Urol Clin N Am 11(2):327–336.
28. Lee WR, Hanks GE, Schultheiss TE, Corn BW, Hunt MA (1995). Localized prostate cancer treated by external-beam radiotherapy alone: serum prostate-specific antigen — driven outcome analysis. J Clin Oncol 13(2):464–469.
29. Epstein JI, Carmichael M, Partin AW, Walsh PC (1993). Is tumor volume an independent predictor of progression following radical prostatectomy? A multivariate analysis of 185 clinical stage B adenocarcinomas of the prostate with 5 years of followup. J Urol 149:1278–1281.
30. Rogers E, Ohori M, Kassabian VX, Wheeler TM, Scardino PT (1995). Salvage radical prostatectomy: outcome measured by serum prostate specific antigen levels. J Urol 104–110.
31. Pontes JE, Montie J, Klein E, Huben R (1993). Salvage surgery for radiation failure in prostate cancer. Cancer 71(Suppl 3):976–980.

Medical Advances

11. The chemoprevention of prostate cancer and the prostate cancer prevention trial

Otis W. Brawley and Ian M. Thompson

The impact of prostate cancer is substantial, and this fact is often cited as the reason for aggressive screening for and aggressive treatment of the disease. There are, of course, significant uncertainties regarding the efficacy of both prostate cancer screening and prostate cancer treatment [1]. Indeed, both are active areas of investigation, and the goal of reducing prostate cancer morbidity and mortality continues to elude modern medicine. An approach deserving consideration is the chemoprevention of prostate cancer.

The term *Chemoprevention* was originally coined by Sporn et al. [2] in 1976. The term is defined as the use of specific natural or synthetic chemical agents to reverse, suppress, or prevent carcinogenic progression to invasive cancer [3]. While the chemoprevention of cancer may be a relatively new concept, the concept of using a drug to prevent a chronic disease is not new. Treatment of hypertension is, in essence, chemoprevention of cardiovascular and renal disease. Similarly, medical treatment of hypercholesterolemia is chemoprevention of cardiovascular disease. Advances in the understanding of the molecular and cellular biology of carcinogenesis have made chemoprevention of several cancers a real possibility [3].

This chapter describes current leads in prostate cancer chemoprevention and the Prostate Cancer Prevention Trial (PCPT) [4–6]. The PCPT, which began in the fall of 1993, is sponsored by the National Cancer Institute and coordinated by the Southwest Oncology Group. Its primary purpose is to determine whether prolonged 5-alpha-reductase inhibition will decrease an individual's risk for development of prostate cancer or progression of small indolent cancers to larger potentially aggressive ones.

Biological basis of cancer chemoprevention

The strategy of chemoprevention is strongly linked to the concept that carcinogenesis is a multistage process involving initiation, promotion, and progression [3,7]. Carcinogenesis begins with a genetic alteration called initiation. Initiation can occur due to a hereditary genetic alteration or acquired genetic damage due to the action of physical, viral, or chemical carcinogens.

Pienta, K.J., (ed.), DIAGNOSIS AND TREATMENT OF GENITOURINARY MALIGNANCIES. Copyright

Promotion is the part of the process leading to phenotypical change of cells and ultimately to loss of replication control, metastasis, and invasiveness. Progression is the portion of the process in which cancerous cells form malignant tumor with increased morphologic change.

The key concept in cancer chemoprevention is that cancer can be prevented or controlled through interference with the factors causing cancer initiation, promotion, or progression [7]. Cancers ideal for chemoprevention are those with long promotion phases. Prostate cancer is a disease with a high histologic prevalence and a low rate of clinical progression, and it occurs at older ages, when competing causes of mortality are high. Delaying the promotion or progression of a prostatic tumor for just a few years can have significant positive impact.

Potential chemopreventive agents generally have antimutagenic, antioxidant, or antiproliferative activity. Compounds that stop cancer progression or metastases can in some instances serve the same purpose as chemopreventive agents. Agents under active pre-clinical and clinical investigations include initiation inhibitors that induce enzymes that detoxify carcinogens (oltipraz, the flavonoids, and isothiocynanates); antioxidants that scavenge reactive oxygen species (N-acetylcysteine); and inhibitors of enzymes that activate carcinogens (butylated hyroxyanisole). Agents that inhibit promotion include those that inhibit DNA synthesis and cellular proliferation, such as the non-steroidal anti-inflammatory agents, calcium, and selenium. Inhibitors of angiogenesis may also have chemopreventive properties (thalidomide).

Cancer chemoprevention is not yet established in clinical practice. Before a chemoprevention strategy can become standard practice, evidence of its benefit must be gathered from well-designed clinical trials. Chemoprevention trials are usually large, long term, randomized, placebo controlled, and double blind. The size and design of chemoprevention trials often allow for the assessment of drugs for prevention of multiple cancers and study of endpoints beyond cancer. Several clinical chemoprevention trials have been completed in the fields of the upper aerodigestive tract, colon, skin, bladder, breast, and cervical cancers, with surprising and useful results [3,7]. A number of trials will be ongoing into the twenty-first century. Chemoprevention has attracted great interest. If it is to be developed most economically, the strategies tested should target the most common cancers and those at high risk for these cancers.

Prostate cancer: is it a preventable disease?

Populations and cultures around the world have highly variable prostate cancer mortality rates [8]. In addition, it has been noted that Japanese and Chinese men who migrate from Asia to the United States and adopt American habits have a higher prostate cancer mortality rates and risk of prostate cancer death than men in their native country [9–12]. These studies suggest that an environmental influence acquired when adopting American habits or lost when giving up Japanese habits is a causal cofactor or promoter of clinically significant prostate cancer. Removal of the acquired promoter influence or adoption of the antipromoter influence might prevent prostate cancer.

The promotional influences on prostate cancer apparently act over a period of years. Autopsy studies of men dying of trauma and heart disease find that multiple small microscopic foci of prostate cancer are common in early to midadulthood [13]. This finding suggests that promotional influences act over a prolong period and that the window of opportunity for inhibiting cancer promotion is decades long.

Potential approaches for prostate cancer prevention

Difluoromethylornithine (DFMO)

The human prostate is unusual in that benign hyperplasia characterized by cell proliferation and growth is common with age among Western populations. Benign prostatic hyperplasia is amazingly rare in Asian populations, where prostate cancer rates are also low [11,12]. Polyamines are important in cell proliferation and differentiation. Normal cell proliferation is associated with increased synthesis of putrescine, spermidine, and spermine. Depletion of these agents prevents the completion of the S-phase of the cell cycle [14]. Perhaps associated with its tendency for hyperplasia, the benign prostate contains very high concentrations of polyamines and of polyamine synthetic enzymes such as ornithine decarboxylase (ODC), the rate-limiting enzyme in polyamine synthesis. Difluoromethylornithine (DFMO) is an irreversible inhibitor of ODC. In rats, DFMO causes a reduction in prostate weight without effect on other organs. DFMO also inhibits growth of the Dunning R3327 rat prostate carcinoma in vitro and in vivo [15]. There are several small human chemoprevention trials to assess DFMO in bladder and prostate cancer prevention.

Diet

One of the most obvious differences between cultures is diet, and the relationship of diet and prostate cancer has been of great interest [8,16–20]. The dietary factor most widely studied is dietary fat intake. Populations with diets high in fat do have higher relative risks for prostate cancer mortality [21–28]. A number of studies have shown that populations with diets high in fiber and presumably lower in fat are associated with lower incidences of prostate cancer [29–37]. The protective effect of a low-fat diet may lie in its alteration of circulating androgen levels. Reduction of dietary fat intake leads to reduction in urinary and serum androgens.

An evaluation of dietary modification in the form of a low-fat diet would take decades, involve thousands of men, and be difficult to do in a controlled clinical trial. A low-fat diet can, however, be advocated without definitive proof of prostate cancer prevention because of its known collateral health benefits.

Vitamins

Diets rich in vitamin A from plant sources are associated with decreased prostate cancer risk [34,38–40]. It has also been suggested that the intake of vitamin A from animal sources may increase risk [33,35,41,42]. It is likely that there is a lower fat content in the diets of men with high plant vitamin A intake and a higher fat content in the diets of men with high animal vitamin A intake. Although the fat issue cannot be separated from the vitamin A issue, these studies and others have been used to support the study of retinoids (natural and synthetic analogues of vitamin A) as potential prostate cancer chemopreventive agents. There are animal data suggesting that retinoids have prostate cancer chemopreventive activity, and some small human trials have started to assess the effects of the retinoid fenretinide (4-HPR) on human prostate pathologies [43,44].

Population studies suggest that there is a correlation between low levels of vitamin D and increased risk of clinical prostate cancer [45]. There are also some laboratory data suggesting that vitamin D analogues may have some prostate cancer chemopreventive activity. Human study of vitamin D as a chemopreventive has been hampered by the hypercalcemic efforts of vitamin D and its analogues, but interest continues.

The Alpha-tocopherol/Beta-carotene Lung Cancer Prevention Trial was recently completed in Finland. It had the surprising finding that men randomized to alpha-tocopherol (vitamin E) had a one third reduction in prostate cancer when compared to those taking placebo. This trial, which was not designed to study prostate cancer prevention, randomized 28,000 male smokers, age 50 to 69 at entry, to alpha-tocopherol (vitamin E), beta-carotene, and/or placebo in a randomized, 2×2 factorial design. Surprisingly, there was a statistically significant increase in lung cancer incidence and mortality in those receiving beta-carotene after a median follow-up of 6.1 years. This trial demonstrates the importance of testing chemoprevention hypotheses before their widespread implementation, since the results stand in contrast to the predicted outcome. Investigation of these surprising trial results continues. Alpha-tocopherol clearly merits further study as a prostate cancer preventive agent.

Hormonal therapy

Androgenic stimulation is important to prostate biology. Castration of males in childhood and early adulthood prevents benign prostatic hyperplasia and prostate cancer [46,47]. Removal of androgenic stimulation leads to a decrease in prostate weight. Castration has been utilized in treatment of severe prostatism for nearly a century [48]. The hormonal sensitivity of prostate cancer has been exploited in treatment since 1941 [48].

It has been suggested that populations with greater androgenic stimulation of the prostate may be more prone to develop clinically significant prostate cancer [49,50]. Studies testing this hypothesis vary widely in their results, because such studies are difficult [49]. Androgens other than testosterone may be responsible for androgenic stimulation of the prostate, and serum androgen levels may not correlate with intraprostatic androgen activity. Several studies have found no difference in baseline circulating testosterone level in prostate cancer patients when compared to controls [51–54]. Other studies have found a positive correlation between androgen levels and prostate cancer risk. Barrett-Connor and colleagues studied 1008 men for 14 years and found a positive dose–response correlation for plasma androstenedione level and the development of prostate cancer [55]. Meikle et al. observed a higher sex hormone binding globulin level in men with prostate cancer when compared to controls and noted a higher testosterone conversion rate in patients with prostate cancer [56].

While studies of hormonal differences in men with prostate cancer yield unclear results, differences in mean androgenic activity among populations may explain varying risks of prostate cancer mortality. Ross et al. observed a higher circulating testosterone concentration in African-American men when compared to white American men [57]. African-American men have a twofold increased prostate cancer mortality rate in comparison to white Americans. Ross and colleagues have also found higher levels of 3-alpha, 17-beta-androstenediol glucuronide and androsterone glucuronide in black and white American men when compared to Japanese men, who are at very low risk for prostate cancer mortality [58]. 3-Alpha, 17-beta-androstenediol glucuronide and androsterone glucuronide are thought to be markers for 5-alpha-reductase activity.

The role of dietary fat in the etiology of human prostate cancer can be linked to the concept that androgenic stimulation causes prostate cancer. The populations with higher androgen levels also have higher average amounts of fat in their diet [20]. It is theorized that high levels of dietary fat cause higher bioavailability and production of sexual hormones [59–61]. Precise mechanisms are not well defined, but it is known that plasma concentrations of fatty acids are responsive to dietary fat, and these levels, in turn, do correlate with concentrations of bioavailable sex steroids [62]. Fatty acids inhibit binding of gonadal steroids to serum sex hormone-binding globulin, causing greater bioavailable of gonadal hormones [63]. In addition, a low-fat, high-fiber diet decreases the enterohepatic circulation of gonadal hormones, resulting in increased fecal excretion of gonadal hormones and possibly lowering serum levels [64].

In animal models, androgens promote cell proliferation and inhibit prostate cell death [65]. Almost all animal models of prostate carcinogenesis require exogenous androgen administration to induce prostate cancer [66,67]. While the precise role of androgens in the etiology of human prostate cancer is unclear, the above facts taken as a whole suggest that prostate cancer can be prevented if androgenic reduction, inhibition, or blockade can be applied. Most hormonal treatments that remove androgens or block their cellular effects have side effects that significantly limit the usefulness of these treatments as chemopreventives. A key point in prostate cancer biology makes possible tolerable reduction in androgenic stimulation of the prostate. The more potent and major androgen in the normal prostate is dihydrotestosterone (DHT) and not testosterone [68,69]. The enzyme 5-alpha-reductase within the prostate converts testosterone (T) to the more potent dihydrotestosterone (DHT) (figure 11-1). This enzyme can be blocked with minimal toxicity.

In humans, DHT promotes development of prostate cells, benign prostatic hyperplasia (BPH), and possibly serves as a promoter for prostate cancer. An observation of nature documents the key role that 5-alpha-reductase-2 and

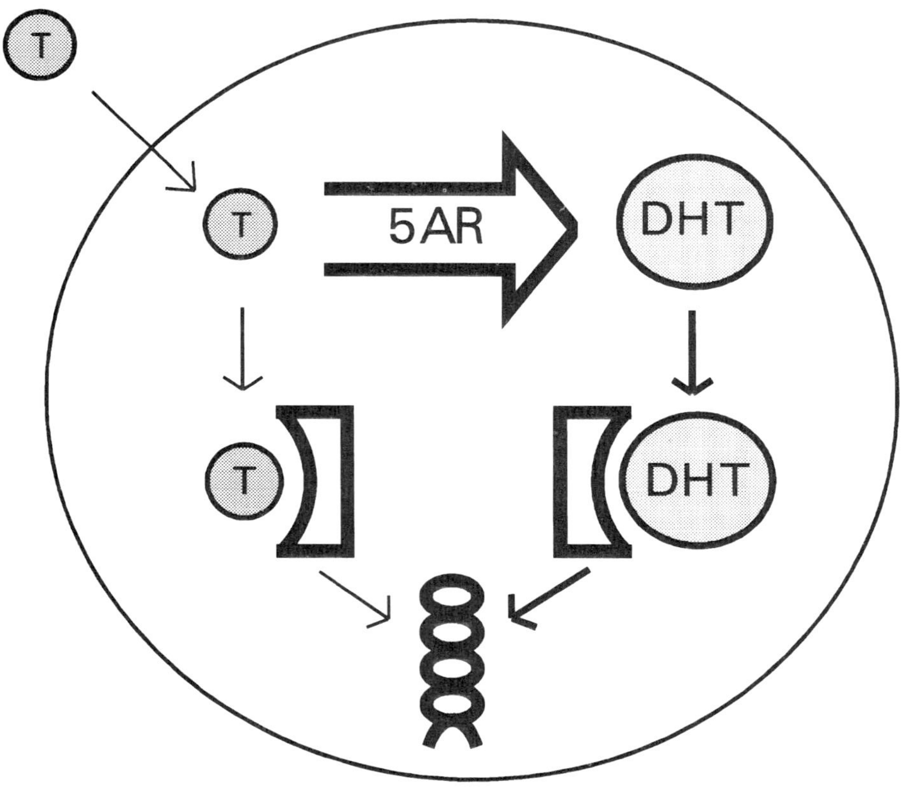

Figure 11-1. 5-alpha-reductase in the prostate cell. Testosterone (T) secreted by the adrenal or testes enters the prostate and is converted by 5-alpha-reductase (5AR) to the more potent dihydrotestosterone (DHT). This conversion occurs with very high efficiency in the normal male.

DHT plays in prostate development and prostate cancer [70,71]. Males with inherited homozygous 5-alpha-reductase deficiency are pseudohermaphrodites with a female or ambiguous external genitalia until puberty. The normal increase in T production at puberty induces development of a small phallus and virilization. After puberty, individuals with the enzyme deficiency usually become morphologically and functionally normal males, although they never develop acne or male pattern baldness. Men deficient in 5-alpha reductase have underdeveloped prostates and do not develop prostate cancer even though they maintain normal serum testosterone levels after puberty. No other illnesses are associated with 5-alpha-reductase deficiency, and females with the inherited enzyme deficiency have no known medical sequelae [41,70].

The enzyme 5-alpha-reductase is a nuclear-membrane-bound NADPH-dependent delta-3-ketosteroid 5-alpha-oxidoreductase. Its primary function is to convert testosterone to DHT [69,72]. DHT is 8 to 10 times more potent an androgen than testosterone [68,69]. 5-Alpha-reduction amplifies the androgenic effect of testosterone. There are two 5-alpha-reductase isoenzymes: 5-alpha-reductase-1 is present in low levels in a number of tissues, and 5-alpha-reductase-2 is found in androgen-sensitive cells of the skin, liver, and prostate [41]. The testes and adrenal glands secrete T into the bloodstream. In the normal prostate, a substantial fraction of T diffusing into 5-alpha-reductase-containing cells is irreversibly converted to DHT. Inhibitors of 5-alpha-reductase greatly reduced intraprostatic DHT levels and thus androgenic stimulation of the prostate without the severe systemic effects of systemic androgen blockade.

The recent availability of a well-tolerated 5-alpha-reductase inhibitor, finasteride, means that the prevention of prostate cancer may be possible [73]. Finasteride (Proscar) was approved by the U.S. F.D.A. in 1992 for the treatment of benign prostatic hyperplasia [73]. Preclinical and clinical studies demonstrate that seven days of finasteride, 5 mg daily, causes a 70% decrease in serum DHT levels with an 8% to 10% increase in serum testosterone. This dosing causes intraprostatic DHT levels to decrease by greater than 90% and T levels to increase by a factor of 5 to 7. Finasteride therapy causes an estimated overall decrease in androgenic stimulation of the prostate of more than 75% [69,72].

5-alpha-reductase inhibition and prostate cancer

A cancer-preventive manipulation need not have antitumor activity in order to be effective. There are, however, data showing that 5-alpha-reductase inhibitors have some antitumor activity. Several studies using prostate tumor in tissue culture or rodent implant models have demonstrated that 5-alpha-reductase inhibitors can inhibit and prevent the progression of some prostate cancers [42,74]. PC3 and DU145 are relatively androgen-insensitive human prostate cancer cell lines. In tissue culture, finasteride causes dose-dependent growth inhibition of these cell lines [75]. This activity suggests that finasteride may be interfering with additional autocrine mechanisms to sustain growth [75]. It is also conceivable that these cell lines are not relatively androgen insensitive but actually hypersensitive to androgen stimulation (and therefore frugal in its use of androgen). The human prostate cancer PC-82 is a moderately differentiated human prostatic adenocarcinoma cell line. Its growth in mice is inhibited when 5-alpha-reductase inhibitors are administered. Enzyme inhibitors also suppress growth of implanted hormone-sensitive Dunning R-3327G rat prostate tumor [76–78].

Available rodent carcinogenesis models are not ideally suited for testing the finasteride cancer prevention hypothesis. Most of these models involve pulse doses of a chemical carcinogen followed by chronic administration of high doses of androgens [61,67]. The exogenous androgen can override the androgen reduction effect of finasteride. The fact that androgen administration is necessary to promote prostate cancer development in laboratory animals is in itself supportive of the theory that decreasing androgenic stimulation can lower prostate cancer risk. Tsukamoto and colleagues have demonstrated that finasteride therapy prevents prostate cancer in the F344 rat model [79]. In this study, rats were administered an initiator and chronic low-dose testosterone propionate therapy. Rats administered finasteride or the androgen blocker casodex had a lower rate of prostate cancer development when compared to controls [79].

In a human trial involving men with stage D prostate cancer, finasteride induces a small decline in PSA. The clinical significance of this decline is unknown, but it does indicate some anticancer activity [80]. Andriole and colleagues [81] evaluated the long-term effect of finasteride versus placebo on serum prostate-specific antigen levels of men with measurable serum PSA after prostatectomy. Patients treated with finasteride had a delayed increase in PSA compared with placebo, and there was also the suggestion of fewer recurrences. Among those with recurrence, there was no effect on initial response to subsequent hormonal therapies. These data suggest that finasteride has a tumor suppression effect and is unlikely to adversely affect the success of future therapies [81].

An effective cancer chemopreventive agent must be administered in a tolerable fashion and have minimal side effects, if any. An agent with other gains (benefits beyond cancer prevention) is desirable. Finasteride has few side effects [72,82,83]. It is widely used throughout the world; indeed, over a million men in the age group at risk for prostate cancer take the drug daily to treat benign prostatic hyperplasia.

The prostate cancer prevention trial

The Prostate Cancer Prevention Trial (PCPT) was designed by a multidisciplinary group of scientists convened by the Division of Cancer Prevention and Control of the National Cancer Institute. The trial began accruing subjects in the fall of 1993 and has accrued remarkably well. The hypothesis of the trial is that a prolonged finasteride-induced decrease in androgenic stimulation of the prostate will inhibit or retard the progression of prostate cells through the carcinogenic process, resulting in a decreased period prevalence of diagnosed prostate cancer.

The PCPT is a randomized placebo controlled trial involving 18,000 men, aged 55 or above in good health (figure 11-2) [5,6]. Each subject will be treated

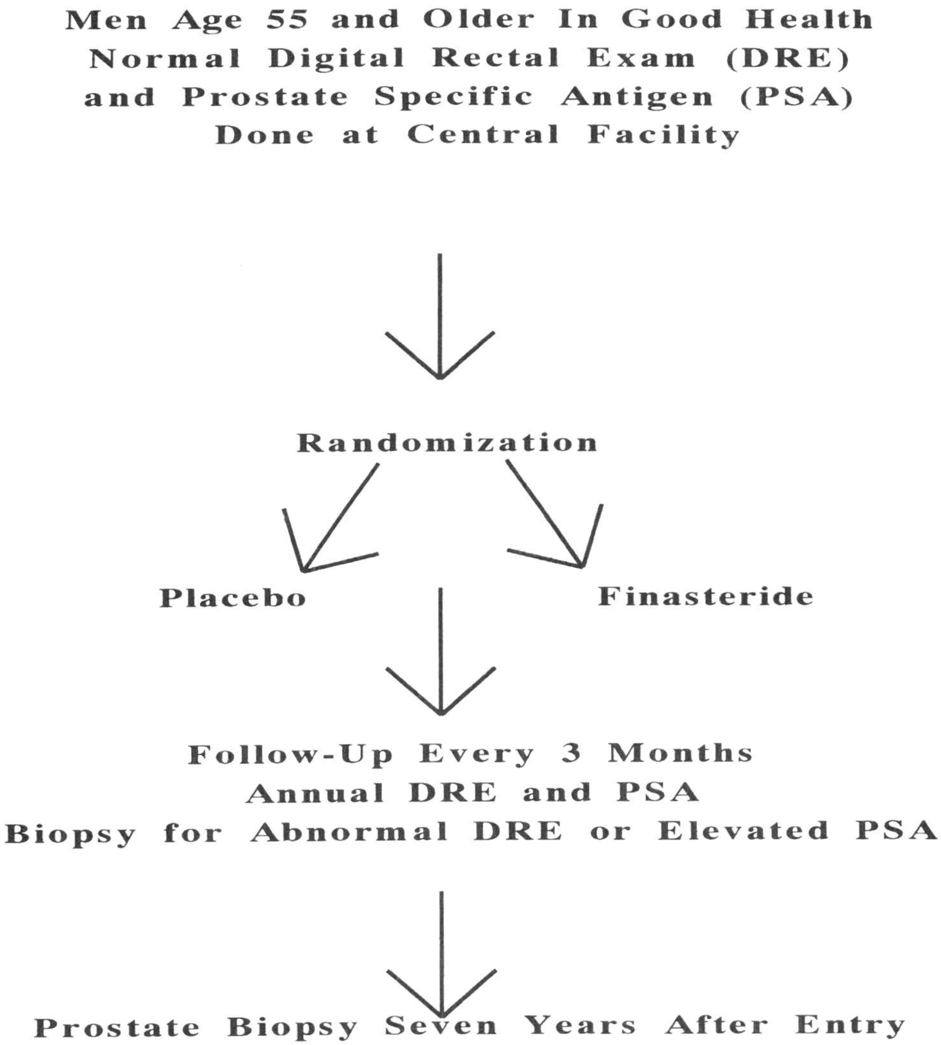

Figure 11-2. The Prostate Cancer Prevention Trial Schema. All men are treated with finasteride (5 mg/day) or placebo for a period of seven years. All patients receive yearly assessment for development of prostate cancer. All who have not been diagnosed with prostate cancer at the end of the treatment period will receive a sextant biopsy of the prostate.

for seven years. The actual trial will span approximately ten years, with all participants followed for life. Prostatic digital rectal examination must not be suggestive of malignancy. Subjects can have an enlarged prostate, but should not have symptoms of prostatism so severe that a transurethral resection of the prostate (TURP) is thought necessary in the near future. PSA must be less than 3.0 ng/ml (by Hybritech, normal is usually considered less than 4.0 ng/ml). These requirements are an attempt to be as sure as possible that men entering the trial do not have prostate cancer.

Subjects undergo digital rectal examination and serum PSA on an annual basis. Because finasteride decreases serum PSA and there are concerns about interassay PSA variability, all PSAs are analyzed at a central laboratory, and corrected numerical values are reported to patients and physicians. An algorithm has been worked out to minimize the risk of a detection bias (to assure that both arms of the study have an equal number of blind sextant prostatic biopsies to evaluate for malignancy due to PSA abnormality) [84]. To further assure as little bias as possible, all subjects are asked to undergo transrectal ultrasound and prostate biopsy after seven years on study. The trial design has a 90% power to detect a 25% reduction in prostate cancer period prevalence.

This trial allows for more than just assessment of finasteride in the prevention of cancer. It allows for the prevention of benign prostatic hypertrophy (BPH) and prevention of the need for a transurethral resection of the prostate. This study will yield information on prostate cancer screening, particularly the use of changing PSA over time in men on finasteride and in the placebo groups. There is some evidence that 5-alpha-reductase inhibition may increase the specificity of PSA screening for prostate cancer [85,86]. Annual serum samples are being preserved so that promising future tests may be evaluated. The trial is also an opportunity for biologists to obtain tissue and history, thereby enhancing the opportunity to understand benign and malignant prostate pathologies.

The future

As our abilities to find more and more prostate cancer continue, the need for effective prostate cancer prevention will increase. The PCPT is the first large-scale prostate cancer chemoprevention study. While basic research may ultimately provide reliable intermediate biomarkers that can make large clinical trials unnecessary in the future, the concept of chemoprevention is here to stay.

Note

1. The opinions expressed herein are those of the authors and do not necessarily reflect those of the Departments of the Army, Defense, or Health and Human Services.

References

1. Woolf SH (1995). N Engl J Med 333:1401–1405.
2. Sporn MB, Dunlop NM, Newton DL (1976). Fed Proc 35 1332–1338.
3. Lippman SM, Benner SE, Ki Hong W (1994). J Clin Oncol 12:851–873.
4. Feigl P, Blumenstein B, Thompson IM, Crowley J, Wolf M, Kramer BS, Coltman C, Brawley OW, Ford LG (1995). Controlled Clin Trials 16:150–163.
5. Brawley OW, Ford LG, Thompson IM, Perlman JA, Kramer BS (1994). Cancer Epidemiol Biomarkers Prev 3:177–182.
6. Thompson IM, Feigl P, Coltman C (1995). In Chemoprevention of Prostate Cancer with Finasteride, DeVita V, Hellman S, Rosenberg S (eds), vol. 5, pp. 57–76.
7. Sporn MB (1991). Cancer Res 51:6215–6218.
8. Pienta KJ, Esper PS (1993). Ann Intern Med 118:793–803.
9. Meikle AW, Smith JA (1996). Urol Clin North Am 17:709–718.
10. Shimizu H, Ross RK, Bernstein L, Yatani R, Henderson BE, Mack TM (1991). Br J Cancer 963–966.
11. Muir CS, Nectoux J, Staszewski J (1991). Acta Oncol 30:133–140.
12. Flanders WD (1984). Prostate 5:621–629.
13. Sakr WA, Haas GP, Cassin BF, Pontes JE, Crissman JD (1993). J Urol 150:379–385.
14. Heby O (1981). Differentiation 19:1–20.
15. Heston WDW, Kadmon D, Lazan (1982). Prosate 3:383–389.
16. Dunn JE (1975). Cancer Res 35:3240–3245.
17. Haenszel W, Kurihoro M (1969). J Natl Cancer Inst 40:43–68.
18. Yu H, Harris RE, Gao R, Wynder EL (1991). Int J Epidemiol 20:76–81.
19. Muir CS, Nectoux J, Staszewski J (1991). Acta Oncol 30:133–140.
20. Pienta KJ, Esper PS (1993). J Natl Cancer Inst 85:1538–1541.
21. Kolonel LN, Nomura AMY, Hinds MW, Hirohata T, Hankin JH, Lee J (1983). Cancer Res 43:(Suppl)2397–2402.
22. Lew EA, Garfinkel L (1979). J Chron Dis 32:563–576.
23. Severson RK, Grove JS, Nomura AM, Stemmerman GN (1988). Br Med J 297:713–715.
24. Kaul L, Heshmat MY, Kovi J, Jackson MA, Jackson AG, Jones GW (1987). Nutr Cancer 9:123–128.
25. Severson RK, Nomura AMY, Grove JS, Stemmermann GN (1989). Cancer Res 49:1857–1860.
26. Berg JW (1975). Cancer Res 35:3345–3350.
27. Armstrong B, Doll R (1975). Int J Cancer 15:617–631.
28. Rose DP, Boyar, AP, Wynder EL (1986). Cancer 58:2363–2371.
29. Rotkin ID (1977). Cancer Treat Rep 61:173–180.
30. Hutchinson GB (1976). Semin Oncol 3:151–159.
31. Slattery ML, Schumacher MC, West DW, Robinson LM, French TK (1990). Am J Clin Nutr 52:752–757.
32. Snowdon DA, Phillips RL, Choi W (1984). Am J Epidemiol 120:244–250.
33. Mettlin C, Selenskas S, Natarajan N, Huben R (1989). Cancer 64:605–612.
34. Mills PK, Beeson WL, Phillips RL, Fraser GE (1989). Cancer 64:598–604.
35. Hirayama T (1979). Natl Cancer Inst Monogr 53:149–155.
36. Heshma MY, Kaul L, Kovi J, Jackson MA, Jackson AC, Jones GW (1985). Prostate 6:7–17.
37. Ohno Y, Yoshida O, Oishi K, Yamabe H, Schroeder F (1988). Cancer Res 48:1331–1336.
38. Kolonel LN, Hinds MW, Nomura AMY, Hankin JH, Lee J (1985). Natl Cancer Inst Monogr 69:137–142.
39. Graham S, Haughey B, Marshall J, et al. (1983). J Natl Cancer Inst 70:687–692.
40. Kolonel LN, Yoshizawa CN, Hankin JH (1988). Am J Epidemiol 127:999–1012.
41. Anderson S, Berman DM, Jenkins EP, Russell DW (1991). Nature 354:159.
42. Kadoham N, Karr JP, Murphy GP, Sandberg AA (1984). Cancer Res 44:4947–4954.
43. Pollard M, Luckert PH. Sporn MB (1996). Cancer Res 51:3610–3611.

44. Slawn K, Kadmon D, Park SH (1996). Cancer Res 53:4461–4465.
45. Schwartz GG, Hulka BS (1990). Anticancer Res 10:1307–1312.
46. Wynder ER, Mabuchi K, Whitmore W (1971). Cancer 28:344–368.
47. Hovenian MS, Deming CL (1948). Surg Gynecol Obstet 86:29–35.
48. Huggins C, Hodges CV (1941). Cancer Res 1:293–297.
49. Ross RK (1990). Proc Annu Meet Am Assoc Cancer Res 31:457–458.
50. Montie JE, Pienta KJ (1994). Urology 43:892–899.
51. Meikle W, Stanish WM (1982). J Clin Endocrinol Metab 54:1104–1108.
52. Ghanadian R, Puah KM, O'Donohue EPM (1979). Br J Cancer 39:696–699.
53. Hammond GL, Kontturi M, Vihko R (1978). Clin Endocrinol 9:113–121.
54. Comstock GW, Gordon GB, Hsing AW (1993). Cancer Epidemiol Biomarkers Prev 2:219–221.
55. Barrett-Connor E, Garland C, McPhillips JB, Khaw KT, Wingard DL (1990). Cancer Res 50:169–173.
56. Meikle AW, Smith JA, Stringham JD (1987). Prostate 10:25–31.
57. Ross RK, Berstein L, Judd H, Hanisch R, Pike M, Henderson B (1986). J Natl Cancer Inst 76:45–48.
58. Ross RK, Berstein L, Lobo RA, Shimizu H, Stanczyk FZ, Pike M (1992). Lancet 339:887–889.
59. Hamalainen E, Adlercreutz H, Puska P (1984). J Steroid Biochem 20:459–464.
60. Coffey DS (1979). Geneva Int Union Against Cancer 48:4–23.
61. Noble RL (1959). Cancer Res 19:1125–1139.
62. Bruning PF, Bonfrer JMG (1989). Cancer Res 46:2606–2609.
63. Street C, Howell RJS, Perry L (1989). Acta Endocrinol 120:175–179.
64. Pusater DJ, Roth WT, Ross JK, Shultz TD (1990). Am J Clin Nutr 51:371–377.
65. Kyprianou N, Isaacs JT (1988). Endocrinology 122:552–562.
66. Nobel RL (1977). Cancer Res 37:1929.
67. Shirai T, Tamano S, Kato T, Iwasaki S, Takahashi S, Ito N (1991). Cancer Res 51:1264–1269.
68. Grino P, Griffin J, Wilson J (1990). Endocrinology 126:1165–1172.
69. Geller J (1990). J Clin Endocrinol Metab 71:1552–1555.
70. Petersen RE, Imperato-McGinley J, Gautier T, Sturla E (1977). Am J Med 62:170–191.
71. Imperato-McGinley J, Guerrero L, Gautier T, Petersen RE (1974). Science 186:1213–1215.
72. McConnell JD, Wilson J, George FW, Geller J, Pappas F, Stoner E (1992). J Clin Endocrinol Metab 74:505–508.
73. Gormley G, Stoner E, Bruskewitz R, et al. (1992). N Engl J Med 327:1185–1191.
74. Petrow V, Padilla GM, Mukherji S, Marts SA (1984). J Pharm Pharamacol 36:352–353.
75. Bologna M, Muzi P, Biordi L, Pestuccia CV (1992). Current Therapeut Res 5:799–813.
76. Damber JE, Bergh A, Daehlin L, Petrov V, Landstrom M (1992). Prostate 20:187–190.
77. Lamb JC, English H, Levandoski PL, Rhodes GR, Johnson RK, Isaacs JR (1992). Endocrinology 130:685–694.
78. Brooks JR, Berman C, Nguyen H (1991). Prostate 18:215–227.
79. Tsukamoto S, Adaza H, Imada S, Koiso K, Tomoyuki S, Ideyama Y, Kudo M (1995). J Natl Cancer Inst 87:842–843.
80. Presti JC, Fair WR, Andriole G, Sogani PC, Seidman FD, Ng J, Gormley G (1992). J Urol 148:1201–1204.
81. Andriole G, Lieber MD, Smith JA, et al. (1995). Urology 45:491–497.
82. Stoner E, The Finasteride Study Group (1994). Urology 43:284–294.
83. Rittmaster R (1994). N Engl J Med 330:120–125.
84. Thompson IM, Coltman C, Brawley OW, Ryan A (1995). Semin Urol 13:122–129.
85. Guess HA, Heyse JF, Gormley G (1993). Prostate 22:31–37.
86. Stoner E, Round E, Ferguson D, Gormley G, The Finasteride Study Group (1994). J Urol 151:1296–1300.

12. Total androgen blockade for prostate cancer: the end does not justify the means

Milind Javle and Derek Raghavan

It has been known for more than two centuries that the growth of the normal prostate and of its malignancies is dependent upon hormonal function [1,2]. More recently, the application of this knowledge to the management of advanced prostate cancer has been rationalized, building upon the Nobel-prize-winning observation that castration or the administration of estrogens causes regression of advanced prostate cancer in dogs [3,4]. The physiology of prostatic growth is summarized in figure 12-1 [5].

Testosterone, the dominant stimulus for prostatic growth, is converted to dihydrotestosterone (DHT) within prostate cells by 5α-reductase. Testosterone and DHT bind to the androgen receptor and, in turn, this complex interacts with DNA, leading to increased protein synthesis. Adrenal androgens are also converted to testosterone and DHT in the prostate, and it is believed that they also may contribute to the stimulation of growth of prostatic tissues. However, there is also evidence against the importance of adrenal androgens in this context — for example, patients with hypogonadotrophic hypogonadism do not have normal prostate development, despite the presence of adrenal androgens.

In advanced or metastatic disease, depending upon the criteria of assessment of outcome [6,7], tumor shrinkage can be achieved in 50% to 70% of cases in response to bilateral orchiectomy, the administration of systemic estrogens, the use of analogues of luteinizing hormone-releasing hormone (LHRH), or by combinations of some of these approaches (combined androgenic blockade) [8–10].

Combined androgenic blockade

Combined androgenic blockade (CAB), in which central inhibition of androgen production (i.e., medical or surgical orchiectomy) is combined with peripheral blockade of circulating androgens (e.g., the use of flutamide or cyproterone acetate to block the function of adrenal androgens) has arisen largely from the work of Labrie and colleagues, who have reported objective tumor regression in nearly 100% of cases of prostate cancer in preclinical

Pienta, K.J., (ed.), DIAGNOSIS AND TREATMENT OF GENITOURINARY MALIGNANCIES.

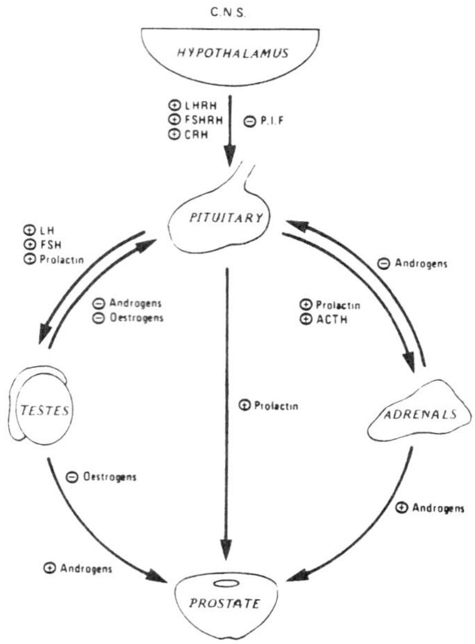

Figure 12-1. Physiology of hormonal therapy of prostate cancer. (From Raghavan and Lange in Shearman (RP), *Clinical Reproductive Endocrinology*, Churchill Livingstone, London, 1985, p. 736.

models and then in clinical trials [11,12]. While extremely important in concept, this work has been questioned subsequently because of the inability of other investigators to duplicate the very high reported response rates. Nevertheless, these studies have given rise to a generation of subsequent studies of combined androgenic blockade.

Perhaps one of the most important studies to test this concept, and certainly the most widely cited in the literature, was reported by Crawford and colleagues [13] for North American Intergroup. In this randomized clinical trial, 300 patients with metastatic prostate cancer were allocated to treatment with leuprolide and placebo, and 303 received leuprolide and flutamide. Progression-free survival was 13.8 and 16.9 months, respectively, and the median survival times were 28.3 and 35.6 months, respectively. When viewed in the context of the overall life expectancy of patients with advanced prostate cancer, this result, despite its statistical significance, is not viewed as clinically of great importance. However, of interest, in a *retrospective* subset analysis, it was noted that a more substantial difference in outcome was seen among patients with good performance status and minimal metastatic disease (i.e., bone metastases confined to the axial skeleton and/or lymph node involvement). In this small subgroup, at 96 months of follow-up, there was a 29-month difference in progression-free survival and a 19-month difference in median total survival in favor of the CAB arm [14]. In addition to the small numbers in this subset, it should also be noted that in the whole trial, the complete response rate to CAB was 7.9%, compared to 7.1% after monotherapy, suggesting that the major biological impact was derived among the patients who sustained partial objective responses (35.7% with CAB; 28.2% after monotherapy); in fact, it seems unlikely that, with similar complete response rates, a difference in the frequency of partial remission would have a particularly important biological impact on any disease. Notwithstanding the above, Crawford and others have interpreted the results of the Intergroup study as supporting the importance of the role of CAB and have launched another randomized trial in patients with less advanced disease to assess the impact of CAB. The results are awaited with interest.

By contrast, several other randomized trials have been reported in which the authors have interpreted their data to show no significant role for CAB. For example, in the first report of a trial conducted by the European Organization for the Research and Treatment of Cancer (EORTC), Keupens et al. found no difference in outcome for patients randomized to receive orchiectomy alone versus those who received goserelin plus flutamide [15]. However, of interest, a later analysis of this study suggested a survival advantage for CAB, particularly in a subset analysis of patients with minimal disease [16]. In our view, substantially different results of a randomized trial in two closely spaced consecutive reports, in a disease with a relatively long natural history, calls into question the power and accuracy of that study.

Similar studies have been effected by the Danish Prostatic Cancer Group (orchiectomy vs. goserelin vs. goserelin plus flutamide) [17], the International Prostate Cancer Study Group (goserelin vs. goserelin plus flutamide) [18], and the Italian Prostatic Cancer Project Study Group (goserelin vs. goserelin plus flutamide) [19]. None of these has shown an important difference in outcome, especially when total survival was considered as the primary endpoint. Less clearly defined are differences in disease-free survival, although this endpoint can be influenced substantially by the methodology employed to detect relapse [7].

The Australian Prostate Cancer Study Group [20] compared the use of bilateral orchiectomy plus flutamide vs. bilateral orchiectomy plus placebo. Although this trial accrued only 222 patients, and was interpreted as showing no significant difference in response rate (45% and 56%, respectively) or relapse-free survival, the patients treated with bilateral orchiectomy plus flutamide had a shorter median overall survival (23 months) than those treated by combined androgenic blockdade (31 months), but this difference did not achieve statistical significance. Similarly, the time points at which 25% and 75% of deaths had occurred were not significantly different in this trial.

Perhaps one of the most strident arguments against the impact of CAB is the recent meta-analysis published by the International Prostate Trialists' Collaborative Group [21]. In this analysis of all the registered randomized clinical trials comparing CAB with monotherapy, more than 5000 deaths had occurred. Dalesio and colleagues reported a remarkable lack of difference in end results when the whole group was considered, despite small differences in favor of CAB in some of the constituent trials (see figure 12-2) [21].

Finally, in considering whether to recommend CAB, the toxicity of the regimen should be considered. Although many patients in the various clinical trials were able to tolerate this regimen for periods measured in years, it should not be forgotten that flutamide can cause gastrointestinal side effects, including nausea, diarrhea, and occasionally hepatitis. It has been suggested that some of the newer analogues, such as biclutamide, will be better tolerated and will thus allow the true impact of CAB to be realized (as a function of improved patient compliance). If it is found that biclutamide is more active than flutamide, it is possible that an improved outcome will be achieved by this approach. However, it seems unlikely that amelioration of a relatively modest profile of toxicity, in the absence of enhanced anticancer activity, will have a major impact on survival in this context.

Another consideration is cost-effectiveness. The annual cost of flutamide was reported as $2500 per patient [22]. If one considers the major 'positive' trial [13], with a median survival of just under three years from CAB compared to 28 months for monotherapy, the cost per year of life saved was more than $12,000 [22]. While it is difficult to place a specific value on human life, we must be aware of the ongoing reduction of health resources available, and it will become increasingly important to define the presence or absence of real,

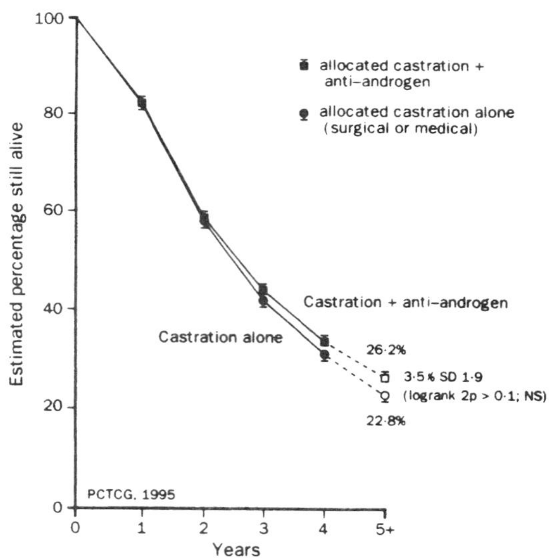

Figure 12-2. Survival in 22 randomised prostate cancer trials: MAB vs castration alone. 5710 patients, 3283 deaths. In the first year there were 475 deaths out of 2512 person-years in the MAB group (logrank O-E = −6.0, variance = −196.1, NS) versus 498/2561 in the controls. In the second year there were 594/1778. (From Prostate Cancer Trialists' Collaborative Group, *Lancet*, 1995, 346: 265–269.

quantifiable benefit when additional therapies are being considered for routine use.

Finally, it is not surprising to find only a modest impact from CAB, compared to monotherapy, when one considers the broader context of prostate cancer, a malignancy that is composed of diverse constitutive elements that include hormonally sensitive and nonresponsive elements.

Heterogeneity of prostate cancer: impact on the outcome of hormone therapy

There is clear evidence from preclinical models and some clinicopathological studies that diverse populations of tumor cells, with different morphological and functional characteristics, are present within individual deposits of cancer at the time of first presentation. This finding is further manifested by the range of histologic, ultrastructural, hormone receptor, growth factor receptor, and flow cytometric features present in human biopsy specimens [23–28].

Of particular importance is the demonstration of coincidental subpopulations of cells with classical adenocarcinomatous features intermingled with cells that exhibit neurocrine differentiation [29,30], features of small cell undifferentiated carcinoma [24,30,31] and even the presence of cells that actually represent transitional cell carcinoma [32]. It thus has seemed unlikely that any one procedure would permanently control these disparate tumor cell populations, at least in the setting of advanced disease [6].

The factors that regulate growth, differentiation, tumor progression, and response to treatment in prostate cancer have not been defined, although candidate genes being studied include Rb, ras, p53, bcl, neu, erbB-2 and those governing expression of the androgen receptor, TGF-beta, and other growth factors [33–39]. The ability to identify these more accurately and to define prognostic determinants with greater specificity will allow more appropriate selection of aggressive therapy for localized disease with greater metastatic potential as well as more precise management of patients with advanced disease.

Furthermore, since the apparent genetic instability of the tissues that comprise adenocarcinoma of the prostate will tend to confound simple strategies of management of advanced disease, some understanding of the molecular biology of this complex disease is essential. Several genetic alterations have been proposed in prostate cancer, ranging from allelic loss to point mutations and changes in DNA methylation. The mutated phenotype is known to play a role in carcinogenesis [40]. Mutations in oncogenes, the genes involved in DNA repair, and tumor suppressor genes have been proposed as possible mechanisms leading to tumorigenesis. Three studies have documented low-frequency *ras* gene mutations in prostate cancer [41–43], although two Japanese studies have shown that mutations of *ras* occur in both latent and clinically manifest disease [44,45], implying racial differences in the evolution of this disease.

Cytogenetic analysis has revealed aberrations of several chromosomes in association with the genesis of prostate cancer, including 7q, 8, 10, and 16 [46–48]. Furthermore, mutations have been identified in the suppressor genes, P53 and Rb, located respectively on chromosomes 17 and 13 [49,50]. Of particular interest, p53 mutations appear to be relatively uncommon in primary prostate cancer and are seen frequently in bone metastases, implying that mutation of p53 may be a late event in the generation of prostate cancer [51,52].

Hypermethylation of CpG sequences (associated with the 5′ regulatory region of the gene) is associated with gene inactivation. Hypermethylation at polymorphic locus D17S5 on chromosome 17p13.3 has been associated with colonic and bronchogenic cancers. This has also been demonstrated in prostate cancer cell lines [53], suggesting that there may be a tumor suppressor gene on chromosome 17p that is separate from p53.

Thus, the broad range of genetic anomalies associated with prostate cancer appears likely to be intimately involved in the constitutive heterogeneity of function of prostate cancer, and in turn to create a more complex target for therapeutic endeavors.

Future strategies for treatment of advanced prostate cancer

For the management of advanced disease, alternative strategies have already been explored, including the use of first-line cytotoxic chemotherapy [54] and the combination of cytotoxic chemotherapy with endocrine treatment (chemoendocrine therapy) [55,56]. The use of first-line cytotoxic chemotherapy has not been successful in improving outcomes, and despite encouraging objective response rates with chemoendocrine therapy, randomized clinical trials have either demonstrated no survival benefit [57] or, in one study without clearly defined randomization, only a modest difference in outcome in favor of chemoendocrine treatment [58]. The problem may also be that the traditionally available cytotoxic agents are simply not very active against prostate cancer. Recently, several innovative cytotoxic treatments have been assessed for advanced prostate cancer, including suramin [59], mitoxantrone [60], and oral cyclophosphamide [61], each of which appears to be demonstrating substantial anticancer activity. It may be that the incorporation of such agents into the treatment of advanced cancer may make significant contributions to the prolongation of patient survival.

However, in view of our current concepts regarding tumor progression, with the consequent alterations in tumor characteristics between early-stage and advanced disease, it appears quite possible that systemic therapy could be much more effective in the treatment of early-stage disease than in metastatic disease, lending support to the concept of the early introduction of systemic therapy into the management of prostate cancer.

There are two situations in which CAB is likely to have a continued role in routine management: 1) for patients who are about to commence treatment with LHRH agonists (to avoid the phenomenon of tumor flare that arises from the transient agonist phase of testosterone production after the initial administration of the LHRH agonist); and 2) for cases of documented production of significant androgenic steroids from the adrenal glands, where either peripheral blockade (with flutamide or biclutamide) or central reduction of steroid production (by aminoglutethimide or ketoconazole) may have a role. Otherwise, it seems unlikely that CAB will have any major role in the routine management of advanced prostate cancer in the future. Whether there is some specific benefit for CAB in the management of 'minimal' metastatic disease will become clear upon the completion of the current Intergroup trial. In the absence of convincing data, our standard approach is to recommend bilateral orchiectomy for advanced disease or initial CAB for patients who refuse orchiectomy, with cessation of flutamide after the initial agonist phase. The provocative report by the Southwest Oncology Group [57] of an apparent survival benefit from estrogens compared to orchiectomy in an assessment of chemoendocrine therapy requires further testing. Finally, the exploration, in well-structured clinical trials, of the combination of cytotoxic chemotherapy and hormonal manipulation may produce a real improvement in the results of treatment of advanced prostate cancer, rather than the statistically significant but clinically unimportant impact of combined androgenic blockade.

References

1. Hunter J (1786). Observations on Certain Parts of the Animal Oeconomy. Bibliotheca osteriana: London.
2. Cabot AT (1896). The question of castration for enlarged prostate. Ann Surg 24:265–309.
3. Huggins C, Hodges CV (1941). Studies on prostatic cancer. I. The effect of castration, of estrogen and of androgen injection on serum phosphatases in metastatic carcinoma of the prostate. Cancer Res 1:293–297.
4. Scott WW, Menon M, Walsh PC (1980). Hormonal therapy of prostatic cancer. Cancer 45:1929–1936.
5. Raghavan D, Lange PH (1985). Endocrine aspects of genitourinary neoplasia. In Shearman RP (ed), Clinical Reproductive Endocrinology. Churchill Livingstone: Edinburgh, London, Melbourne, New York, pp. 727–752.
6. Raghavan D (1988). Non-hormone chemotherapy for prostate cancer: principles of treatment and application to the testing of new drugs. Semin Oncol 15:371–389.
7. Raghavan D, Tannock IF (1989). Clinical trials in genitourinary oncology: What have they achieved? In Smith PH (ed), Combination Therapy in Urological Malignancy. Springer Verlag: London, Berlin, pp. 225–253.
8. Leuprolide Study Group (1984). Leuprolide versus diethylstilbestrol for metastatic prostate cancer. N Engl J Med 311:1281–1286.
9. Goldenberg L, Bruchovsky N (1986). Hormonal manipulation for advanced prostate cancer — conventional approaches. In Raghavan D, Scher HI, Leibel S, Lange PH (eds), Principles and Practice of Genitourinary Oncology. J.B. Lippincott: Philadelphia.
10. Crawford ED, Eisenberger MA, McLeod DG, et al. (1989). A controlled trial of leuprolide with and without flutamide in prostatic carcinoma. N Engl J Med 321:419–424.

11. Labrie F, Dupont A, Belanger A, et al. (1982). New hormonal therapy in prostatic carcinoma: combined therapy with LHRH agonist and antiandrogen. Clin Invest Med 5:267–275.
12. Labrie F, Dupont A, Belanger A, et al. (1985). Combination therapy with flutamide and castration (LHRH agonist or orchiectomy) in advanced prostate cancer: a marked improvement in response and survival. J Steroid Biochem 23:833–841.
13. Crawford ED, Eisenberger MA, McLeod DG, et al. (1989). A controlled trial of leuprolide with and without flutamide in prostatic carcinoma. N Engl J Med 321:419–424.
14. Denis L, Murphy GP (1993). Overview of phase III trials in combined androgenic treatment in patients treated with metastatic prostate cancer. Cancer 12(Suppl):3888–3895.
15. Keuppens F, Denis L, Smith P, et al. (1990). Zoladex and flutamide versus bilateral orchiectomy. A randomized phase III EORTC 30853 study. Cancer 66:1045–1057.
16. Denis L, Carneiro de Moura JL, Bono A, et al. Goserelin acetate and flutamide versus bilateral orchiectomy: A phase III EORTC trial (30853). Urology 42:119–130.
17. Iversen P, Christensen MG, Friis E, et al. (1990). A phase III trial of zoladex and flutamide versus orchiectomy in the treatment of patients with advanced carcinoma of the prostate. Cancer 66:1058–1066.
18. Tyrell C, Altwein J, Klippel F, et al. (1991). A multicenter randomized trial comparing the luteinizing hormone-releasing hormone analogue goserelin acetate alone and with flutamide in the treatment of advanced prostate cancer. J Urol 146:1321–1326.
19. Boccardo F, Pace M, Rubagotti A, et al. (1993). Goserelin acetate with or without flutamide in the treatment of patients with locally advanced or metastatic prostate cancer. Eur J Cancer 29A:1088–1093.
20. Marshall V, Thompson P, Raghavan D, et al. (1992). First report of Australian multicenter randomized prostate cancer trial: flutamide does not add to the effect of orchiectomy for metastatic prostate cancer. Proc Am Assoc Cancer Res 33:220.
21. Prostate Cancer Trialists' Collaborative Group (1995). Maximum androgen blockade in advanced prostate cancer: an overview of 22 randomised trials with 3283 deaths in 5710 patients. Lancet 346:265–269.
22. McLeod DG, Moul JW (1995). Controversies in the treatment of prostate cancer with maximal androgen deprivation. Surg Clin North Am 4:345–359.
23. Noble RL (1980). Development of androgen-stimulated transplants of Nb rat carcinoma of the dorsal prostate and their response to sex hormones and tamoxifen. Cancer Res 40:3551–3554.
24. Van Haaften Day C, Raghavan D, Russell P, et al. (1987). Xenografted small cell undifferentiated cancer of the prostate: possible common origin with prostatic adenocarcinoma. Prostate 11:271–279.
25. Horoszewicz JS, Leong SS, Kawinski E, et al. (1977). LNCaP model of human prostatic carcinoma. Cancer Res 43:4049–4058.
26. Bichel P, Frederiksen P, Kjaer T, et al. (1977). Flow microfluorometry and transrectal fine needle biopsy in the classification of human prostatic carcinoma. Cancer 40:1206–1211.
27. Ronstrom L, Tribukait B, Esposti PL (1981). DNA pattern and cytological findings in fine-needle aspirates of untreated prostatic tumors A flow-cytofluorometric study. Prostate 2:79–88.
28. Pittman S, Russell PJ, Jelbart ME, et al. (1987). Flow cytometric and karyotypic analysis of a primary small cell carcinoma of the prostate: a xenografted cell line. Cancer Genet Cytogenet 26:165–169.
29. Davis NS, diSant'Agnese PA, Ewing JF, Mooney RA (1989). The neuroendocrine prostate: characterization and quantitation of calcitonin in the human prostate gland. J Urol 142:884–888.
30. Scher HI, Logothetis CJ (in press). Chemotherapy of advanced prostate cancer. In Raghavan D, Scher HI, Leibel S, Lange PH (eds), Principles and Practice of Genitourinary Oncology. J.B. Lippincott: Philadelphia.
31. Jelbart ME, Russell PJ, Russell P, Raghavan D (1988). The biology and management of small

cell undifferentiated carcinoma of the prostate. In Williams CJ, Krikorian J, Raghavan D (eds), Textbook of Uncommon Cancer. Wiley-Liss: London, pp. 249–262.
32. Montie JE, Wood DP Jr, Venderburg S, et al. (1990). The significance and management of transitional cell carcinoma of the prostate. Semin Urol 7:262–268.
33. Carter BS, Epstein JI, Isaacs WB (1990). Ras gene mutations in human prostate cancer. Cancer Res 50:6830–6832.
34. Mellon K, Thompson S, Charlton RG, et al. (1992). p53, c-erbB-2 and the epidermal growth factor receptor in the benign and malignant prostate. J Urol 147:496–499.
35. Harper ME, Goddard L, Glynne-Jones E, et al. (1993). An immunocytochemical analysis of TGF-α expression in benign and malignant prostatic tumors. Prostate 23:9–23.
36. Myers RB, Oelschlager D, Srivastava S, Grizzle WE (1994). Accumulation of the p53 protein occurs more frequently in metastatic than in localized prostatic adenocarcinomas. Prostate 25:243–248.
37. Rinker-Schaeffer CW, Partin AW, Isaacs WB, Coffey DS, Isaacs JT (1994). Molecular and cellular changes associated with the acquisition of metastatic ability by prostatic cancer cells. Prostate 25:249–265.
38. Brooks JD, Bova GS, Isaacs WB (1995). Allelic loss of the retinoblastoma gene in primary human prostatic adenocarcinomas. Prostate 26:35–39.
39. Taplin M-E, Bubley GJ, Shuster TD, et al. (1995). Mutation of the androgen-receptor gene in metastatic androgen-independent prostate cancer. N Engl J Med 332:1393–1398.
40. Nowell P (1976). The clonal evolution of tumor cell progression: a review. Science 194:3074–3079.
41. Gumerlock PH, Poonamalle UR, Meyers FJ, et al. (1991). Activated ras alleles in human prostate cancer are rare. Cancer Res 51:1632–1637.
42. Moul JW, Freidrichs PA, Lance RS (1992). Infrequent ras oncogene mutations in human prostate cancer. Prostate 20:327–338.
43. Isaacs WB, Bova GS, Moton RA, et al. (1994). Molecular biology of prostate cancer. Semin Oncol 21:514–521.
44. Konishi N, Enomoto T, Buzard G, et al. (1992). K ras activation and ras p21 expression in latent prostate carcinoma in Japanese men. Cancer 69:2293–2299.
45. Anwar K, Nakakuki K, Shiraishi T, et al. (1992). Presence of ras oncogene mutations and human papilloma virus DNA in human prostate carcinoma. Cancer Res 52:5991–5996.
46. Atkin NB, Baker MC (1985). Chromosome studies of five cancers of the prostate. Hum Genet 70:359–364.
47. Kunimi K, Bergerheim USR, Larssson I-L, et al. (1991). Allelotyping of human prostatic adenocarcinoma. Genomics 11:530–536.
48. Natt E, Magenis RE, Zimmer J, et al. (1989). Regional assignment of the human loci for uvomorulin and chymotrypsinogen B with the help of two overlapping deletions on the long arm of chromosome 16. Cytogenet Cell Genet 50:145–148.
49. Bookstein R, Shew J, Chen P (1990). Suppression of tumorigenicity of human prostate carcinoma cells by replacing a mutated Rb gene. Science 247:712–715.
50. Bookstein R, Rio P, Madreperia S, et al. (1990). Promoter deletion and loss of retinoblastoma gene expression in human prostate carcinoma. Proc Natl Acad Sci USA 87:7762–7767.
51. Visakorpi T, Kallioniemi OP, Heikkinen A, et al. (1992). Small subgroup of aggressive highly proliferative prostatic carcinomas defined by p53 accumulation. J Natl Cancer Inst 84:883–887.
52. Bookstein R, MacGrogan D, Milsenbeck SG, et al. (1993). p53 is mutated in a subset of advanced stage prostate cancer. Cancer Res 53:3369–3373.
53. Morton RA, Bova GS, Isaacs WB (1993). Hypermethylation of chromosome 17p 13.3 in human adenocarcinoma of the prostate. J Urol 149:376.
54. Seifter EJ, Bunn PA, Cohen MH, et al. (1986). A trial of combination chemotherapy followed by hormonal therapy for previously untreated metastatic carcinoma of the prostate. J Clin Oncol 4:1365–1373.

55. Citrin DL, Hogan TF, Davis TE (1983). Chemohormonal therapy of metastatic prostate cancer: a pilot study. Cancer 52:410–414.
56. Eisenkraft S, Huben RP, Pontes JE (1984). Orchiectomy and chemotherapy with estramustine, cis-platinum, cyclophosphamide, and 5-fluorouracil in newly diagnosed prostate cancer with bone metastases. Urol 23(Suppl):51–53.
57. Osborne CK, Blumenstein B, Crawford ED, et al. (1990). Combined versus sequential chemo-endocrine therapy in advanced prostate cancer: final results of a Southwest Oncology Group Study. J Clin Oncol 8:1675–1682.
58. Kubota Y, Nakada T, Imai K, et al. (1995). Chemo-endocrine therapy in patients with stage D2 prostate cancer. Prostate 26:50–54.
59. Myers C, Cooper M, Stein C, et al. (1992). Suramin: a novel growth factor antagonist with activity in hormone-refractory metastatic prostate cancer. J Clin Oncol 10:881–889.
60. Raghavan D, Pearson B, Coorey G, et al. (1989). Management of hormone-resistant prostate cancer: experience at Royal Prince Alfred Hospital. In Johnson DE, Logothetis CJ, von Eschenbach AC (eds), Systemic Therapy for Genitourinary Cancers, Year Book Medical Publishers: Chicago, London, pp. 245–250.
61. Raghavan D, Cox K, Pearson B, et al. (1993). Oral cyclophosphamide for the management of hormone refractory prostate cancer. B J Urol 72:625–628.

13. Therapy for hormone-resistant prostate cancer: no longer a myth

Daniel P. Petrylak and Bassam Abi-Rashid

Androgen ablation, initially effective in 80% of patients with advanced prostate cancer, does not cure. In 1996, it is estimated that 41,500 men will die from hormone-resistant metastatic prostate cancer, ranking it the second leading cause of cancer death in the United States [1]. Past options for patients who fail androgen ablation were limited, with most cytotoxic agents being ineffective or having minimal antitumor activity. Two reviews of chemotherapy for hormone-refractory prostate cancer found response rates of 6.5% (95% [confidence intervals] (CI), 5.6%–7.4%) [2] and 8.7% (95%CI, 6,4%–9.0%) [3], respectively, in 1683 and 1001 adequately treated patients. Despite such dismal results, progress in treatment of hormone-refractory prostate cancer has occured in the three years since the last review. The use of human prostate cancer cells in vitro and in vivo animal models to evaluate drug synergy has identified promising new drugs and combinations for evaluation in phase II trials. Durable responses, in some cases lasting more than one year, have been observed in patients treated with these therapies. Significant progress has also been achieved in the management of cancer pain. Along with these treatment advances, important observations have been made regarding the clinical behavior of metastatic prostate cancer, which have had direct implications not only for identifying active drugs, but also for trial methodology. The use of tumor markers to measure response, as well as the recognition of potentially confounding factors (e.g., flutamide withdrawal and the use of corticosteroids) have allowed for more rapid and precise evaluation of these drugs and have also helped to set the standard for future trials. This article reviews some of the more promising developments in the evaluation and treatment of hormone-resistant prostate cancer.

Response evaluation

Bone is the sole site of metastases in 80% to 90% of patients with hormone-resistant prostate cancer. The inherent shortcomings of using bone scans and plain films to assess antitumor response in osteoblastic bone lesions have forced investigators to search for other measures of outcome. Bidimensional

Pienta, K.J., (ed.), DIAGNOSIS AND TREATMENT OF GENITOURINARY MALIGNANCIES.

measurements in bone are difficult to obtain, even with current MRI technology. Measurable soft tissue disease has been used as a clinical trial endpoint, but only 20% of men present with such metastatic lesions, thereby slowing trial accrual. Soft tissue metastases may also exhibit different biological behavior; responses in measurable lesions can be accompanied by discordant disease progression in bone. Unfortunately, pain and quality of life scales do not differentiate analgesic from cytotoxic drug action. Inclusion of quality of life and pain scales, in addition to measurement of pain medication use, can be used to assess osseous response. These parameters can be used separately or along with measurable disease to assess drug activity.

Declines in serum tumor markers such as prostate-specific antigen (PSA), while of proven value in monitoring patients for relapse after radical prostatectomy or radiation therapy, have been evaluated as surrogate measures of response in hormone-refractory patients. A rise in serum PSA after local therapy clearly indicates relapse. However, in assessing response to a cytoxic agent, the converse may not necessarily indicate an active drug. Declines in serum PSA may not only be the result of tumor cell death; decreased expression due to dedifferentiation, or the direct effect of drug on tumor cell PSA synthesis, can result in serum PSA declines. Despite these concerns regarding the validity of using PSA as a trial endpoint in androgen-resistant patients, declines in PSA have correlated with clinical response to hormonal and cytotoxic treatment [4] as well as with survival. A multivariate analysis [5] of 110 patients from seven clinical trials revealed that any 50% decline in PSA after cytotoxic therapy and a decline in the natural logarithm of LDH were the two most significant parameters in predicting survival. In contrast, Eisenberger analyzed PSA declines at four weeks after suramin therapy, and declines greater than 50% did not portend longer survival [••]. These disparate observations highlight the fact that the optimal time for the measurement of PSA after cytotoxic therapy has yet to be established. Moreover, further difficulties in interpreting PSA declines may result from the class of agents being studied. Responding patients may manifest different temporal patterns of PSA expression after being treated with a cytostatic, cytotoxic, or differentiating agents. Since PSA expression is increased with differentiation in prostate cancer tissue specimens, one would expect the PSA to actually rise with respect to therapy, since each therapeutic approach may have a different pattern of PSA response. Prospective studies are warranted to validate these observations and to define the optimal times for measurement.

Two variables were unrecognized during the initial design of some clinical trials: the effects of flutamide withdrawal and the independant activity of corticosteriods. Patients whose serum PSA is rising despite total androgen blockade will, upon cessation of flutamide, manifest a decline in PSA approximately 40% [6] of the time. The duration of this withdrawal response is generally short, and may be specific not only to flutamide but also to other antiandrogens [7]. Corticosteriods, used to aid patients in the management of bone pain, can also induce PSA responses in some patients and can also cause regression of soft tissue disease [8]. Therefore, these variables must also be accounted for in the review of previous clinical trials, as well as in future trial designs.

Suramin

Suramin, a polysulfonated napthylurea, has been studied extensively in hormone-resistant prostate cancer patients. Synthesized, in the 1900s as an antitrypanosomitid, interest in suramin as an antiretroviral and anticancer agent was rekindled when it was found to inhibit reverse transciptase and growth of fresh tumor specimens from colonic, endometrial, renal, and prostatic tissues [9]. In prostate cancer cell lines, the effect of suramin is concentration dependent, stimulating tumor growth at 100 ug/mL yet inhibiting growth above 200 ug/mL. The antitumor activity of suramin had been attributed to several potential mechanisms: inhibition of glycolysis [10], topoisomerases I and II [11], peptide growth factor binding [12], protein kinase C [13], and lysosomal enzymes.

Initial studies in prostate cancer patients demonstrated durable responses, complicated by moderate and sometimes severe toxicity. Myers et al. [14] administered suramin by continuous infusion to obtain a target dose level of 300 ug/ml at the end of a 14-day period, with repeat cycles every eight weeks. Despite toxicities that included Guillain-Barre syndrome, coagulopathy, and fatigue, lasting responses were seen in soft tissue and bone. PSA decline of more than 50% and more than 75% were noted in 55% and 34% of treated patients, respectively. Awareness from these early trials that severe toxicities were observed at more than 300 ug/mL, in addition to in vitro observations of cell inhibition at 200–300 ug/ml, has led investigators to optimize dosing by using adaptive control with computer simulations to rapidly attain therapeutic levels. Using this technique, Eisenberger [15] et al. administered suramin, initially at a dose of 1 gram/m^2 by bolus followed by subsequent boluses to maintain targeted plasma ranges of 200–300, 175–275, and 150–250 ug/ml. Responses were observed in each cohort; of 31 evaluable patients, 24 had a greater than 50% reduction in PSA after suramin therapy. Soft tissue responses were noted in 50% of patients with measurable disease. Pain improvement, as measured by a decrease in narcotic administration, was noted in 83% of patients treated. It is unclear whether this improvement is due to an analgesic effect of suramin, separate from its antitumor properties. Toxicities such as renal and hepatic insufficiency and sensory or motor neuropathy were observed, as in the continuous infusion trial; however, coagulopathy was uncommon when suramin was given by bolus administration. Further experience in dosing suramin has led to several fixed bolus schedules targeting different plasma concentrations, which can be safely administered without adaptive control. Disparate results, however, have been observed, with some groups reporting PSA responses of more than 50% in 60% to 75% of patients [16,17], and others reporting a 12% rate of PSA decline [18], using a similar dosing schedule. These discrepancies are difficult to rectify; however, they may be partially explained by patient populations with different characteristics.

Suramin induces adrenal insufficiency, necessitating concomitant administration of corticosterids from the onset of therapy. Although these doses are only sufficient to replace physiological adrenal function, nonetheless, their administration still may interfere with assessment of response. Two studies addressed this issue [19,20], first by withdrawing flutamide in patients who progressed on total androgen ablation, and then administering hydrocortisone. In one study, patients received hydrocortisone concomitant with flutamide withdrawal, and in the second, hydrocortisone was administered after patients failed flutamide withdrawal. Patients who progressed on hydrocortisone were then treated with suramin administered by bolus. Combining data from these two studies, 12 of 55 (18%, 95% CI = 12%–35%) responded to suramin, as evidenced by a greater than 50% decline in serum PSA. The durations of PSA responses were short, with one group reporting median time to progression of 2.6 months and the second group reporting a duration of response of 4 to 21 weeks. Noteably, soft tissue responses were not observed in either trial. These studies suggest that suramin has independent activity, albeit limited. Further investigations are required to ascertain whether the observed response rates are primairly due to hydrocortisone, or if any clinical synergy exists between hydrocortisone and suramin: earlier administration of cortisone may alter the biology of the tumor, thus making it less sensitive to therapy. Increased expression of antiapoptosis protein BCL-X has been observed after steriod administration in leukemic cell lines [21] and may have a role in prostate cancer response. Further clinical information on the role of steriods and potential clinical synergy may be clarified by the ongoing randomized Parke-Davis trial of suramin + hydrocortisone versus hydrocortisone alone.

Estramustine-based combinations

Estramustine phosphate, an estradiol linked by a carbamate ester to a nornitrogen mustard, was originally thought to have two modes of action, since cleavage of estramustine by prostate cells yields estrogenic and alkylating moieties [22]. Lack of myelosuppression in patients treated with estramustine argues against its action as an alkylating agent, since in vitro studies do not demonstrate DNA damage; rather, estramustine arrests mitosis [23]. Estramustine exerts its antitumor effect by binding to microtubular-associated proteins (MAPS), hindering microtubule assembly [24], interfering with nuclear matrix proteins, and inhibiting collagenase secretion [25], as well as glutathione transferases. Estramustine may also increase intracellular drug concentration through inhibition of p-glycoprotein [26], a transmembrane efflux pump associated with the multidrug resistance phenotype. In vitro studies have also demonstrated synergy between estramustine and etoposide [27], as well as estramustine and taxol.

Oral etoposide is marginally active when used singly in patients with hormone-resistant prostate cancer. Hussein observed two partial responses in 24 men treated with etoposide 50 mg/m^2/day for 21 days. PSA declines of short duration ranging between 19% and 68% of baseline were observed in 7 of 24 patients [28]. In a limited study by Crawford [29], 3 of 7 patients treated with 20 days of etoposide 50/mg/m^2/day had a greater than 50% decline in PSA. Significantly, etoposide combined with estramustine results in clinical synergy. Pienta et al. [30] administered estramustine 15 mg/kg/day with etoposide 50 mg/m^2/day in 42 patients with hormone-resistant disease. In patients with measurable soft tissue disease, three patients demonstrated a complete response in lymph nodes and lung. Three partial responses were observed in liver, skin, and lymph nodes. PSA declines of greater than 50% and greater than 75% were observed in 52% and 21% of patients treated, respectively. The overall median survival of these patients was 44 weeks, with responding patients surviving significantly longer than nonresponders. Of note, the single-agent activity of oral estramustine as measured by a 50% decline in serum PSA is 21%, with an overall PR rate of 14% [31].

The most thoroughly studied combination is estramustine and vinblastine. Estramustine is administered at dosages of 10 mg/kg/day orally and vinblastine 4–6 mg/m^2/week given as an intravenous bolus. Four studies have been published in 94 evaluable patients with 26% of patients with soft tissue disease demonstrating a response 32–35. PSA declines of 50% and 75% were noted in 45% and 25% of treated patients, respectively. Pain was reduced in 48% of all patients treated in one study and in 68% of responding patients in a second. Toxicities attributed to this combination included gastrointestinal discomfort, leucopenia, and peripheral neuropathy.

A second approach to microtubule inhibition is the combination of estramustine with taxol. In vitro studies evidence synergy when taxol is combined with estramustine against the DU145 hormone-resistant human cancer cell line [36]. Activity is detectible at concentrations even as low as 1 nM, which is approximately 100-fold lower than achievable plasma levels. Administration of taxol by a continuous infusion of 120 mg/m^2 over 96 hours, in combination with estramustine 10 mg/kg/day, resulted in serum PSA declines of 50% and 75% in 65% and 35% of patients treated, respectively [37]. Three partial responses were observed in seven patients with soft tissue disease. Toxicity was tolerable. Indeed, taxol has minimal clinical activity when administered as a single agent. The Hoosier Oncology Group treated 23 men with hormone-resistant prostate cancer with taxol [38] administered over 24 hours at dosages of 135–175 mg/m^2. PSA declines greater than 50% of baseline values were not observed in 21 adequately treated patients, though one patient demonstrated a complete response in cervical lymph nodes. It is unclear whether these differences in response are due to the synergy of estramustine combined with taxol or to different infusion schedules of taxol (96 hours vs. 24

hours). Clearly, further studies are warranted to more fully evaluate these observations.

Ketoconazole: combination therapy and derivatives

Ketoconazole, an azole used as an antifungal agent, has been extensively evaluated in hormone-resistant prostate cancer. In one study, 20% of men treated with ketoconazole and hydrocortisone had a prolonged PSA response [39]. In general, an analogue of ketoconazole, liarozole, has been shown to reduce PSA by greater than 50% in 50% of treated patients [40] with hormone-resistant prostate cancer. These drugs are known to prolong the metabolism of retinoic acid, and patients who respond to liarozole manifest symptoms of vitamin A overload, such as chelosis and dry skin.

Observation of in vitro synergy between ketoconazole and doxorubicin in the DU145 prostate cancer cell line justified a phase II trial of this combination in androgen-independent prostate cancer. Sella et al. [41] treated 39 men with ketoconazole 400 mg PO TID and with weekly doxorubicin 20 mg/m^2 by continous infusion given over 24 hours. Hydrocortisone was only administered for clinical adrenal insufficiency. Of 38 evaluable patients, 21 had a 50% or greater decrease in PSA, with 7 of 12 patients with soft tissue metastases evoking a partial response. Patients were not observed for flutamide withdrawal; however, in those patients who did not receive prior flutamide, the response rate was 75%. Median survival was 15.5 months in all treated patients, 17.3 months in those patients who had a PSA response, and 11.6 months in patients who did not respond.

Summary

In conclusion, there have been impressive efforts to identify new cellular targets for the treatment of hormone-refractory disease. It appears that in some cases, survival may be extended; however, further prospective trials are necessary to confirm these observations.

Acknowledgments

We would like to thank Dr. Julie Wong for helpful comments in the preparation of this manuscript.

References

1. Parker SL, Tong T, Bolden S, Wingo PA (1996). Cancer statistics 1996. CA 46:5–28.
2. Eisenberger M, Kennedy P, Abrams J (1987). How effective is cytotoxic chemotherapy for disseminated prostatic carcinoma. Oncology 2:59–69.

3. Yagoda A, Petrylak D (1993). Cytotoxic chemotherapy for advanced hormone resistant prostate cancer. Cancer 71:1098–1109.
4. Fossa SD, Paus E (1994). Reduction of serum prostate-specific antigen during endocrine or cytotoxic treatment of hormone resistant prostate cancer. Eur Urol 26:29–34.
5. Kelly WK, Scher HI, Mazumadar M, Vlamis V, Schwartz M, Fossa SD (1993). Prostate-specific antigen as a measure of disease outcome in metastatic hormone-refractory prostate cancer. J Clin Oncol 11:607–615.
6. Scher HI, Kelly WK (1993). Flutamide withdrawal syndrome: its impact on clinical trials in hormone refractory prostate cancer. J Clin Oncol 11:1566–1572.
7. Small EJ, Carrol PR (1994). Prostate-specific antigen decline after casodex withdrawal: evidence for antiandrogen withdrawal syndrome. Urology 43:408–410.
8. Storlie JA, Buckner JC, Wiseman GA, Burch PA, Hartmann LC, Richardson RL (1994). Prostate specific antigen levels and clinical response to low-dose dexamethasone for hormone-refractory metastatic prostate carcinoma. Proc Am Soc Clin Oncol 13:235.
9. Taylor CW, Lui R, Fanta P, Salmon SE (1992). Effects of suramin on in vitro growth of fresh human tumors. J Natl Cancer Inst 84:489–494.
10. Fantini J, Rognoni JB, Roccabianca M (1989). Suramin inhibits cell growth and glycolytic activity and triggers differentiation of human colonic adenocarcinoma cell clone HT29-D4. J Biol Chem 264:10282–10286.
11. Yamazaki H, Dilworth A, Myers CE, Sinha BK (1993). Suramin inhibits DNA damage in human prostate cancer cells treated with topoisomerase inhibitors in vitro. Prostate 23:25–26.
12. Myers C, Cooper M, Stein C (1992). Suramin: a novel growth factor antagonist with activity in hormone-refractory metastatic prostate cancer. J Clin Oncol 10:881–889.
13. Hensey CE, Boscobonoinik D, Azzi A (1989). Suramin, an anti-cancer drug, inhibits protein kinase C and induces differentiation in neuroblastoma cell clone NB2A. FEBS Left 58:156–158.
14. Myers C, Cooper M, Stein C, LaRocca R, Walther MM, Weiss G, Trepel J, Linehan WM (1992). Suramin: a novel growth factor antagonist with activity in hormone refractory metastatic prostate cancer. J Clin Oncol 10:881–889.
15. Eisenberger MA, Renyo LM, Jordrell DI, Sinibaldi VJ, Tkaczuk KH, Sridhara R, Zuhowski EG, Lowitt MH, Jacobs SC, Egorin MJ (1994). Suramin, an active drug for prostate cancer: interim observations in a phase I trial. J Natl Cancer Inst 85:594–597.
16. Eisenberger MA, Sinibladi V, Renyo L, Sridhara R, Jordrell D, Zuhowski E, Tkaczuk K, Lowitt MH, Hemady R, Jacobs S, VanEcho D, Egorin M (1995). Phase I and clinical evaluation of a pharmacologically guided regimen of suramin in patients with hormone-refractory prostate cancer. J Clin Oncol 13:2175–2186.
17. Kobayshi K, Vokes EV, Vogelzang NJ, Janisch L, Soliven B, Rattain M (1995). Phase I study of suramin given by intermittent infusion without adaptive control in patients with advanced cancer. J Clin Oncol 13:2196–2207.
18. Kelly WK, Scher HI, Mazumdar M, Pfister D, Curley T, Leibertz C, Cohen L, Vlamis V, Dnistrian A, Schwartz M (1995). Suramin and hydrocortisone: determining drug efficacy in androgen-independent prostate cancer. J Clin Oncol 13:2214–2222.
19. Kelly WK, Curley T, Leibretz C, Dnistrian A, Schwartz M, Scher HI (1995). Prospective evaluation of hydrocortisone and suramin in patients with androgen independent prostate cancer. J Clin Oncol 13:2208–2213.
20. Dawson NA, Cooper MR, Figg WD, Headlee DJ, Thibault A, Bergan RC, Steinberg SM, Sausville EA, Myers CE, Sartor O (1995). Antitumor activity of suramin in hormone-refractory prostate cancer controlling for hydrocortisone treatment and flutamide withdrawal. Cancer 76:453–462.
21. Lotem J, Sachs L (1995). Regulation of bcl-2. bcl-XL, and bax in the control of apoptosis by hematopoietic cytokines and dexamethasone. Cell Growth Differ 6:647–653.
22. Kadohama N, Kirdani RY, Murphy GP (1988). Estramustine phophate: metabolic aspects related to its action in prostate cancer. J Urol 119:235.

23. Eklov S, Nilsson S, Larson A, Bjork P, Hartley-Asp B (1992). Evidence for a non-estrogenic cytostatic effect of estramustine on human prostatic carcinoma cells in vivo. Prostate 20:43–50.
24. Dallof B, Billstrom A, Cabral F, Hartley-Asp B (1993). Estramustine depolymerizes microtubules by binding to tubulin. Cancer Res 53:4573–4581.
25. Wang M, Stearns ME (1988). Blocking of collagenase secretion by estramustine during in vitro tumor cell invasion. Cancer Res 48:6262–6271.
26. Speicher LA, Barone LR, Chapman AE, Hudes GR, Laing N, Smith CD, Tew KD (1994). P-glycoprotein binding and modulation of the multidrug resistant phenotype by estramustine. J Natl Cancer Inst 6:688–694.
27. Pienta KJ, Lehr JE (1993). Inhibition of prostate cancer growth by estramustine and etoposide: evidence for interaction at the nuclear matrix. J Urol 149:1622–1625.
28. Hussain MH, Pienta KJ, Redman BG, Cummings GD, Flaherty LE (1994). Oral etoposide in the treatment of hormone-refractory prostate cancer. Cancer 74:100–103.
29. Crawford ED, Daneshgari F, Mejeski SA (1992). Etoposide in the treatment of hormone-refractory advanced carcinoma of the prostate, Semin Oncol 19:53–57.
30. Pienta KJ, Redman B, Hussain M, Cummings G, Esper P, Appel C, Flaherty L (1994). Phase II evaluation of oral estramustine and oral etoposide in hormone-refractory adenocarcinoma of the prostate. J Clin Oncol 10:2005–2012.
31. Yagoda A, Smith JA, Soloway MD (1991). Phase II study of estramustine phosphate in advanced hormone-refractory prostate cancer with increasing prostate specific antigen levels. Proc Am Urol Assoc.
32. Hudes GR, Greemberg R, Krigel RL, Fox S, Scher R, Litwin S, Watts P, Speicher L, Tew K, Comis R (1992). Phase II study of estramustine and vinblastine, two microtubule inhibitors, in hormone-refractory prostate cancer. J Clin Oncol 11:1754–1761.
33. Seidman AD, Scher HI, Petrylak D, Smart T, Dershaw DD (1992). Estramustine and vinblastine: use of prostate specific antigen as a clinical trial endpoint for hormone refractory prostatic cancer. J Urol 147:931–934.
34. Amato R, Logothetis C, Dexus F (1991). Preliminary results of phase II trial of estramustine and vinblastine for patients with progressive hormone-refractory prostate carcinoma. Proc Am Assoc Cancer Res 32:186.
35. Atiq O, Lewis B (1994). Treatment of hormone-refractory prostate adenocarcinoma with estramustine and vinblastine chemotherapy. Proc Am Soc Clin Oncol 13:240.
36. Speicher L, Barone L, Tew KD (••). Combined antimicrotuble activity of estramustine and taxol in human prostatic carcinoma cell lines. Cancer Res 52:4433–4440.
37. Hudes GR, Obasaju C, Chapman A, Gallo J, McAleer C, Greemberg R (1995). Phase I study of paclitaxel and estramustine-preliminary activity in hormone-refractory prostate cancer. Semin Oncol 22:6–11.
38. Roth BJ, Yeap BT, Wilding G, Kasimis B, McLeod D, Loeher P (1993). Taxol in advanced, hormone-refractory carcinoma of the prostate. Cancer 72:2457–2460.
39. Gerber GS, Chodak GW (1991). Prostate specific antigen for assessing response to ketoconazole and prednisone in patients with hormone-refractory metastatic prostate cancer. J Urol 144:1177–1179.
40. Mahler C, Verhelst J, Dennis L (1993). Ketoconazole and liarozole in the treatment of advanced prostate cancer. Cancer 71:1068–1073.
41. Sella A, Kilborn R, Amato R, Bui C, Zukiwski A, Ellerhost J, Logothetis C (1994). Phase II study of ketoconazole combined with weekly doxorubicin in patients with androgen-independant prostate cancer. J Clin Oncol 12:683–688.

14. Renal, bladder, and prostate cancers: gene therapy

Michael A. Carducci and Jonathan W. Simons

Human gene therapy has emerged as a major research endeavor in experimental therapeutics for cancer. Gene therapy as clinical research is still in its earliest stages. Nevertheless, in the past three years, over 200 peer-reviewed manuscripts in human gene therapy have been published. Furthermore, 120 clinical protocols of human gene therapy have gained approval of the Recombinant DNA Advisory Committee (RAC) of the National Institutes of Health (NIH) since the treatment of the first patient with human gene therapy in 1990. Currently, over 14 clinical trials of therapeutic gene transfer in the treatment of urologic malignancies are underway worldwide, and more are under active development or pending approval (Table 14-1).

As was the case for research in recombinant cytokines in hematopoesis and monoclonal antibodies in previous decades, media attention on the potential of basic research in gene therapy has far exceeded the clinical results of gene therapy research to date. Despite this, it is likely that new knowledge acquired from gene therapy research will be applied to the twenty-first-century practice of urological oncology. The reason for this is becoming obvious. The ability to direct therapy using discrete genes as drugs allows molecular characterization and dissection of new therapeutic pathways. The identification and further study of antineoplastic mechanisms of action, driven by gene therapy research, virtually guarantees broader and novel approaches to systemic therapy for cancers in comparison with the current modalities, which center around classes of drugs screened for their antiproliferative effects. As described below, gene therapy research may be more the means to the end than an end in itself for future cancer pharmacology.

Definition of gene therapy

Gene therapy can be defined as the introduction of a normal or modified gene into human cells to treat a genetic or acquired disease with the information encoded in the therapeutic DNA molecule [1]. In cancer therapy, the strategy is to prevent, ameliorate, or eliminate neoplasia by altering the genetic characteristics of cells and alter therapeutically the diseased phenotype of neoplastic

Pienta, K.J., (ed.), DIAGNOSIS AND TREATMENT OF GENITOURINARY MALIGNANCIES.

Table 14-1. Approved human gene therapy trials in urological oncology

Cancer type	Gene	Vector	Ex vivo	In vivo	PI
Prostate	gIFN + IL-2	Retroviral	+		Gansbacher
Prostate	Anti-c-myc	Retroviral		+	Steiner
Prostate	TK	Adenoviral		+	Scardino
Prostate	GM-CSF	Retroviral	+		Simons
Prostate	PSA	Pox	+		Chen
Prostate	IL-2	AAV-plasmid	+		Paulson
Renal	IL-2	Retroviral	+		Gansbacher
Renal	GM-CSF	Retroviral	+		Simons
Renal	GM-CSF	Retroviral	+		Tokyo Institute of Med.
Renal	HLA-B7	Liposome		+	Figlin
Renal	HLA-B7/B2	Liposome		+	Vogelsang
Renal	HLA-B7/B2	Liposome	+		Fox

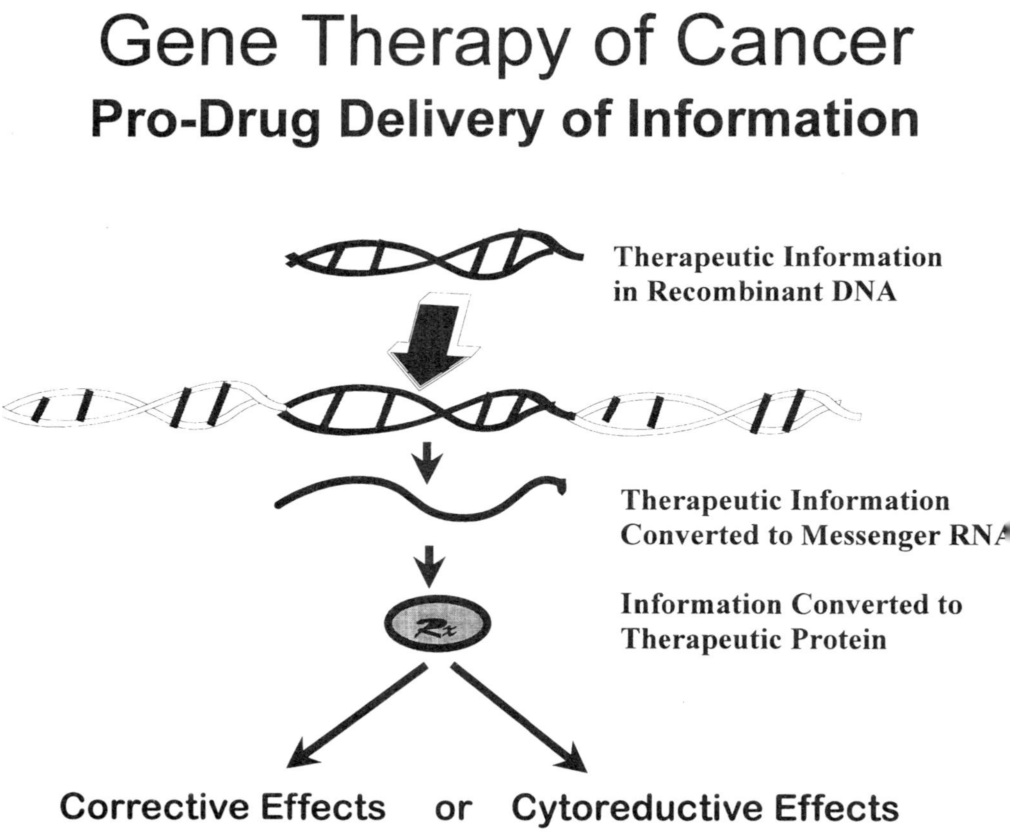

Figure 14-1. ••.

cells. The genetic modification can be performed either ex vivo or in vivo depending on the strategy. At its essence, gene therapy is a prodrug delivery strategy. The therapeutic information encoded in the transferred DNA molecule is converted to the desired therapeutic protein via transcription to messenger RNA and translation to protein (figure 14-1).

Watson and Crick identified the double helical structure of DNA [2,3], allowing scientists to understand how information coded by DNA could be replicated and also be accurately turned into protein. Fundamental discoveries by geneticists, biochemists, and molecular biologists in the past three decades have led to a number of principles that underpin all gene therapy strategies. A central principle is that the genetic code for all amino acids is known and thus the DNA molecule can be engineered to generate any therapeutic protein (including novel proteins designed by humans). Two major areas of research concern the design of human gene transfer systems (vector development) and identification of therapeutic genes for the therapy.

Vector development

Without gene transfer vectors that are efficient in transferring the therapeutic information, there cannot be a clinically meaningful gene therapy. Methods of efficient gene transfer emerged after new discoveries in three areas of molecular biology research in the 1970s and early 1980s. These three areas involved 1) the observation that tumor viruses achieve oncogenic transformation by stable integration of viral DNA into the chromosomal DNA of human cells; 2) the development of quantitative methods to study effective ways to transfer (transfect) DNA into mammalian cells; and 3) the explosive advances in recombinant DNA technologies, which allowed isolation of large amounts of pure gene sequences in little time [4].

Vectors are engineered DNA or RNA sequences that encode sites into which genes of interest can be cloned. The therapeutic gene of interest is usually placed downstream of a promoter sequence for RNA polymerase. This placement allows for expression of the messenger RNA of the therapeutic gene after the vector enters the cell targeted for therapy. Promoter sequences control the expression of downstream genes and thus serve as a critical engineering element of therapeutic gene therapy. In many applications of gene therapy, the target cell may already have copies of the therapeutic human gene being transferred; however, expression of the native copies of this gene may have been inactivated or reduced as a consequence of differentiation, or may have been mutated in carcinogenesis.

In the biosphere, viruses have succeeded in efficient gene transfer for over a billion years. Viral vectors remain the foundation for most gene therapy research. However, both physical and viral methods are being modified genetically to improve vector entry. Physical methods such as microscopic gold bullets of DNA fired from a gene gun, direct microinjection, electroporation, calcium phosphate transfection, liposomal encapsulation, and dextran precipitation are often less efficient but are well established for plasmid DNA transfer. In addition, physical methods are currently less efficient in getting stable DNA transfer relative to replication-defective viral vectors [5].

Efficacy of vectors is influenced by the efficiency of transfection. High-efficiency transfection is defined as the ability of a vector to insert the gene of interest into a large number of target cells (1 in 2 cells = 50% efficiency, for instance). Like dosing a drug, the copies of the transferred gene per treated cell can be quantitated by Southern blots. The therapeutic aim is to successfully induce expression of the gene of interest in most of those cells. This aim is in contrast to traditional in vitro gene transfer, which can be achieved for experimental purposes using electroporation, direct injection of DNA, or calcium phosphate precipitation and which transfect only a small number of cells (1 in 10,000) [6].

With the need for high-efficiency gene transfer, three current methods for vectors to enter target cells are available for clinical applications: engineered viruses that are indiscriminate in target cell preference; engineered viruses that enter only specific tissues/cells; and the physical method of DNA constructs packaged in liposomes that biophysically fuse and deliver DNA, which survives the lysosome to enter the cell cytoplasm [6]

Transfection and transduction (protein expression from the transfected vector) can be accomplished with a variety of vectors that are DNA viruses or retroviruses that have been rendered replication-defective via genetic engineering, minimizing their potential for causing viral infection in humans [6–11]. The different types of such constructs that are available are listed in table 14-2, and several properties define the potential limitations and advantages of each vector system [6]. First, retroviral vectors and adeno-associated virus (AAV) vectors have the property of mediating gene transfer via stable insertion of the gene of interest into the chromosomal DNA of the treated cells. As the target DNA is replicated, so too is the inserted therapeutic gene embedded in the chromosomal DNA. Thus, transduction with these vectors may be durable, with the gene of interest expressed long-term in the target cell as well as its progeny. For corrective gene therapy, this result is critical for maintenance of the corrected cell phenotype over the lifetime of the patient.

Gene transfer mediated by adenovirus, vaccinia (pox viruses), and liposomal constructs, in contrast, is generally episomal: the transferred gene is expressed without actual integration of the gene into the target cell chromosomal DNA. Until further engineering, these vector systems are better suited for clinical applications requiring transient expression of transferred therapeutic genes. For cytoreductive gene therapy, transient tumoricidal gene expression is thought desirable in maintaining a high therapeutic index (high cancer cell kill/low normal tissue toxicity). One special family of vectors under development for clinical trials that show tissue specificity are herpes viruses, which can infect nonreplicating neural cells [7].

Although retroviral vector-mediated gene transfer can be durable, the inac-

Table 14-2. Characteristics of vectors for clinical gene transfer

Vector	Stable gene expression	Ex vivo role	In vivo role	Current advantages	Current limitations
Retrovirus	+	+	+/−	High-efficiency genomic integration	Requires target cell mitosis; potential recombinant retrovirus
Adeno-associated virus (AAV)	+/−	+	?	High stable titer readily attainable	Deletions on integration
Adenovirus	−	+	+	High titer; accepts large DNA constructs	Potential antivector immunity and replication in vivo
Vaccinia	−	+	+	High titer	Antivector immunity and replication in vivo
Liposomal DNA	−	+	+	Ease of production, safety features	Low efficiency
Naked DNA	+	?	?	Long-term expression	Low efficiency
Herpes Simplex Virus	+	+	?	Ease of production	Tropism restricted

tivation of viral titer from complement activation when given intravenously has so far limited its potential for direct intravenous in vivo gene transfer to diseased cells [12]. These constructs appear better suited for ex vivo gene transfer into cells that are then returned to the patients. Retroviral vectors also require target cell proliferation for integration; gene transfer will succeed only in dividing cells [13]. The possibility of pathogenic mutagenesis during chromosomal insertion of the vector and the difficulty in isolating high titers of retrovirus for clinical use are further limitations associated with this vector system [6].

Some AAV vectors appear to mediate durable genetic transduction and are themselves sufficiently stable for potential direct in vivo gene transfer [14,15]. However, integration of AAV genomes into target cell DNA appears less efficient than the best retroviral vectors, and has been associated with a tendency toward inactivation via deletions or rearrangements during gene transfer. Adenovirus and vaccinia vectors can readily transfer genes directly in vivo, but expression of the transferred genes is transient.

Adenoviral vectors have the capacity to transfer large DNA sequences (in the range of tens of thousands of base pairs) compared with other viral vector systems. In concept, several therapeutic genes can be delivered simultaneously using these vectors. Adenovirus vectors have been chosen for transmembrane regulatory gene transduction in cystic fibrosis gene therapy clinical trials; these vectors are attractive since they can efficiently infect nondividing respiratory epithelial cells in vivo. The replication-defective virus particles are amenable to purification and concentration without significant loss of transduction activity. The extensive viral genomic machinery that allows transfer of large sequences of DNA in adenovirus vectors is not without potential cost: these vectors induce antiviral vector antibodies, activate T-cell and macrophage responses, and are potentially limiting prospects for long-term intermittent therapy with this vector in sensitized individuals [16]. Likewise, vaccinia vectors also can induce antiviral vector antibodies, and these vectors are limited currently by their propensity to induce lysis of target cells [17]. However, vaccinia viral vectors are highly immunogenic and may serve as excellent platforms to present antigen genes to the patient immune system.

Sophisticated genetic manipulation is required to render viral vectors most likely to be nonpathogenic. For example, a retroviral vector in intensive cancer clinical trials in genitourinary oncology is MFG; it is derived from a mouse leukemia virus. To render this virus replication defective (and thus nonpathogenic and useful as a vector), genes encoding the pathogenic viral products gag and pol were excised. A 'packaging cell line' that produces the gag and pol products is required for final assembly of the retroviral vector for gene transfer [9]. In some adenovirus vectors, portions of the E1 oncoprotein viral sequences are similarly deleted for increased likelihood of clinical safety [8]. Moreover, to engineer virus-derived vectors, it is not sufficient to merely delete sequences important for viral replication. For clinical use, the absence of potential homologous recombination events leading to replication-competent viral particles must also be tested. Issues in the molecular design of vectors contribute to the preclinical regulatory review by the NIH Recombinant DNA Advisory Committee (RAC) as well as the FDA.

Currently, no single vector possesses all the desirable properties of every therapeutic application of cancer gene therapy. Some clearly advantageous properties of human gene therapy vectors include permanence of transduction, target tissue specificity, high efficiency of in vivo direct gene transfer, fidelity of gene expression levels over time, and capacity for transfer of large DNA sequences. In choosing a vector system for a clinical application in genitourinary cancer research, the relative importance of these performance characteristics is considered. These properties must be evaluated in the context of the therapeutic principle being tested.

Two human gene therapy strategies are currently under clinical or preclinical development for the treatment of urological cancers. The first strategy is *corrective* gene therapy; this is the replacement or inactivation of defective copies of genes in preneoplastic or neoplastic cells with genes that are used to slow or reverse the loss of growth control pathways. The second strategy is *cytoreductive* gene therapy and includes treatment strategies based on the common goal of selectively killing malignant cells.

Corrective strategies of gene therapy for genitourinary cancers

Cancer pathogenesis has a genetic basis, and the disease is clearly the product of the interaction of epigenetic factors and genetic alterations, where a series of genetic abnormalities accumulate in a cell, resulting in neoplasia [18]. Corrective gene therapy is directed at preventing or reversing steps in the pathophysiology of the disease by insertion of a gene into diseased tissue, which corrects a critical pathway in neoplasia. Gene therapy for inborn errors of metabolism serves as the paradigm. For example, treatment of cystic fibrosis (CF) by insertion of wild-type CF genes into bronchial epithelial cells of CF patients is the therapeutic goal. Several inherited urological cancer syndromes are now identified. In particular, the VHL gene in renal cell carcinoma, the WT-1 and TW-2 genes in Wilm's tumors, and p53 mutations in CIS bladder cancer are identifiable targets for gene therapy [19–25]. There is a widening list of potential mutated tumor suppressor genes that might be 'corrected' in urological cancers by in vivo gene therapy of precancerous lesions. Multiple genes may need correction. Four to six genetic alterations are estimated to be necessary to generate most genitourinary cancers, whether by point mutations, deletions, translocations, rearrangements, or amplification [24]. These genetic changes cause a dysfunction of the growth control mechanisms of the transformed stem cells that proliferate in organ homeostasis. The molecular targets of carcinogenesis in urological cancers are still being defined, cancer type by cancer type. Thus potential targets for corrective gene therapy include oncogenes, tumor suppressor genes, apoptosis genes, methylation of transcription control elements, activated mutator genes, dysregulated transcription factors (in the nucleus), nuclear matrix genes, growth receptors (at the cell membrane), signaling enzymes such as G proteins, cell adhesion molecules, tyrosine kinases, and protein kinases [19–27].

In addition to correcting mutant genes by replacement with a wild-type gene, an alternative corrective approach involves transfer of antisense DNA to block effects of overexpressed or mutated oncogenes or genes that block cancer cell apoptosis. Another strategy to affect the aberrant expression of oncogenes is through the use of hammerhead ribozymes, such as that developed by Curiel et al. Using a recombinant adenovirus, the inserted gene cassette contains an H-ras ribozyme for use against neoplastic cells possessing a mutant H-ras oncogene [28].

In theory, affected GU-tract stem cells, in the setting of known diagnosed inheritance of a GU cancer syndrome, could be treated by transfer of wild-type genes prior to onset of clinical disease. Genetic testing on a wide scale will clearly allow identification of at-risk patients in family cancer syndromes. One potentially attractive aspect of bladder cancer gene therapy, in particular, is the possibility of delivering corrective genes, for example, wild-type retinoblastoma or p53 genes, through cystoscopically directed intravesical instillation [29]. The bladder is also attractive as an organ site for translation to clinical evaluation of corrective gene therapy strategies. Through cystoscopy, biopsy, and PCR, efficiency of gene transfer in vivo can be easily measured and therapeutic effects monitored.

At least three limitations in corrective gene therapy of urological cancers exist currently. Firstly, corrective gene therapy requires ultimately that 100% of cancer cells be corrected, or inevitably malignant clones can expand and metastasize. Currently, in vivo gene-transfer efficiencies by intravenous administration or local administration are under 10% of cancer cells with a single treatment. Secondly, correcting one genetic defect in a multistep process of genetic hits may not be sufficient once the cancer has produced a fully invasive and metastatic clone. Thus precancerous lesions, which may be microscopic and undetectable clinically, appear the most likely lesions to respond to treatment. Corrective gene therapy may be tested as an active strategy for cancer *prevention in situ* in the future. Lastly, a number of target genes for correction, for example the chromosome 9p locus and hereditary prostate cancer gene for bladder cancer and prostate cancer, respectively, have not yet been identified.

Cytoreductive strategies of gene therapy for genitourinary cancers

In addition to reversing genetic mutations, cancer gene therapy also permits the local (paracrine) delivery of therapeutic agents to kill neoplastic cells. The tumoricidal effects can be driven from therapeutic information in the DNA molecule either through activation of antitumor T-cell killing or directly by tumoricidal proteins.

The most thoroughly evaluated form of cytoreductive cancer gene therapy involves stimulation of an antitumor immune response against a malignancy by vaccinating affected patients with genetically modified tumor cells (figure 14-1). Tumor cells are removed at surgery from the patient, are placed into tissue culture, and are genetically transduced with a gene for immunostimulatory cytokines. The gene-modified tumor vaccine is then irradiated to prevent subsequent tumor growth and reinjected into the patient. Cells mediating an antitumor immune response are activated due to the presence of immunostimulatory gene products made by the transduced tumor vaccine cells in close proximity to tumor-specific antigens present on the vaccine tumor cell surface. These immune mediator cells, including T cells, natural killer cells, and antigen-presenting cells, can then circulate and eradicate or slow the growth of distant micrometastases (figure 14-2). Ex vivo gene transfer into the tumor cells is required, since the tumor cells alone do not make sufficient immunostimulatory gene products to act as an effective vaccine. This form of cancer gene therapy — cytoreductive gene therapy — already shows clear promise in preclinical testing and is maturing into clinical trials currently [30–34].

Over 30 immunostimulatory genes that modulate the immune responses have been screened for use in gene-modified tumor vaccine strategies of gene

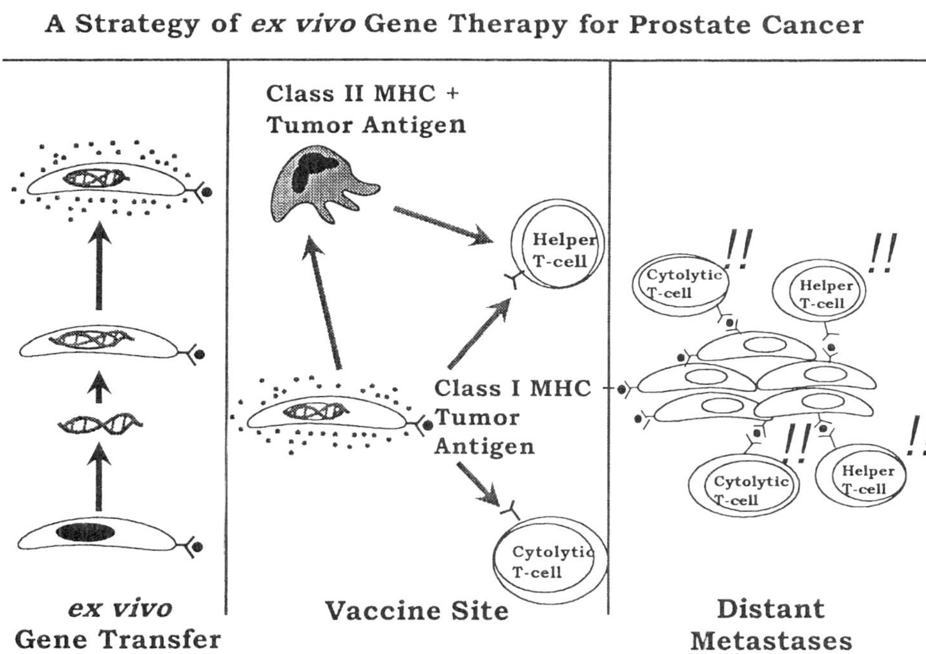

Figure 14-2. ••

therapy (Dranoff, personal communication). The original report using this strategy showed induction of antitumor effect in nude mice via vaccination of tumor cells transduced to secrete IL-2; this study aimed to achieve nonspecific (T-cell-independent) antitumor effect by producing significant systemic levels of IL-2 [35]. Fearon and colleagues then demonstrated that a tumor-specific, T-cell-mediated immune response could be augmented by vaccination of tumor cells of the same origin as treated cells after transduction with IL-2 [36]; such vaccination protected animals from subsequent tumor challenge [37]. Gamma interferon was shown to promote protection against subsequent tumor challenge as well [38]. Other cytokines, including IL-4, IL-6, and GM-CSF, were then shown to have the ability to eliminate microscopic tumor cell deposits when mouse tumor cells were transduced with the respective cytokine genes and when these cytokine-secreting tumors were then used as therapeutic vaccines [39–48].

A second direction in cytoreductive gene therapy under clinical development is transfer of tumoricidal drug susceptibility genes [49–57]. This strategy is an undeveloped area in urological cancer gene therapy. A simple definition of cytoreductive or 'suicide' gene therapy is selective cancer cell killing by expression of a cytotoxic gene, delivered by a vector, which when expressed directs the killing of the cell from inside the cell. The cancer cell must be transduced in order to express the cytotoxin gene. Selective cancer cell killing can be a consequence of 1) selective tropism of the vector for cancer versus normal cells, 2) cancer-specific transcription promoters versus normal tissue promoters to express the cytotoxin, cDNA, or 3) selective cytotoxicity of the toxin to cancer cells versus normal cells. Critical in this approach is the bystander effect. The bystander effect is the killing of cancer cells by an activated cytotoxin gene that is several cell diameters away from the transduced cell. This bystander effect amplifies the low efficiency of actual gene transfer into measurable shrinkage of solid tumors in rat models [52].

Currently, the most widely used suicide gene approach has been using the herpes simplex virus thymidine kinase (HSV-tk) gene in brain tumors and other tumors [58,59]. No published data exist on this approach in preclinical urologic cancer. The most relevant animal model, an experimental rat brain tumor model, has been studied using ganciclovir administered intraperitoneally [58]. Ganciclovir has a high affinity for HSV-tk, which phosphorylates ganciclovir to a monophosphate form. Cellular GMP-kinase then phosphorylates the monophosphate form of ganciclovir to a triphosphate form. This triphosphate form of ganciclovir is toxic to cells through its high affinity (Km = 1.5uM) for DNA polymerase. Therefore, ganciclovir-triphosphate is toxic to any cell in S-phase of the cell cycle. Since not all cells will be cycling at the same time, a few percent escape the immediate toxic effects of ganciclovir-triphosphate [59,60].

Introduction of the HSV-tk gene has been conducted via adenoviral or retroviral vectors [60]. A dramatic and significant antitumor effect occurs after exposure of the cells to ganciclovir. Apparently, not all tumor cells must incorporate the suicide gene [52,61,62]. Noninfected tumor cells can be eradicated via the bystander effect. The bystander effect has been hypothesized to be due to 1) transfer of the HSV-tk enzyme through vesicles, 2) transfer of toxic molecules through gap junctions, 3) transfer of hydrolases or other enzymes associated with programmed cell death that may be induced to nearby cells, 4) upregulating immune recognition secondary to killing of affected cells, and 5) tissue or tumor ischemia due to integration of the HSV-tk gene upon cell death to adjacent cells [62]. To date, close cell-to-cell contact is required for the bystander effect to work. The bystander effect is an attractive feature of retroviral strategies, since retroviruses are unable to infect all cells of a tumor.

Unfortunately, the HSV-tk gene for prostate cancer is unlikely to be highly effective, since the growth fraction of prostate cancer is minimal and typically less than 2% of cells at any time [63]. Isaacs has shown that prostate cancer progression is due to loss of programmed cell death pathways rather than increased mitotic rates. High mitotic rates are required for sensitivity to HSV-tk and ganciclovir [63]. In this respect, bladder cancer, with its higher mitotic rate and its clinical sensitivity to S-phase cell cycle chemotherapy (MVAC, for example), is an obvious target for this form of therapy. Still, the pathways of cell death in the bystander effect need molecular dissection for improving efficacy. The bystander effect may also lead to increased toxicity by harming local, normal cells. Although this approach has been fairly extensively studied in animal models of brain tumors and mesothelioma, it has not yet been critically tested in the treatment of preclinical models of urological malignancies or taken yet to clinical trials.

A modification of cytoreductive gene therapy involves tissue-specific expression of drug susceptibility genes or cell toxins [6,64]. Vectors are being constructed that contain tissue-specific promoters that restrict expression of the transferred cytotoxic gene. Prostate cancer is a potentially optimal target for such approaches. By designing a construct with a gene of interest whose expression is controlled by the PSA promoter and regulatory sequences, only cells that normally express PSA would express the transferred therapeutic gene product. Pilot studies have examined this approach by evaluating expressions of luciferase (a 'reporter' gene that encodes a readily assayed gene product) transcribed downstream from a human PSA promoter sequence after transfection of human prostate cancer cell lines in vitro [64]. This confers an element of specificity to prostate cell killing using gene therapy.

Lastly, using tissue- or cancer-cell-specific promoters, a high concentration of tumoricidal proteins may be obtained locally via gene transfer when systemic administration would be too toxic. For example, recombinant tumor necrosis factor (rTNF) has been actively explored in gene therapy for its tumoricidal properties and its ability to engender antitumor immune responses. TNF has produced encouraging antitumor responses in mice, but the maximal tolerated dose in humans is 40-fold less than the doses that are required to elicit this response in mice [65]. Local high concentration via rTNF gene transfer and secretion by transduced cell appear promising.

Translation to clinical trials

Special ethical considerations and safety considerations are still involved in the evaluation of human gene-therapy clinical trials. Somatic-cell gene therapy has now been achieved in over 100 patients and appears to have gained acceptance as not having any extra a priori hazards than any other form of experimental therapy. The theoretical risk of the spread of recombinant, pathogenic, new human viruses is evaluated in every gene transfer trial, and all trials involving viral vectors require additional patient testing for detection of any recombinant virus in patients. Currently, germline and enhancement genetic engineering of tissues are being carried out in laboratory and farm animals. The technical ability to attempt human application of these techniques clearly exists [66]. Since the Holocaust, however, political policy discussions of gene therapy research clearly distinguish between somatic cell therapy and germ-cell manipulation and its eugenics implications. Currently, human germ-cell gene transfer is not sanctioned by the National Institutes of Health Recombinant DNA Advisory Committee, which oversees all United States human gene therapy research.

As depicted in table 14-1, cytoreductive strategies involving antitumor immune responses have been directed at renal cell carcinoma. A more diversified set of approaches is being directed at prostate cancer. The generation of antitumor immune responses by use of ex vivo gene-transduced vaccines is being applied. In addition, the use of gene therapy in vivo is being explored via antisense and suicide gene strategies. The in vivo treatment of bladder cancer with alternative vector systems is imminent in several institutions with target genes for corrective therapy, including p53 and Rb.

Clinical results to date

Limited data exist to date from the early cohort of human gene therapy clinical trials. Many early studies focused on simply achieving measurable gene transfer. This is no longer a scientific or clinical objective that alone justifies clinical research. The principle of human gene transfer is clearly established. All GU oncology gene therapy trials completed or currently underway are phase I studies. Efficacy testing in phase II studies is now commencing. The real test of gene therapy as a new form of cancer pharmacology is just beginning.

Gene therapy is unlikely to efface the need for multimodality approaches to the reduction of morbidity and mortality of urological cancers. If past performance predicts future behavior, however, the rapid discoveries in this area of molecular medicine can be predicted to have a great impact on the practice of genitourinary oncology in the twenty-first century. Current approaches — especially vector systems — will likely appear like outmoded prototypes of technology, like obsolescent software. Yet, the new principles of molecular therapeutics utilized in gene therapy strategies have clear potential to be reduced to practice.

References

1. Kelley WN (1994). The impact of gene therapy on medicine and society: gene therapy for neoplastic diseases. Ann NY Aced Sci 76:12–19.
2. Watson JD, Crick FH (1953). Molecular structure of nucleic acids. A structure for doexyribose nucleic acid. Nature 171:737–738.
3. Watson JD, Crick FH (1953). Genetic implications of the structure of deoxyribo nucleic acid. Nature 171:737–738.
4. Tolstoshev P (1993). Gene therapy, concepts, current trials and future directions. Annu Rev Pharmacol Toxicol 32:573–596.
5. Sikora K (1994). Genes, dreams, and cancer. Br Med J 308:1217–1221.
6. Mulligan R (1993). The basic science of gene therapy. •• 260:926–932.
7. Johnson P, Miyanohara A, Levine F, Cahill T, Friedmann T (1992). Cytotoxicity of a replication-defection mutant of herpes simplex virus type 1. J Virol 66:2952–2965.
8. Jones N, Shenk T (1979). Isolation of adenovirus type 5 host range deletion mutants defective for transformation to rat embryo cells. Cell 17:683–689.
9. Danos O, Mulligan R (1988). Safe and efficient generation of recombinant retrovirus with amphotropic and ecotropic host ranges. Proc Natl Acad Sci USA 85:6460–6464.
10. Miller A (1990). Retrovirus packaging cells. Hum Gene Ther 1:5–14.
11. Kozarsky K, Wilson J (1993). Gene therapy: adenovirus vectors. Curr Opinion Genet Dev 3:399–503.
12. Cornetta K, Moen R, Culver K, Morgan R, McLacherlin J, Sturm S, Selegue J, London W, Blaese R, Anderson W (1990). Amphotropic murine leukemia retrovirus is not an acute pathogen for primates. Hum Gene Ther 1:15–30.
13. Roe T, Reynolds T, Yu G, Brown P (1993). Integration of murine leukemia virus DNA depends on mitosis. EMBO J 12:2099–2108.
14. Kotin RM, Siniscalco M, Samulski R, Zhu X, Hunter L, Laughlin C, McLaughlin S, Muzyczka N, Rocchi M, Berns K (1990). Site-specific integration of adeno-associated virus. Proc Natl Acad Sci USA 87:2211–2215.
15. Muzyczka N (1992). Use of adeno-associated virus as a general transduction vector for mammalian cells. Curr Top Microbiol Immunol 158:97–129.
16. Anderson W (1992). Human gene therapy. Science 256:808–813.
17. Moss B, Flexner C (1987). Vaccinia virus expression vectors. Annu Rev Immunol 5:305–324.
18. Culver KW, Blaese RM (1994). Gene therapy for cancer. TIG 10(5):174–178.
19. Friend SH, Bernards R. Rogeli S, Weinberg RA, Rapaport JM, Albert DM, Dryja TP (1986). A human DNA segment with properties of the gene that predisposes to retinoblastoma and osteosarcoma. Nature 323:643–646.
20. Latif F, Tory K, Gnarra J, et al. (1993). Identification of the von Hippel–Lindau disease tumor suppressor gene. Science 260:1317–1320.
21. Baker SJ, Fearon ER, Nigro JM, Hamilton SR, Preisinger AC, Jessup JM, van Tuinen P, Ledbetter DH, Barker DF, Nakamura Y, et al. (1989). Chromosome 17 deletions and p53 gene mutations in colorectal carcinomas. Science 244:217–221.
22. Fearon ER, Vogelstein B (1990). A genetic model for colorectal tumorigenesis. Cell 61:759–767.

23. Rose EA, Glaser T, Jones C, et al. (1990). Complete physical map of the WAGR region of 11p13 localizes a candidate Wilm's tumor gene. Cell 60:495–508.
24. Carter BS, Ewing CM, Ward WS, Treiger BF, Aalders TW, Schalken JA, Epstein JL, Isaacs WB (1990). Allelic loss of chromosome 16q and 10q in human prostate cancer. Proc Natl Acad Sci USA 87:8751–8755.
25. Presti JC Jr, Reuter VE, Galan T, Fair WR, Cordon-Cardo C (1991). Molecular genetic alterations in superficial and locally advanced human bladder cancer. Cancer Res 51:5405–5409.
26. Yang C, Cirielli C, Capogrossi MC, Passaniti A (1995). Adenoviirus-mediated wild-type p53 expression induces apoptosis and suppresses tumorigenesis of prostatic tumor cells. Cancer Res 55:4210–4213.
27. Kleinerman DI, Zhang WW, Lin SH, Nguyen TV, von Eschenback AC, Hseih JT (1995). Application of a tumor suppressor (C-CAM1)- expressing recombinant adenovirus in androgen-independent human prostate cancer therapy: a preclinical study. Cancer Res 55:2831–2836.
28. Feng M, Cabrera G, Deshane J, Scanlon KJ, Curiel DT (1995). Neoplastic reversion accomplished by high efficiency adenoviral-mediated delivery of an anti-ras ribozyme. Cancer Res 55:2024–2028.
29. Werthman P, Drazan K, Csete M, Bullington D, Zhang W, Rosenthal J, Shaked A (1994). Adenoviral-mediated transfer of human p53 tumor suppressor gene to rat bladder in vivo. J Urol 151:389A.
30. Sanda M, Ayyagari S, Jaffee E, Epstein J, Clift S, Cohen L, Drannoff G, Pardoll D, Mulligan R, Simons J (1994). Demonstration of a rational strategy for human prostate cancer gene therapy. J Urol 151:622–628.
31. Vieweg J, Rosenthal F, Bannerji R, Heston W, Fair W, Gansbacher B, Gilboa E (1994). Immunotherapy for prostate cancer in the Dunning rat model: use of cytokine gene modified tumor vaccines. Cancer Res 54:1760–1765.
32. Carducci MA, Ayyagari SR, Sanda MG, Simons JW (1995). Gene therapy for human prostate cancer: translational research in the hormone refractory Dunning prostate cancer model. Cancer 75:2013–2020.
33. Golumbek PT, Lazenby AJ, Levitsky HI, Jaffee LM, Karasuyama H, Baker M, Pardoll DM (1991). Treatment of established renal cancer by tumor cells engineered to secrete interleukin-4. Science 254:713–716.
34. Dranoff G, Jaffee E, Lazenby A, Golumbek P, Levitsky H, Brose K, Jackson V, Hamada H, Pardoll D, Mulligan RC (1993). Vaccination with irradiated tumor cells engineered to secrete murine granulocyte-macrophage colony-stimulating factor stimulates potent, specific, and long-lasting antitumor immunity. Proc Natl Acad Sci USA 90:3539–3543.
35. Bubenik J, Voitenok NN, Kieler J, Prassolov VS, Chumakov PM, Bubenikova D, Simova J, Jandlova T (1988). Local administration of cells containing an inserted Il-2 gene and producing IL-2 inhibits growth of human tumors in nu/nu mice. Immunol Lett 19:279–282.
36. Fearon ER, Pardoll DM, Itaya T, Golumbek P, Levitsky HI, Simons JW, Karasuyama H, Vogelstein B, Frost P (1990). Interleukin-2 production by tumor cells bypasses T helper function in the generation of an antitumor response. Cell 60:397–403.
37. Gansbacher B, Zier K, Daniels B, Cronin K, Bannerji R, Gilboa E (1990). Interleukin-2 gene transfer into tumor cells abrogates tumorigenicity and induces protective immunity. J Exp Med 172:1217–1224.
38. Gansbacher B, Bannerji R, Daniels B, Zier K, Cronin K, Gilboa E (1990). Retroviral vector-mediated gamma-interferon gene transfer into tumor cells generates potent and long lasting antitumor immunity. Cancer Res 50:7820–7825.
39. Porgador A, Tzehoval E, Katz, A, Vadai E, Revel M, Feldman M, Eisenbach L (1992). Interleukin 6 gene transfection into Lewis lung carcinoma tumor cells suppresses the malignant phenotype and confers immunotherapeutic competence against parental metastatic cells. Cancer Res 52:3679–3686.

40. Cordon-Cardu C, Fuks Z, Drobnjak M, Moreno C, Eisenbach L, Feldman M (1991). Expression of HLA-A,B,C antigens on primary and metastatic tumor cell populations of human carcinomas. Cancer Res 51:6372–6380.
41. Sanda M, Simons J, Pardol D, Restifo N (1993). Human prostate cells escape immunity via reversible heterogeneous defects in antigen processing. J Urol 149:374A.
42. Hock H, Dorsch M, Kunzendorf U, Uberla K, Qin Z, Diamanstein T, Blankenstein T (1993). Vaccinations with tumor cells genetically engineered to produce different cytokines: effectivity not superior to a classical adjuvant. Cancer Res 53:714–716.
43. Steiner M, Barrack E (1992). Transforming growth factor-B1 overproduction in prostate cancer: effects on growth in vivo and in vitro. Mol Endocrinol 6:15–25.
44. Connor J, Bannerji R, Saito S, Heston W, Fair W, Gilboa E (1993). Regression of bladder tumors in mice treated with interleukin-2 gene-modified tumor cells. J Exp Med 177:1127–1134.
45. Moody B, Lazenby A, Ewing C, Isaacs W (1994). Interleukin-2 transfected prostate cancer cells generate a local anti-tumor effect in vivo. Prostate 24:244–251.
46. Levitsky H, Lazenby A, Hayashi R, Pardoll D (1994). In vivo priming of 2 distinct antitumor effector populations: the role of MHC class-I expression. J Exp Med 179:1215–1224.
47. Sanda M, Carducci M, Ayyagari S, Kim W, Cohen L, Mulligan R, Pardoll D, Simons J (1994). Gene therapy for human prostate cancer: efficacy in animal models and feasibility for human trials. J Urol 151:492A.
48. Belldegrun A, Tso C, Sakata T, et al. (1993). Human renal carcinoma line transfected with interleukin-2 and/or interferon alpha gene(s): implications for live cancer vaccines. J Natl Cancer Inst 85:207–216.
49. Furman P, McGuirt P, Keller P, Fyfe J, Elion G (1980). Inhibition by acyclovir of cell growth and DNA synthesis of cells biochemically transformed with herpes virus genetic information. Virology 102:420–430.
50. St Clair M, Lambe C, Furman P (1987). Inhibition by ganciclovir of cell growth and DNA synthesis of cells biochemically transformed with herped virus genetic information. Antimicrob Agents Chemother 31:844–849.
51. Mattews T, Boehme R (1988). Antiviral activity and mechanism of action of ganciclovir. Rev Infect Dis 10 (Suppl 3):S490–S494.
52. Freeman S, Abboud C, Whartenby K, Packman C, Koeplin D, Moolten F, Abraham G (1993). The 'bystander effect': tumor regression when a fraction of the tumor mass is genetically modified. Cancer Res 52:5274–5283.
53. Culver K, Ram Z, Wallbridge, S, Ishii H, Oldfield E, Blaese R (1992). In vivo gene transfer with retroviral vector-producer cells for treatment of experimental brain tumors. Science 256:1550–1552.
54. Moolten F, Wells J (1990). Curability of tumors bearing herpes thymidine kinase genes transferred by retroviral vectors. J Natl Cancer Inst 82:297–300.
55. Smythe W, Hwang H, Amin K, Eck S, Davidson B, Wilson J, Kaiser L, Albelda S (1994). Use of recombinant adenovirus to transfer the herpes simplex virus thymidine kinase (HSTtk) gene to thoracic neoplasms: an effective in vitro drug sensitization system. Cancer Res 54:2055–2059.
56. Caruso M, Panis Y, Gagandeep S, Houssin D, Salzmann J, Klatzmann D (1993). Regression of established macroscopic liver metastases after in situ transduction of a suicide gene. Proc Natl Acad Sci USA 90:7024–7028.
57. Takamiya Y, Short M, Ezzeddine Z, Moolton F, Breakefield X, Martuza R (1992). Gene therapy of malignant brain tumors: a rat glioma line bearing the herpes simplex virus type 1-thymidine kinase gene and wild type retrovirus kills other tumor cells. J Naurosci Res 33:493–503.
58. Ram Z, Culver KW, Walbridge S, Blaese RM, Oldfield EH (1993). In situ retroviral-mediated gene transfer for the treatment of brain tumors in rats. Cancer Res 53:83–88.
59. Culver KW, Van Gilder J, Link CJ, Carlstrom T, Buroker T, Yuh W, Koch K, Schabold K,

et al. (1994). Gene therapy for the treatment of malignant brain tumors with in vivo tumor transduction with the herpes simplex thymidine kinase gene/ganciclovir system. Hum Gene Ther 5:343–379.

60. Chen SH, Shine HS, Goodman JC, Grossman RG, Woo SL (1994). Gene therapy for brain tumors: regression of experimental gliomas by adenovirius mediated gene transfer in vivo. Proc Natl Acad Sci USA 91:3057–3059.
61. Bi WL, Parysek LM, Warnick R, Stambrook, PI (1993). In vitro evidence that metabolic cooperation is responsible for the bystander effect observed with HSV-tk retroviral gene therapy. Hum Gene Ther 4:725–731.
62. Ram Z, Walbridge S, Shawker T, Culver KW, Blasese RM, Oldfield EH (1994). The effect of thymidine kinase transduction and ganciclovir therapy on tumor vasculature and growth of 9L gliomas in rats. J Neurosurg 81:256–260.
63. Isaacs JT, Landniu PI, Berges R, Martikainen P, Kyprianou N, English HF (1992). Androgen regulation of programmed cell death of normal and malignant prostate cells. J Androl 13:455–484.
64. Taneja S, Gelldegrun A, Dardashti K, Cohan P, Dekernion J, Pang S (1994). Construction of a prostate specific antigen promoter-driven gene transfer vector: a novel strategy for target specific gene therapy in prostate cancer. J Urol 151:491A.
65. Fujiwara T, Grimm E, Roth J (1994). Gene therapeutics and gene therapy for cancer. Curr Opinion Oncol 6:96–105.
66. Anderson W (1992). Editorial: uses and abuses of human gene transfer. Hum Gene Ther 3:1–2.

15. The role of immunotherapy in urologic malignancies

Yousif A. Abubakr and Bruce G. Redman

A proposed mechanism for the progression of cancer is the failure or overwhelming of the immune surveillance system[1]. That some form of immune recognition does indeed occur against malignant cells in patients has been shown by numerous investigators [2–7]. Our inability to effectively manipulate the immune response against neoplasia represents more a lack of knowledge about immune antitumor interactions than a lack of antitumor immunity. Immunotherapeutic strategies for the treatment of cancer include both active and passive approaches. Active immunotherapy can be achieved by immunizing the host against either tumor, modified tumor, or tumor-associated antigens. The passive approach includes monoclonal antibody therapy, the transfer to the host of sensitized cells capable of mediating antitumor responses, and administration of various cytokines.

Despite the need for more knowledge about tumor immunity, advances have been made against urologic malignancies with two forms of immunotherapy. Bacillus Calmette-Guerin (BCG) has become a standard in the prevention of recurrence and treatment of early-stage bladder cancer while interleukin-2 (IL-2) remains the only approved agent for the treatment of advanced renal cell carcinoma (RCC) in the United States. We will review in this chapter the current status of immunotherapy of urologic malignancies and offer some thoughts about future options.

Immunotherapy of renal cell carcinoma

Interferons

Interferons have immunomodulatory properties that can augment cellular cytotoxicity and enhance the expression of a variety of surface antigens [8]. As a class of agents, interferons have also exhibited direct antiproliferative properties that also may be responsible for their clinical activity, and as such they cannot be considered as true biologic response modifiers such as IL-2. Interferons have exhibited antitumor activity against a variety of malignancies, including RCC.

Pienta, K.J., (ed.), DIAGNOSIS AND TREATMENT OF GENITOURINARY MALIGNANCIES.

Quesada et al. were the first to report objective responses in 5 of 19 (20%) patients with metastatic RCC treated with partially purified human leukocyte interferon-α (IFN) [9]. Several trials have, subsequently, confirmed the activity of both the partially purified and recombinant forms of IFN against RCC [10–14]. The vast majority of responses are partial responses. A response rate of 14% was found in 465 patients treated in phase II and III trials utilizing various doses and schedules of IFN [15]. The overall median survival of patients treated with IFN (11.4 months) has not been dramatically different from that of untreated patients with metastatic RCC.

The optimal dose and schedule of IFN-α are not known. Responses have been reported at all dose levels investigated. High-does regimens (more than 20 MU) exhibit treatment-limiting toxicities, while low-dose regimens (less than 3 MU) are probably less effective. A regimen of 5–10 MU per M^2 subcutaneously of recombinant IFN-α 3–5 times a week or daily is the most commonly used dose and schedule in clinical trials. Experience with IFN-β and-γ is more limited in the treatment of RCC, but responses are generally similar to or lower than IFN-α [16–18]. Factors that may predict for responsiveness to IFN-α in metastatic RCC include male sex, excellent performance status (ECOG 0–1), and lung and lymph node only metastases [19].

The toxicity of interferons, though common, is reversible upon discontinuation or dose modification. Flu-like symptoms are the most common adverse effects, occurring in 75% to 100% of patients. Fatigue and asthenia associated with chronic administration, occurs in up to 45% of the patients and can be dose limiting. Skin rash, gastrointestinal complaints, leukopenia, thrombocytopenia, and hepatic enzyme abnormalities are frequently encountered toxicities. Less common toxicities include central nervous system, renal, and cardiac toxicities and are dose-related, occurring at doses more than 18 MU.

IFN-α as a single agent has not impacted greatly on the natural history of patients with metastatic RCC. Selection of patients with favorable prognostic features for response to IFN (i.e., lung and lymph node metastases, good performance status) leads to better therapeutic results.

Interleukin-2 (IL-2)

IL-2 is the first true biologic response modifier (BRM) to enter clinical trials, since it has no direct antitumor activity. IL-2 stimulates T-cell proliferation, activates cytotoxic responses in T-cells, and induces and augments non-MHC-restricted CTL killing [20]. The U.S. Food and Drug Administration (FDA) has approved IL-2 for clinical use in metastatic RCC based on the ability of high-dose bolus infusions of IL-2 to induce durable remissions in a minority of patients [21–23].

High-dose IL-2

High-dose IL-2 regimens [20,21] consist of a dose of 600,000 to 720,000 IU/kg of IL-2 administered as an intravenous bolus over 15 minutes every eight hours for up to 14 doses. The same treatment is repeated in 7 to 10 days to complete one cycle of therapy. Individual doses are omitted rather than delayed for toxicity. The same treatment course may be repeated in responding patients in 12 weeks.

The major limiting factor to the more widespread use of high-does IL-2 is the intensity of its associated toxicity. IL-2 induces the activation and proliferation of T-lymphocytes and natural killer cells, with the production of various cytokines including tumor necrosis factor, interleukin-6, and interferon-γ. The production of these cytokines is felt to be responsible for most of the toxic effects of IL-2, but the cytokines may also be involved in the therapeutic activity of this agent.

Rosenberg et al. summarized the NCI experience using high-dose IL-2 in the treatment of metastatic RCC [23]. Of 149 petients, 10 (7%) had complete remission and 20 (13%) had partial remission, for an overall response rate of 20%. Patients with visceral metastases had similar response rates to those with lung or lymph node sites of metastases. The median duration of response for partial responders was 22 months (range 4-69+ months). The median duration of response for those achieving complete remissions has not been reached, with 7 of 10 remaining in remission 7+ to 76+ months. These results have been duplicated by many other investigators using similar high-dose regimens.

The capillary leak syndrome manifesting as hypotension and fluid retention remains the major dose-limiting toxicity of high-dose IL-2 regimens. Reversal of the hypotension with vasopressors and judicious fluid management while at the same time avoiding fluid overloads that can result in pulmonary edema are the basic management principles of high-dose IL-2 regimens.

Reversible renal dysfunction manifested as oliguria and elevation of serum creatinine may result from the hypotension and resultant decreased renal perfusion seen with IL-2 therapy. Nausea, vomiting, diarrhea, purutic skin rash, and hepatic enzyme elevation are other reversible toxicities associated with IL-2.

Central nervous system toxicity can occur in up to 20% of patients. The spectrum of central nervous system toxicity ranges from somnolence to frank psychosis. The onset of confusion is an indication to stop therapy immediately. Cardiac toxicity can manifest as myocardial ischemia or infarction, myocarditis, dysrhythmias, or pericardial effusion. Supraventricular tachyarrhythmias are more common than ventricular dysrhythmias. Screening of potential candidates for IL-2 therapy with complete cardiac evaluation including stress testing has dramatically reduced the number of fatal cardiac events. Hypothyroidism or hyperthyroidism may result as a long-term delayed toxicity of IL-2 therapy. The occurrence of thyroid dysfunction has been correlated with responses to IL-2 by some but not all investigators.

High-dose IL-2 therapy has significant morbidity (albeit reversible) and requires hospitalization with occasional intensive care unit support. Older patients and patients with pre-existing cardiopulmonary disease are not candidates for high-does IL-2 therapy. Because of this, numerous reports of phase I and II trials of low-dose IL-2, either by continuous infusion or subcutaneous injection, in metastatic RCC have appeared in the literature [24,25]. Different doses and schedules of administration have been utilized. Representative results [26–32] are shown on table 15-1. Though the response rates in these trials vary, they appear to be comparable to the response rates obtained with high-dose IL-2. However, it is unclear at this time whether the duration of responses to low-dose regimens will be comparable to the duration of response achieved with high-dose regimens.

A phase III randomized study of high-dose (720,000 IU/kg) versus an intermediate-dose (720,000 IU/kg) IL-2 by bolus administration showed comparable complete response rates (3% vs. 7%) and partial responses (8% vs. 17%), respectively [33]. Randomized trials of high- versus low-dose IL-2 therapy with longer follow-up are needed to determine the optimal dose and schedule of IL-2 as a single agent in metastatic RCC.

Table 15-1. Results of low-dose IL-2 therapy

Investigator [ref]	Dose (IU)	Route	No. of pts.	Response: Complete (%)	Response: Partial (%)
Whitehead [26]	3–30 × 10^6 IU/M^2/d × 5 d per week	SQ	15	0 1 minor response	0
Marumo [27]	1 × 10^6 IU/d	IV/SQ	11	2 (18)	1 (9)
Lissoni [28]	9 × 10^6 IU/M^2 × 2 d then 1.8 × 10^6 IU/M^2 q12° 5 d/wk	SQ	13	0	4 (31)
Sleijfer [29]	9–18 × 10^6 IU/d 5 d/wk × 6 wks	SQ	26	2 (8)	4 (15)
Stoter [30]	3 × 10^6 IU/M^2 5 d/wk, 2 ×/month × 2 month, then monthly	CIV	18	1 (6)	2 (11)
Stein [31]	0–16 × 10^6 IU 5 d/wk × 8 wks	SQ	9	0 (0)	2 (22)
Leahy [32]	22 × 10^6 IU/M^2 5 d/wk × 2 wks	SQ or CIV	12	1 (8)	0

Abbreviations: IU, international units; IV, intravenous; SQ, subcutaneous; CIV, continuous intravenous infusion; d, day; wk, week.

IL-2 Combination therapy

In experimental murine tumor models, the combination of IL-2 and IFN-α has synergistic antitumor effects [34]. However, extensive immunological evaluations of patients participating in a phase I clinical trial of IL-2 and the combination of IL-2/IFN-∝ showed no difference in the immune parameters evaluated [35]. A number of phase I and II trials of combination therapy with IL-2 and IFN have been published. The goal of most of these trials was to decrease the toxicity of IL-2 therapy and to improve the efficacy in an outpatient treatment program. Severe fatigue, weight loss and elevation of serum creatinine to above 2 mg/dl were the major toxicities encountered. Different doses and treatment schedules have been investigated. Response rates have been less than or similar to those obtained with high dose IL-2 therapy. Table 15-2 shows the results of representative trials of combination IL-2 and IFN-α therapy in metastatic RCC [36–42].

IL-2 and IFN-∝ have also been combined with chemotherapy in the treatment of metastatic RCC. Though chemotherapy is ineffective in the treatment of RCC, several preclinical reports have shown that 5-fluorouracil (5FU) has immunomodulatory effects, especially when combined with IL-2 and IFN-∝ [43]. Two clinical trials using different doses and schedules of 5FU/IL-2/IFN-∝ have reported response rates of 40% to 50% [44,45]. These preliminary results are encouraging and are being evaluated in larger numbers of patients to confirm the activity of these regimens and better define response duration.

Adoptive cellular therapy

Adoptive cellular therapy is a process whereby autologous lymphocytes are 'activated' exvivo and transfused back into the patient. Various types of adoptive cellular therapy have been reported in the treatment of metastatic RCC. Lymphokine-activated killer (LAK) cells, tumor-infiltrating lymphocytes (TILs), autolymphocyte therapy (ALT), and CD8+ selected lymphocytes have all been evaluated in the treatment of RCC, and none has shown superior antitumor activity to that of IL-2 alone [46,47]. Current investigations of adoptive cellular therapy are directed toward developing a more potent effector cell by using gene transfection strategies or 'arming' cells with bispecific monoclonal antibodies.

Monoclonal antibody therapy

The monoclonal antibody G250 (MoAbG250) recognizes a tumor-associated antigen (TAA) that is abnormally expressed in RCC and not in normal kidney or most normal tissues [48]. MoAbG250 is expressed in about 75% of primary RCC. In a phase I/II trial of escalating doses of 131 I-labeled MoAbG250 in metastatic RCC, 21 patients have been treated. The maximum dose given was

Table 15-2. Representative trial of combination IL-2 and IFN

Investigator [ref]	Dose & Schedule	Route	No of pts.	Response Complete (%)	Partial (%)
Atozpodien [36]	IL-2: 9×10^6 IU/M^2 q 12° $\times$ 2 d then 1.8×10^6 IU/M^2 q 12° $\times$ 6 wks	SQ	14	2 (14)	3 (22)
	IFN: 5×10^6 IU/M^2	SQ			
Mittelman [37]	IL-2: 3×10^6 IU/M^2/d $\times$ 4 days	CIV	15		
	IFN: 5×10^6 IU/M^2/d $\times$ 4 days, treatment repeated weekly $\times$ 4	IM		2 (13)	2 (13)
Besana [38]	IL-2: 9–18 $\times 10^6$ IU/M^2/d $\times$ d 1–5 IFN: 9×10^6 IU/d, d 8–28 SQ	CIV	17	1 (6)	5 (29)
Lipton [39]	IL-2: 3–12 $\times 10^6$ IU/M^2/d 4–5 d/wk $\times$ 4 wks	CIV	39	6 (15)	7 (18)
	IFN: 3–12 $\times 10^6$ IU/M^2/d 2–5 d/wk $\times$ 4 wks	IM			
Bergmann [40]	IL-2: 18×10^6 IU/M^2 IV bolus, plus 18×10^6 IU/M^2 SQ QOD	IV and SQ	36	2 (6)	7(19)
	IFN: 10×10^6 IU/M^2 QOD for 14 days, q 6 wks $\times$ 4	SQ			
Ravund [41]	IL-2: 18×10^6 IU/M^2/d $\times$ 2 days, then 3.6×10^6 IU/M^2/d for 5 d/wk $\times$ 6 wks	SQ	38	1 (3)	6 (18)
	IFN: 5×10^6 IU/tiw	SQ			
Atzpodien [42]	IL-2: 20×10^6 IU/M^2 tiw, wks 1 & 4–5 $\times 10^6$ IU/M^2, tiw wks 2,3,5,6	SQ SQ			
	IFN: 6×10^6 IU/M^2/wk 1 & 4 6×10^6 IU/M^2 tiw wks 2,3,5,6	SQ	152	9 (6)	29 (19)

Abbreviations: IU, international units; d, day; wk, week; tiw, three times a week; civ, continuous intravenous infusion; sq, subcutaneous.

90 mCi/m^2. Grade IV thrombocytopenia was seen at doses above 75 mCi/m^2. Reversible hepatic enzyme elevation was seen in most patients, probably due to MoAbG250 accumulation in the liver. There were no major responses; however, three minor responses were reported. In a companion imaging study, G250 localized specifically to sites of RCC, with lesions as small as 8 mm visualized [49]. A chimerized MoAbG250 is being developed with which multiple treatments may become feasible in the future.

Immunotherapy of bladder cancer

BCG therapy for superficial bladder cancer

Since Morales et al. [50] published their initial report of the efficacy of intravesical BCG therapy in preventing bladder cancer recurrences, several other reports have confirmed their results [51–55]. BCG is not directly cytotoxic to bladder cancer cells. It acts by inducing a local inflammatory reaction in the bladder mucosa and a delayed hypersensitivity-type reaction. The first step is the attachment of the bacteria to the bladder wall. Fibronectin plays an important role in this step [56]. This is followed by internalization of BCG, which is followed by the expression of delayed hypersensitivity [57,58]. A polysaccharide capsule produced by the metabolically active bacterium is the primary means of interaction between BCG and the vesical mucosa [56].

The effector mechanisms of the antitumor response are immunologic and nonspecific. A variety of cytokines with known antineoplastic effects are produced in response to BCG administration and are detected in the urine. These include interferon gamma, interleukin-1 interleukin-2, and tumor necrosis factor [59,60].

Several strains of BCG from various manufacturers have been used for intravesical therapy. Considering the genetic variability and the differences in dosing, the results with BCG therapy, with few exceptions, have been remarkably consistent. The dose and schedule of BCG therapy are not agreed upon. An initial induction phase of six weekly treatments is universally accepted but not deemed optimal. BCG therapy beyond the six-week induction course is controversial, and there is no solid evidence supporting any specific maintenance regimen. Multiple nonrandomized studies have suggested that some form of maintenance therapy is beneficial [53,61,62]. Options for further therapy include three additional treatments at three months, six additional treatments, monthly treatments for two years, or 1 to 3 treatments over 3 to 6 months for 1 to 2 years. A randomized trial from the Southwest Oncology Group has shown a consistent benefit of one maintenance regimen in disease-free survival [63]. Patients with CIS or recurrent high-grade T1 tumors not responding to a single six-week course of BCG may benefit from an additional six-week course of BCG [64]. Morales et al. used a combination of intravesical therapy and intradermal inoculations in their original report; however, subsequent work by Lamm et al. [65] led to the elimination of the intradermal route, which does not contribute to the efficacy of intravesical BCG.

The optimal dose per installation of BCG is not determined. Morales used a dose of 120 mg in his original protocol for reasons of convenience. There have been no well-designed dose–response studies. Subsequently lower doses of 60 mg and 27 mg of BCG have been tested [65–67] and were shown to be effective; however, side effects were not reduced significantly. The effective number of viable organisms was determined by Bast to be in the range of 10^6–10^8 colony-forming units (CFU) [68]. Lamm et al. found the optimal number to be 10^7 CFU, irrespective of the BCG strain studied [69].

There are three clinical situations for which intravesical BCG therapy has been shown to be effective. Multiple studies of primary CIS of the bladder have shown that BCG therapy can eradicate disease in 70% of patients, with well over half remaining free of recurrence at five years. Primary CIS of the bladder is an aggressive form of superficial bladder cancer, with an average incidence of subsequent invasive disease of 54% (78% in symptomatic patients or those with extensive disease) [70]. Because of these results, BCG is considered the treatment of choice for primary CIS of the bladder.

BCG is also used for prophylaxis in those patients at high risk of recurrence after definitive transurethral resection of superficial bladder cancer. This group of patients include those with a history of recurrent superficial bladder cancer, T1 tumors (especially if multiple), high-grade Ta tumors, and multifocal CIS. Multiple phase II studies have shown the effectiveness of intravesical BCG in reducing tumor recurrences, and randomized controlled studies have confirmed these results [51,55,71–73]. Tumor progression defined as muscle invasion or metastases is significantly decreased and survival improved in those high–risk patients receiving prophylactic BCG [51]. The ten-year disease-specific survival rate is 75% for TURN + BCG compared wit 55% for TURB alone [54].

Intravesical BCG has also been used in the small group of patients who have residual superficial disease after transurethral resection. Approximately half of these patients will become disease free after treatment. Intravesical BCG is not indicated in the treatment of muscle-invasive bladder cancer, immunocompromised patients (HIV or drugs), nor patients on anticoagulants or antibiotics that inhibit BCG. Complications of intravesical BCG administration have been reviewed previously [74,75]. Intravesical BCG induces an inflammatory reaction in the bladder. As a result, most patients (about 90%) experience symptoms of dysuria and frequency that typically occur following the third administration and recur with subsequent treatments. A low-grade fever (<101°F) commonly occurs and lasts for 24 hours. Hematuria occurs in about a third of patients and could be severe. Patients experiencing continued hematuria should not be retreated since doing so raises the risk of BCG sepsis. Severe complications occur in less than 5% of treated patients, and include high fever of over 103°F, BCG sepsis, systemic infections, granulomatous prostatitis, epididymitis, orchitis, and renal abscess. BCG sepsis is the most serious complication, although rare, manifesting as high fever with chills, hypotension, confusion, disseminated intravascular coagulation, respiratory failure, jaundice, and leukopenia. Blood cultures are usually negative. Treatment is with isoniazid, rifampin, ethambutol, and prednisone. Patients experiencing severe complications should be given serious consideration of risk versus benefit of further BCG therapy, and usually are not retreated. Patients with mild complications may be retreated with isoniazid prophylaxis.

Immunotherapeutic alternatives to BCG

BCG is remarkably effective in superficial bladder cancer; however, it has significant toxicities. Possibly effective but less toxic alternatives include intravesical interferon, intravesical Keyhole-Limpet Hemocyanin (KLH), and oral bropirimine. A phase I/II trial of intravesical IFN alpha-2b at doses of 50–

1000 million units found a complete response rate of 32% in CIS and 25% in papillary tumors [76]. A randomized study of 10 million versus 100 million units of intravesical IFN alpha weekly for 12 weeks, then monthly for a year, showed complete response in 43% with the higher dose, compared to 5% with the lower dose [77]. Intravesical IFN is nontoxic, and responses were found in patients who failed BCG.

KLH is a high-molecular-weight, highly antigenic glycoprotein derived from the giant keyhole limpet (mollusk). In 1974, Olsson found that intradermal KLH reduced tumor recurrence in patients with superficial bladder cancer [78]. Subsequently, a randomized trial demonstrated that 10 mg of intravesical KLH was better than intravesical mitomycin in reducing tumor recurrences (39% recurrence with mitomycin versus 14% with KLH) [79]. A later randomized trial of 30 mg of intravesical KLH was found to be no better than ethoglucid [80]. KLH is nontoxic, and ongoing trials should clarify its role in superficial bladder cancer.

Bropirimine is a pyrimidinone, with a wide variety of immunostimulatory activities including cytokine release and enhancement of natural killer cell activity. It is active orally and is excreted in the urine in an active form [81]. In a phase I trial of oral bropirimine, 6 of 26 patients with papillary or CIS transitional cell carcinoma of the bladder had a complete response. A subsequent multicenter study found a 50% complete response rate in 54 patients with CIS, 27 of whom had failed BCG [82]. Bropirimine may have a promising role in superficial bladder cancer, particularly for upper tract lesions.

Immunotherapy of prostate cancer

Immunotherapy for prostate cancer has not been adequately tested in the clinical setting. Despite this, innovative research in the field is developing. Monoclonal antibodies and immunotoxins, adoptive immunotherapy, and engineered tumor cell vaccines are the focus of some of these studies. Brinkmann et al. [83] constructed an immunotoxin of the heavy-chain variable region of the monoclonal antibody PR1 fused to a truncated form of pseudomonas exotoxin. The recombinant immunotoxin binds and is cytotoxic to cells containing the PR1 antigen (i.e., prostrate cancer cells and normal prostate cells). gene-transfected tumor cells are also an area of investigation. IL-2-transfected Dunning rat prostate cancer cells initially formed tumors and then regressed spontaneously when injected subcutaneous in syngeneic host [84,85]. Mixtures of IL-2-transfected cells with parental cells also caused tumor regressions locally in rats. This finding indicates that high local IL-2 concentrations induce elimination of the tumor. Adoptive immunotherapy in the Dunning tumor model using IL-2-activated splenocytes and IL-2 caused regression of established tumor and of pulmonary metastases and prolonged the survival of treated animals [86]. In the future, some of these approaches may prove useful in the therapy of prostate cancer.

Future prospects

The bladder and prostate are easily accessible anatomic sites for repeated biopsies and therefore represent ideal organs to test in situ gene-transfection strategies. Several proposed and ongoing phase I trials are evaluating genetically modified tumor cell vaccines. Tumor cells are removed from the body, transduced ex vivo by incorporation of cytokine DNA into the genome, and subsequently reintroduced into the patient. The most common means of gene transfer is the retroviruses, though liposomal delivery and eletroporation are also being investigated. The cytokine genes most commonly transfected are IL-2, GM-CSF, IFN-α, IFN-γ, and less frequently other cytokines. In genitourinary malignancies, phase I and II trials will evaluate autologous tumor cells with transfected GM-CSF, IL-2, IFN-γ, or HLA-B7 CDNA in RCC and prostate cancer.

References

1. Wanderlich JR, Hodes RJ (1991). Biology of cellular immune response. In DeVitta VT, Hellman S, Rosenberg SA (eds), Biologic Therapy of Cancer. JB Lippincott: Philadelphia, pp. 3–21.
2. Klein G, Clifford P, Kleing E, Stjernsward J (1996). Search for tumor specific immune reactions in Burkitt's lymphoma patients by membrane immunofluorescence reaction. Proc Natl Acad Sci USA 55:1628–1635.
3. Morton DL, Malmgren RA, Holmes EC, Ketcham AS (1968). Demonstration of antibodies against human malignant melanoma by immunofluorescence. Surgery 64:233–240.
4. Morton DL, Malgren RA (1968). Human osteosarcomas: immunologic evidence suggesting an associated infection agent. Science 162:1279–1281.
5. Sjögren Ho, Hellstromöm I, Bansal SC (1972). Elution of 'blocking factors' from human tumors capable of abrogating tumor cell destruction by specifically immune lymphocytes. Int J Cancer 9:274–283.
6. Hellström I, Hellström KE (1983). Cell-mediated reactivity to human tumor-type associated antigens: does it exist? J Biol Response Mod 2:310–320.
7. Vanky F, Klein E (1982). Specificity of auto-tumor cytotoxicity exerted by fresh, activated and propagated human T-lymphocytes. Int J Cancer 29:547–553.
8. Kurzrock R, Gutterman Ju, Talpaz M (1991). Interferons α, β, γ: basic principles and preclinical studies. In Devitta VT, Hellman S, Rosenberg SA (eds), Biologic Therapy of Cancer. Philadelphia: JB Lippincott, pp. 247–274.
9. Quesade JR, Swanson DA, Trindade A, Gutterman JU (1983). Renal cell carcinoma: Antitumor effects of leukocyte interferon. Cancer Res 43:940–947.
10. DeKernion JB, Sarna G, Figlin R, Lindner A, Smith RB (1983). The treatment of renal cell carcinoma with human leukocyte alpha interferon. J Urol 130:1063–1066.
11. Kirkwood JM, Harris JE, Vera R, Sandler S, Fischer DS, Khandekar J , Ernstoff MS, Gordon L, Lutes R, Bonomi P, Lytton B, Coblieigh M, Taylor SJ IV (1985). A randomized study of low and high doses of leukocyte alpha-interferon in metastatic renal cell carcinoma: The American Cancer Society Collaborative Trial. Cancer Res 45:863–871.
12. Quesada JR, Rios A, Swanson D, Trown P, Guttermon JU (1985). Antitumor activity of recombinant-derived interferon alpha in metastatic renal cell carcinoma. J Clin Oncol 3:1522–1528.
13. Umeda T, Niijima T (1988). Phase II study of alpha interferon on renal cell carcinoma. Summary of three collaborative trials. Cancer 58:231–235.

14. Vugrin D, Hood L, Taylor W, Laszlo J (1985). Phase II study of human lymphoblastoid interferon in patients with advanced renal cell carcinoma. Cancer Treat Rep 69:817–820.
15. Stahl M, Wilke H-J, Seeber S, Schmoll HJ (1992). Cytokins and cytotoxic agents in renal cell carcinoma: a review. Semin Oncol 19:70–79.
16. Reinhart J, Malspeis Z, Young D, Neidhart J (1986) Phase I/II trial of human recombinant beta interferon serine in patients with renal cell carcinoma. Cancer Res 46:5364–5367.
17. Recombinant human interferon gamma (5-6810), Research group on renal cell carcinoma (1987). Phase II study of recombinant human interferon gamma (5-6810) on renal cell carcinoma. Cancer 60:929–933.
18. Garnick MB, Reich SD, Maxwell B, Coval-Godsmith S, Richie JP, Rudnick SA (1988). Phase I/II study of recombinant interferon gamma in advanced renal cell carcinoma. J Urol 139:251–258.
19. Quesada JR (1989). Role of interferons in the therapy of metastatic renal cell carcinoma. Urology 34:80–83.
20. Rosenberg SA (1993). Principles and applications of biologic therapy. In Devitta VT, Hellman S, Rosenberg SA (eds), Cancer: Principles & Practice of Oncology. JB Lippincott: Philadelphia, pp. 293–324.
21. Rosenberg SA, Lotze MT, Muul LM, Leitman S, Chang AE, Ettinghaussen SE, Matory YL, Skibber JM, Shiloni E, Vetto JT, Seipp CA, Simpson C, Reichert CM (1985). Observations on the systemic administration of autologous lymphokine activated killer cells and recombinant interleukin-2 to patients with metastatic cancer. N Engl J Med 313:1485–1492.
22. Rosenberg SA, Lotze MT, Mmul LM, Chang AE, Avis FP, Leitman S, Linehan WM, Robertson CN, Lee RE, Rubin JT (1987). Patients with advanced cancer using lymphokine-activated killer cells and interleukin-2 or high dose interleukin-2. alone. N Engl J Med 316:889–897.
23. Rosenberg SA, Yang JC, Topalian Sl, Schwartzent ••, Ruber DJ, Weber JS, Parkinson DR, Seipp CA, Einhorn JH, White DE (1994). Treatment of 283 consecutive patients with metastatic melanoma or renal cell cancer using high dose bolus interleukin-2. JAMA 271:907–913.
24. Caligiuri MA, Murray C, Soiffer RJ, Klumpp TR, Seiden M, Cochran K, Cameron C, Ish C, Buchanan L, Perillo D, Smith K, Ritz J (1991). Extended continuous infusion low-dose recombinant interleukin-2 in advanced cancer: prolonged immunomodulation without significant toxicity. J Clin Oncol 9:2110–2119.
25. Phillips JH, Gemlo BT, Myers WW, Rayner AA, Lanier LL (1987). In-vivo and in-vitro activation of natural killer cells in advanced cancer patients undergoing combined recombinant interleukin-2 and LAK cell therapy. J Clin Oncol 5:1933–1937.
26. Whitehead WP, Ward D, Hemingway L, Hemstreet GP III, Bradley E, Konrad M (1990). Subcutaneous recombinant interleukin-2 in a dose escalating regimen in patients with metastatic renal cell carcinoma. Cancer Res 50:6708–6715.
27. Marumo K, Muraki J, Ueno M, Tachibana M, Deguchi N, Baba S, Jitsukawa S, Hata M, Tazaki H (1989). Immunologic study of human recombinant interleukin-2 (low-dose) in patients with advanced renal cell carcinoma. Urology 33:219–225.
28. Lissoni P, Barnis, Ardizzoia A, Crispino S, Paolorossi F, Archili C, Vaghi M, Tancini G (1992). Second line therapy with low-dose subcutaneous interleukin-2 alone in advanced renal cancer patients resistant to interferon-alpha. Eur J Cancer 28:92–96.
29. Sleijer D, •• TH, Janssen RAJ, Buter J, DeVries EGE, Willense PHB, Mulder NH (1992). Phase II study of subcutaneous interleukin-2 in unselected patients with advanced renal cell cancer on an outpatient basis. J Clin Oncol 10:1119–1123.
30. Stoter G, Fossa SD, Rugarli C, Symann M, Jasmin C, Israel L, Bijman JT, Palmer P, Franks CR, Philip T (1989). Metastatic renal cell cancer treated with low-dose interleukin-2. A phase II multicentre study. Cancer Treat Rev 16(Suppl A):111–113.
31. Stein RC, Malkovska V, Morgan S, Galazka A, Aniszewsik C, Roy SE, Shearer RJ, Marsden RA, Beran D, Gordon-Smith EC, Coombes RC (1991). The clinical effects of prolonged treatment of patients with advanced cancer with low dose subcutaneous interleukin-2. Br J Cancer 63:275–278.

32. Leahy MG, Pitfield D, Propert S, Gallagher CJ, Oliver RTD (1992). Phase I study comparing continuous infusion of recombinant interleukin-2 by subcutaneous or intravenous administration. Eur J Cancer 28A(Suppl):1049–1051.
33. Yang JC, Tapalian SL, Parkinson D, Schwartzentruber DJ, Weber JS, Ettinghausen SE, Rosenberg SA (1994). Randomized comparison of high-dose and low-dose intravenous interleukin-2 for the therapy of metastatic renal cell carcinoma. An Interim Report. J Clin Oncol 12:1572–1576.
34. Cameron RB, McIntosh JK, Rosenberg SA (1988). Synergistic antitumor effects of combination immunotherapy with recombinant interleukin-2 and recombinant hybrid alpha-interferon in the treatment of established murine hepatic metastases. Cancer Res 48:5810–5817.
35. Schiller JH, Hanh J, Storer B, Borchert AA, Moore KH, Albertini M, Bechhofer R, Wesley O, Brown RR, Bastin AM, Sondel PM (1992). A direct comparison of immunological and clinical effects of interleukin 2 with and without interferon $\propto$ in humans. Cancer Res 53:1286–1292.
36. Atzpodien J, Körfer A, Franks CR, Poliwoda H, Kirchner H (1990). Home therapy with recombinant interleukin-2 and interferon α-2b in advanced human malignancies. Lancet 335:1509–1512.
37. Mittelman A, Puccio C, Ahmed T, Zeffren J, Choudhury A, Arlin Z (1991). A phase II trial of interleukin-2 by continuous infusion and interferon by intramuscular injection in patients with renal cell carcinoma. Cancer 68:1699–1702.
38. Besana C, Borri A, Bucci E, Citterio G, DiLucca, Fortis C, Matteucci P, Tognella S, Tresoldi M, Baiocchi C, Landonic G, Ghislandi E, Rugarli C (1994). Treatment of advanced renal cell cancer with sequential intravenous recombinat interleukin-2 and subcutaneous α-interferon. Eur J Cancer 30A:1292–1298.
39. Lipton A, Harvey H, Givant E, Hopper K, Lawler J, Matthews Y, Hirsh M, Zeffren J (1993). Interleukin-2 and interferon-alpha-2a outpatient therapy for metastatic renal cell carcinoma. J Immunother 13:122–129.
40. Bergmann L, Fenchel K, Weidmann E, Enzinger Hm, Jan B, Jonas D, Mitrou PS (1993). Daily alternating administration of high-dose alpha-2a-interferon and interleukin-2 bolus infusion in metastatic renal cell cancer. A phase II study. Cancer 72:1833–1842.
41. Ravand A, Negrier S, Cany L, Merrouche Y, LeGuillou M, Blay JY, Clarel M, Gaston R, Oskam R, Phillip T (1994). Subcutaneous low-dose recombinant interleukin-2 and alpha-interferon in patients with metastatic renal cell carcinoma. Br J Cancer 69:1111–1114.
42. Atzpodien J, Lopez Hannienen E, Kirchner H, et al. (1995). Multi-institutional home therapy trial of recombinant human interleukin-2 and interferon alfa-2 in progressive metastatic renal cell carcinoma. J Clin Oncol 13:497–501.
43. Reiter Z, Ozes ON, Blatt LM, Taylor MW (1992). A dual anti-tumor effect of a combination of interferone-alpha or interleukin-2 and 5-fluorouracil on natural killer (NK) cell-mediated cytotoxicity. Clin Immunol Immunopathol 62:103–111.
44. Atzpodien J, Kirchner H, Hanninen EL, Deckert M, Franzke A, Poliwoda H (1994). European studies of interleukin-2 in metastatic renal cell carcinoma. Proc ASCO 13:247 (abstract #773).
45. Sella A, Kilbourn RG, Gray I, Finn L, Zukiwski AA, Ellerhorst J, Amato RJ, Logothetis CJ (1994). Phase I study of interleukin-2 combined with interferon-alpha and 5-fluorouracil in patients with metastatic renal cell cancer. Cancer Biother 9:103–111.
46. Fisher RI, Coltman CA Jr, Doroshow JH, Rayner A, Hawkins MJ, Meir JW, Weirnik P, McMannis JD, Weiss JR, Margolin KA, Gelmo BT, Hoth DF, Parkinson DR, Paletta E (1988). Metastatic renal cell cancer treated with interleukin-2 and lymphokine activated killer cells. A Phase II clinical trial. Ann Inten Med 108:518–523.
47. Rosenberg SA, Lotze MT, Yang JC, Topolian JL, Chang AE, Schwartzentruber DJ, Aebersold P, Leitman S, Linehan WM, Seipp CA, White DE (1993). Prospective randomized trial of high-dose IL-2 alone or in conjunction with lymphokine activated killer cells for the treatment of patients with advanced cancer. J Natl Cancer Inst 85:622–632.

48. Oostenwijk E, Debruyne FMJ, Schalken JA (1995). The use of monoclonal antibody G250 in the therapy of renal cell carcinoma. Semin Oncol 22:34–41.
49. Divgi CR, Bander NH, Welt S, Scott AM, Gulec S, Motzer R, Finn RD, Oosterwijk E, Williams J, Broussard E, Larson SM, Old LJ (1995). Phase I/II trial with I-131 labelled monoclonal antibody (MAB) G250 in metastatic renal cell cancer (RCC). Proc ASCO 14:423 (abstract #1345).
50. Morales A, Eidinger D, Bruce AW (1976). Intracavitary Bacillus Calmette-Guérin in the treatment of superficial bladder tumors. J Urol 116:180–183.
51. Herr HW, Laudone VP, Badalament RA, Oettgen HF, Sogani PC, Freedman BD, Melamed MR, Whitmore WF Jr (1988). Bacillus Calmette-Guérin therapy alters the progression of superficial bladder cancer. J Clin Oncol 6:1450–1455.
52. Lamm DL (1985). Bacillus Calmette-Guérin immunotherapy for bladder cancer. J Urol 134:40–46.
53. Lamm DL, Crawford DL, Crawford ED, Montie JE, Scardino P, Grossman B, Stanisic TH, Smith JA Jr, Sullivan J, Sarsdy MF, Crissman JD, Coltman CA, for the Southwest Oncology Group (1991). A randomized trial of intravesical doxorubicin and immunotherapy with Bacillus Calmette-Guérin for transitional cell carcinoma of the bladder. N Engl J Med 325:1205–1209.
54. Herr HW, Schwalb DM, Ahang ZF, Sogani PC, Fair WR, Whitmore WF Jr, Oettgen HF (1995). Intravesical Bacillus Calmette-Guérin therapy prevents tumor progression and death from superficial bladder cancer: ten year follow-up of a prospective randomized trial. J Clin Oncol 13:1404–1408.
55. Lamm DL (1992). Long-term results of intravesical therapy for superficial bladder cancer. Urol Clin North Am 19:573–580.
56. Morales A, Nickel JC (1992). Immunotherapy of superficial bladder cancer, a developmental and clinical overview. Urol Clin North Am 19:549–556.
57. Ratliff TL, Hudson MA, Catalona WJ (1991). Strategy for improving therapy of superficial bladder cancer. World J Urol 9:95.
58. Becich MJ, Carroll S, Ratliff TL (1991). Internalization of Bacillus Calmette-Gué by bladder tumor cells. J Urol 145:1316–1324.
59. Prescott S, James K, Hargrave TB, Chisolm GD, Smyth JF (1990). Radioimmune assay detection of interferon-gamma in urine after intravesical Evans BCG therapy. J Urol 144:1248–1251.
60. Balbay D, Ozen H, Ozkardes H, Barut A, Bakkaloglu M, Tasar C, Remzi D (1994). Detection of urinary interleukin 2, interleukin 2 receptor, tumor necrosis factor levels in patients with superficial bladder tumors after intravesical BCG immunotherapy. Urology 43:187–190.
61. Haaff EO, Dresner SM, Ratliff TL, Catalona WJ (1986). Two courses of intravesical Bacillus Calmette-Guérin for transitional cell carcinoma of the bladder. J Urol 136:820–824.
62. Kavoussi LR, Terrence RJ, Gillen DP, Hudson MA, Haaff EO, Dresner M, Ratliff TL, Catalona WJ (1988). Results of 6 weekly intravesical Cacillus Calmette-Guérin instillation on the treatment of superficial bladder tumors. J Urol 139:935–940.
63. Lamm DL, Crawford ED, Blumenstein B, Crissman JD, Montie J, Gottesman J, Lowe B, Sarosdy MF, Bohl MF, Weems WL, Grossman HB, Smith JA, Beck TM, Leimert J, Coltman CA (1992). Maintenance BCG immunotherapy of superficial bladder cancer: a randomized prospective Southwest Oncology Group study. J Urol 147:274A (abstract #242).
64. Herr HW (1991). Progression of T1 bladder tumors after intravesical Bacillus Calmette-Guérin. J Urol 145:40–43.
65. Morales A, Nickel JC, Wilson JLW (1992). Dose response of BCG in superficial bladder cancer. J Urol 147:1256–1258.
66. Pagano F, Bast P, Milani C, Meneghini A, Maruzzi D, Garbeglio A (1991). Low dose Bacillus Calmette-Guérin in superficial bladder cancer therapy: is it effective? J Urol 146:32–35.
67. Mack D, Frick J (1995). Low dose Bacillus Calmette-Guérin (BCG) therapy in superficial high risk bladder cancer a phase II study with the BCG strain Connaught Conade. Br J Urol 75:185–187.

68. Bast RC Jr, Zbar B, Borsos T, Rapp HJ (1974). BCG and Cancer I. N Engl J Med 290:1413–1420.
69. Lamm DL, Reichert DF, Harris SC, Lucio RM (1982). Immunotherapy of murine transtional cell carcinoma. J Urol 128:1104–1108.
70. Lamm DL (1992). Superficial bladder cancer, carcinoma in situ. Urol Clin North Am 19:499–509.
71. Lamm DL (1992). Superficial bladder cancer, long term results of intravesical therapy for superficial bladder cancer. Urol Clin North Am 19:573–580.
72. Lamm DL, Griffith JG (1992). Intravesical therapy: does it affect the natural histrory of superficial bladder cancer? (review). Semin Urol 10:39–44.
73. Pagano F, Bassi P, Milani C, Meneghini A, Maruzzi D, Garbeglio A (1991). A low dose Bacillus Calmette-Guérin regimen in superficial bladder cancer therapy: is it effective? J Urol 146:32–35.
74. Lamm DL, Meijden APM Vander, Morales A, Brosman SA, Catalona WJ, Herr HW, Soloway MS, Steg A (1992). Incidence and treatment of complications of Bacillus Calmette-Guérin intravesical therapy in superficial bladder cancer. J Urol 147:596–600.
75. Lamm DL (1992). Complications of Bacillus Calmette-Guérin immunotherapy. Urol Clin North Am 19:562–572.
76. Torti F, Shortliffe L, Williams R, Pitts WC, Kempson RL, Ross JC, Palmer J, Meyers F, Ferrari M, Hannigan J, Spiegel R, McWhirter K, Freiha F (1988). Alpha interferon in superficial bladder cancer: a Northern California Oncology Group study. J Clin Oncol 6:476–483.
77. Glashan R (1990). A randomized controlled study of intravesical alpha-2b interferon in carcinoma in situ of the bladder. J Urol 144:658–661.
78. Olsson CA, Chute R, Rao CN (1974). Immunologic reduction of bladder cancer recurrence rate. J Urol 111:173–176.
79. Jurincic C, Engelmann U, Gasch J, Klippel KF (1988). Immunotherapy in bladder cancer with Keyhole-Limpet hemocyanin: a randomized study. J Urol 139:723–726.
80. Flamm J, Bucher A, Holtl W, Albrecht W (1990). Recurrent superficial transitional cell carcinoma of the bladder: adjuvant topical chemotherapy versus immunotherapy: a prospective randomized trial. J Urol 244:260–263.
81. Rios A, Stringfellow DA, Fitzpatrick FA, Reele SB, Guthnecht GD, Hersh EM (1986). Phase I study of 2-amino-5-bromo-6-phenyl-4(3H)-pyrimidinone (ABPP), an oral interferon inducer in cancer patients. J Biol Respir Modif 5:330–338.
82. Lamm DL (1995). BCG immunotherapy for transitional-cell carcinomal in situ of the bladder. Oncology 9:947–955.
83. Brinkmann U, Gallo M, Brinkmann E, Kunwar S, Pastan I (1993). A recombinant immunotoxin that is active on prostate cancer cells and that is composed of the Fv region of monoclonal antibody PR1 and a truncated form of pseudomonas exotoxin. Proc Natl Acad Sci USA. 90:547–551.
84. Moodry DB, Robinson JC, Ewing CM, Lazenby AJ, Isaacs WB (1994). Interleukin-2 transfected prostate cancer cells generate a local antitumor effect in vivo. Prostate 24:44–51.
85. Vieweg J, Rosenthal FM, Bannerji R, Heston WD, Fair WR, Gansbacher B, Gilboa E (1994). Immunotherapy of prostate cancer in the Dunning rat model: use of cytokine gene modified tumor vaccines. Cancer Res 54:1760–1765.
86. Tjota A, Ahang YQ, Piedmonte MR, Lee CL (1991). Adoptive immunotherapy using lymphokine-activated killer cells and recombinant interleukin-2 in preventing and treating spontaneous pulmonary metasteses of syngeneic Dunning rat prostate tumor. J Urol 146: 177–183.

16. Assessing health-related quality of life in patients with genitourinary malignancies

Mark S. Litwin

The traditional goal in treating patients with cancer has been to maximize their duration of survival. Recent advances in chemotherapy, immunotherapy, surgical technique, and radiation delivery have refined the treatment of urological malignancies so that patients now live longer with their cancers. This is especially true of men with prostate cancer, who often live for many years after the diagnosis. Historically, evaluation of the success of cancer therapies has focused on disease-free survival and other clinical parameters; however, the advent of the medical outcomes movement has generated greater interest in more refined endpoints that are more clinically relevant than alive versus dead, complete response rates, or serum tumor-marker levels.

Health-related quality of life (HRQOL) is one of several variables commonly studied in the field of medical outcomes research. HRQOL encompasses a wide range of human experience, including the daily necessities of life, such as food and shelter, intrapersonal and interpersonal responses to illness, and activities associated with professional fulfillment and personal happiness [1]. Perhaps most importantly, HRQOL involves patients' perceptions of their own health and ability to function in life. The World Health Organization defines health as a 'state of complete physical, mental, and social well-being and not merely the absence of disease' [2]. Since cancer affects both quantity and quality of life, the various components of well-being must be addressed when treating individual patients with cancer and when conducting cancer clinical trials [3]. Despite the commonly held belief that these types of data cannot be collected in large multicenter trials, patient compliance with HRQOL questionnaires is usually high [4].

While *quantity* of life is relatively easy to assess as survival or progression-free interval, the measurement of *quality* of life presents more challenges, primarily because it is less familiar to most clinicians [5]. To quantify these qualitative phenomena, the principles of psychometric test theory are applied. This discipline provides the theoretical underpinnings for the science of survey research. Data are collected with HRQOL surveys, called instruments. Instruments typically contain questions, or items, that are organized into scales. Each scale measures a different aspect, or domain, of HRQOL. Some scales comprise dozens of items, while others may include only one or two items.

Pienta, K.J., (ed.), DIAGNOSIS AND TREATMENT OF GENITOURINARY MALIGNANCIES.

HRQOL instruments may be general or disease-specific. General HRQOL domains address the components of overall well-being, while disease-specific domains focus on the impact of particular organic dysfunctions that affect HRQOL [6]. General HRQOL instruments typically address general health perceptions, sense of overall well-being, and function in the physical, emotional, and social domains. Disease-specific HRQOL instruments for cancer patients focus on more directly relevant domains, such as anxiety about cancer recurrence, nausea from chemotherapy, urinary incontinence from sphincter damage, etc. Since HRQOL may change over time, longitudinal measurement of these endpoints is critical [7,8]. One method recently devised to combine quantity and quality of life in patients with chronic disease is called, 'Time without symptoms of disease and toxicity of treatment (TWiST)' [9]. This technique uses a biometric model to construct a clinically relevant endpoint that incorporates subjective toxicity, time since treatment, and duration of clinical response.

Health-related quality of life instruments

HRQOL instruments are plentiful. Many psychologists, sociologists, health professionals, and statisticians devote their entire professional careers to the activity of developing and statistically validating these surveys. Hence, an abundance of literature exists on general HRQOL, and a significant body of work has been published on HRQOL in cancer patients. Less attention has been paid to HRQOL in patients with urological malignancy; however, this trend is rapidly changing.

One of the earliest predecessors to modern quality of life studies is the Karnofsky performance status scale [10]. Popularized over 40 years ago, this instrument actually is a measure of physical function, not general HRQOL. Scores are determined by clinicians, not by patients. This work laid an important foundation for the HRQOL movement, though it captures only one part of HRQOL. It is reliable and fairly easy to apply [11], but it does not present a complete picture of HRQOL, nor is it based on patient self-report. HRQOL is often confused with functional status and other similar variables. While functional status is one important dimension of HRQOL, it is joined by other aspects of HRQOL such as role function, mental health, vitality, pain, and psychosocial interactions. HRQOL also encompasses the overall sense of satisfaction that an individual experiences in life [12].

Psychometric evaluation of health-related quality of life instruments

The development and validation of new instruments and scales is a long and arduous process. It is not undertaken lightly. Simply drawing up a list of questions that seem appropriate is fraught with potential traps and pitfalls.

For this reason, it is always preferable to utilize established HRQOL instruments.

When scales and instruments are developed, they are first pilot tested to ensure that the target population can understand and complete them with ease. Pilot testing reveals problems that might otherwise go unrecognized by researchers. For example, many terms that are commonly used by medical professionals are poorly understood by patients. This may result in missing data if patients leave questions blank. Furthermore, since many patients with urological malignancy are older and may have poor eyesight, pilot testing often identifies easily corrected visual barriers such as type size and page layout. These problems may also result in missing data and can introduce difficulties in the analysis. Pilot testing is a necessary and valuable part of instrument development. Scales and instruments are also evaluated for the two fundamental statistical properties of reliability and validity.

Reliability refers to how free from measurement error the scale is, i.e., what proportion of a patient's test score is true and what proportion is due to chance variation. Test–retest reliability is assessed by administering scales to patients at two separate time points, typically one month apart. The correlation coefficients between the two scores reflect the stability of responses. Test–retest reliability is most easily assessed when the quality of life domain of interest is not likely to change over short periods of time. Internal consistency reliability is a measure of the similarity of an individual's responses across several items, indicating the homogeneity of a scale [13]. The statistic most often used to quantify the internal consistency, or unidimensionality, of a scale is called Cronbach's coefficient alpha [14]. Generally accepted standards dictate that reliability statistics measured by these two methods should exceed 0.70. It is important to remember that if too long an interval transpires, real change in the variable may artificially deflate test-retest reliability coefficients.

Validity refers to how well the scale or instrument measures the attribute it is intended to measure. Validity provides evidence to support drawing inferences about quality of life from the scale scores. Three types of validity are usually evaluated in new scales and instruments. Content validity, sometimes referred to as face validity, involves a nonquantitative assessment of the scope and completeness of a proposed scale. It is more superficial than other types of validity, and indeed considered by some not to be a true measure of validity at all [15]. Nevertheless, it is almost always included in the early stages of instrument development, even if only as a general review of items by physicians or patients. Criterion validity is a more quantitative approach to assessing the performance of scales and instruments. It requires the correlation of scale scores with future measurable outcomes (predictive validity) and with results from other established tests (concurrent validity). For example, the predictive validity of a new quality of life scale for physical function might be correlated with the number of subsequent physician visits or hospitalizations. Likewise, the concurrent validity of a new sexual function scale might be correlated with objective performance on infusion cavernosometry or nocturnal penile tumescence testing. A new emotional quality of life scale might be correlated with an established mental health index. Generally accepted standards dictate that validity statistics should exceed 0.70.

Construct validity is the most valuable yet most difficult way of assessing a survey instrument. It is difficult to understand, to measure, and to report. This form of validity is often determined only after years of experience with a survey instrument. It is a measure of how meaningful the scale or survey instrument is when in practical use. Often, it is not calculated as a quantifiable statistic. Rather, it is frequently seen as a gestalt of how well a survey instrument performs in a multitude of settings and populations over a number of years. Construct validity is often thought to comprise two other forms of validity: convergent and divergent. Convergent validity implies that several different methods for obtaining the same information about a given trait or concept produce similar results. Evaluating convergent validity is analogous to measuring alternate-form reliability, except that the former is more theoretical and requires a great deal of work, usually by multiple investigators with different approaches. Divergent (discriminant) validity is another theoretically based way of thinking about the ability of a measure to estimate the underlying truth in a given area. For a survey instrument to have divergent validity, it must be shown not to correlate too closely with similar but distinct concepts or traits. This, too, requires much effort over many years of evaluation.

Caveats on the collection of health-related quality of life data

Once an instrument is thoroughly pilot tested and found to be reliable and valid, it must be administered in a manner that minimizes bias. Quality of life data cannot and should not be collected from cancer patients directly by the operating surgeon or treating oncologist or radiotherapist. Patients have an unconscious desire to produce responses that their physicians want to hear [16]. This introduces measurement error. No matter how objective the treating physician may claim to be, it is impossible for her or him to collect statistically meaningful outcomes data through direct questioning. Variations in phrasing, inflection, eye contact, rapport, mood, and other factors are difficult or impossible to eliminate. Data must be gathered by disinterested third parties using established psychometric scales and instruments.

Approaches to the measurement of health-related quality of life

The Southwest Oncology Group (SWOG) has defined the following six principles for HRQOL research in cancer trials: 1) always measure physical functioning, emotional functioning, symptoms, and global quality of life separately; 2) include measures of social functioning and additional protocol-specific measures if resources permit; 3) use patient-based questionnaires; 4) use categorical rather than visual analogue scales; 5) select brief questionnaires, not interviews; and 6) select HRQOL measures with published psychometric properties [17,18].

Using the SWOG guidelines, one can confidently select instruments to assess HRQOL in longitudinal or cross-sectional studies of patients with urological malignancy. The various components of HRQOL should be measured with different scales to assure that each receives adequate attention. Also, it is critical that instruments be self-administered by patients independent of interviewers. Self-assessment of HRQOL frees patient responses from any interviewer bias. Although many instruments utilize visual analogue scales, most quality of life researchers believe that items with specific response sets to choose from provide more accurate information. Longer instruments may yield richer data sets, but they also increase the chance that patients will tire of the survey and provide unreliable or invalid answers. Hence, short instruments are generally preferable when obtaining HRQOL measurements. It is easier and more efficient to use established instruments that have already undergone psychometric validation. When collecting HRQOL data with published instruments, the researcher can then compare the results to other populations with various chronic diseases, including different types of cancer.

It is important to compare results with individuals of the same age without known disease. For example, when measuring sexual function after treatment for prostate cancer, it is more helpful to compare outcomes with age-matched control subjects than with a hypothetical state of perfect sexual function. Since sexual function varies with age, it is critical to maintain the appropriate context of the variable under investigation. This principle holds true with other HRQOL domains as well.

General health-related quality of life instruments

General quality of life instruments have been extensively researched and validated in many types of patients, sick and well. Examples include the RAND Medical Outcomes Study 36-Item Health Survey (also known as the SF-36) [19–24], the Quality of Well-Being scale (QWB) [25–29], the Sickness Impact Profile (SIP) [25,30–32], and the Nottingham Health Profile (NHP) [25,33–37]. Each assesses various components of HRQOL, including physical and emotional functioning, social functioning, and symptoms. Each has been thoroughly validated and tested.

One of the most commonly used general instruments is the RAND 36-Item Health Survey, which was developed during the Medical Outcomes Study, a large-scale, long-term study that examined health-related aspects of daily life in many different types of patients [38]. The survey is a 36-item, self-administered instrument that takes less than ten minutes to complete and quantifies HRQOL in eight multi-item scales that address different health concepts — physical function, social function, bodily pain, emotional well-being, energy/fatigue, general health perceptions, role limitation due to physical problems, and role limitation due to emotional problems. The RAND 36-Item Health Survey is now widely regarded as the gold-standard instrument for the measurement of general HRQOL.

The QWB summarizes three aspects of health status (mobility, physical activity, and social activity) in terms of quality-adjusted life years, quantifying HRQOL as a single number that may range from death to complete well-being. The QWB is contains only 18 items, but it requires a trained interviewer.

The SIP measures health status by assessing the impact of sickness on changing daily activities and behavior. It is self-administered but contains 136 items and can take 30 minutes or longer to complete.

The NHP covers six types of experience with illness — pain, physical mobility, sleep, emotional reactions, energy, and social isolation — by using a series of weighted yes or no items. It contains 38 self-administered items and can be completed fairly quickly.

Cancer-targeted health-related quality of life instruments

Because of the well-documented association of cancer with psychological stress and emotional anxiety, as well as the deficits in activities of daily living that affect patients living with malignancy, cancer-specific quality of life has also been investigated extensively. Numerous instruments have been developed and tested that measure the special impact of cancer on patients' routine activities. Examples include the Cancer Evaluation Rehabilitation System (CARES) [39–42], the Functional Assessment of Cancer Therapy (FACT) [43–47], and the Functional Living Index for Cancer (FLIC) [48,49]. Each has been validated and tested in patients with various types of cancer.

There is less consensus on which cancer instrument best measures cancer-specific HRQOL, but all the instruments focus on similar domains that are of particular concern to patients with cancer. For example, the commonly used CARES Short Form (CARES-SF) is a 59-item, self-administered instrument that measures cancer-related quality of life with five multi-item scales — physical, psychosocial, medical interaction, marital interaction, and sexual function. A large and valuable database of patients with many different tumors, including urological tumors, has been collected by the authors of the CARES. These data are helpful when comparing the experience of prostate cancer patients to that of patients with other types of cancer.

The FACT is usually applied as a two-part instrument that includes a general item set pertaining to all cancer patients (FACT-G) and one of several item sets containing special questions for patients with specific tumors. Each item is a statement that a patient may agree or disagree with across a five-point range. The FACT-G domains include well-being in six areas: physical, social/

family, relationship with doctor, emotional, functional, and miscellaneous. The FACT-G includes 28 items and is self-administered. The authors of the FACT have recently developed two new supplemental disease-targeted HRQOL instruments for patients with bladder or prostate cancer.

The FLIC detects differences in functional states by measuring the physical and emotional quality of cancer patients' daily lives in areas such as coping, fear, depression, pain, nausea, housework, and self-perception. Unlike the other instruments discussed above, the FLIC uses visual analogue scales rather than response sets for its items. A visual analogue scale is a straight line, anchored at each end by phrases that represent the range of a given health state. Patients mark a slash somewhere on the line corresponding to their own perceptions of that variable. Scores are then calculated by measuring the distance from one end of the line to the patient's slash. Visual analogue scales are often used in survey research; however, some patients find this format difficult.

Other instruments, such as the Sexual Adjustment Questionnaire (SAQ) [50], directly address more specific issues with which cancer patients are concerned. The SAQ is a 108-item self-administered tool that has been shown to be reliable and valid in patients with various cancers and in healthy controls. It measures six domains — libido, arousal, activity level, relationships, techniques, and orgasm — used to assess patients before, during, and after cancer treatment.

Health-related quality of life in patients with prostate cancer

Metastatic prostate cancer

Cancer-specific quality of life has been studied in patients with metastatic prostate cancer by Cassileth et al. [51,52], who used established psychometric instruments (including the FLIC) to show changes in HRQOL after treatment. Their work suggests that these men are quite interested in considering quality of life outcomes when selecting specific hormonal therapy. Herr et al. [53] also used established instruments to compare patients receiving hormonal therapy versus observation for metastatic prostate cancer. Their research documented better quality of life scores among patients who elected to defer treatment over those who underwent early intervention. Tannock et al. [54] adapted a series of linear analogue items from an instrument validated in breast cancer patients and applied it along with the established McGill–Melzack pain questionnaire [55] to measure qualitative response to prednisone in patients with symptomatic bone metastases from prostate cancer. Although Tannock et al. did not develop scales, they did measure variables such as fatigue, appetite, anxiety, all of which have been shown to contribute to quality of life in cancer patients. In a recent study of 288 men with prostate cancer, Ganz et al. [56] used the CARES to discriminate between various clinical stages of the disease.

They also demonstrated that among prostate, lung, and colorectal cancer patients, this instrument can be used to document the progressive worsening of quality of life as the cancer advances. These findings were confirmed by Kornblith et al. [57], who used the EORTC Prostate Cancer Quality of Life Questionnaire to survey patients and spouses, demonstrating that as disease progresses, steady HRQOL declines among patients are paralleled by increasing psychological distress among their spouses.

Calais da Silva [58] used a validated EORTC instrument to collect longitudinal data demonstrating wide variations between patients' and investigators' assessments of HRQOL. He rightly implored the research community always to rely exclusively on patient-derived data when examining quality of life in patients with metastatic prostate and other cancers.

Localized prostate cancer

In men treated with radical prostatectomy for early-stage disease, Pedersen et al. [59] carried out a longitudinal study of quality of life changes for 18 months following surgery. The initial distress associated with diagnosis of cancer improved over time, although bother from erectile dysfunction persisted. Overall well-being was minimally affected.

Assessment of prostate-targeted HRQOL in the sexual, urinary, and bowel domains has been documented with a newly established instrument, the UCLA-RAND Prostate Cancer Index. It is a 56-item, self-administered, statistically reliable and valid tool that takes about 20 minutes to complete and that has been shown to be very robust in men with prostate cancer. The UCLA-RAND Prostate Cancer Index was recently used in a large study of men in a managed care population. No differences were seen in general HRQOL when comparing patients who had undergone surgery, radiation, or observation alone for clinically localized prostate cancer or when comparing them to a group of age-matched control subjects without prostate cancer. Among the same patients, significant group differences in HRQOL were identified in the prostate-specific sexual, urinary, and bowel domains [60]. Another study with an early version of the UCLA-RAND Prostate Cancer Index demonstrated that among men treated with surgery or radiation for localized prostate cancer, urinary dysfunction diminished HRQOL much more than did sexual dysfunction. Although negative functional outcomes were found more commonly than the published literature suggests, the bother experienced by these patients did not necessarily correlate with the level of dysfunction [61]. Rieker and colleagues [62] have also used established general HRQOL instruments and newly developed prostate-targeted scales to compare outcomes in men treated with surgery versus radiation for early stage disease. These authors have demonstrated that sexual function and bother have a significant impact on quality of life and are distinct from other dimensions. Herr [63] demonstrated that among men who were incontinent after radical prostatectomy, 26% reported limitations in their usual physical activity and over half experienced moderate to severe emotional distress, but 79% of those evaluated less than five years after surgery said they would choose surgery again, despite their leakage problems. In another well-designed study, Pedersen and colleagues [64] used a validated instrument containing four visual analogue scales (anxiety, voiding disorders, potency, overall assessment) to collect baseline and longitudinal data from men undergoing radical prostatectomy. Overall well-being was not affected in the long term; however, alterations in HRQOL related to sexual function did suffer. Leandri and colleagues [65] reached similar conclusions with an unvalidated, cross-sectional, retrospective survey.

Using a large national Medicare sample, Fowler et al. [66,67] from the Prostate Patient Outcomes Research Team (PORT) used reliable and valid psychometric instruments to document that sexual and urinary dysfunctions are much more common after radical prostatectomy than previously reported. These findings have also been documented by Gburek et al. [68], who reported results from 88 men undergoing surgery, radiation, or both, for early-stage disease. They used a series of new disease-targeted questions on sexual, urinary, and bowel function, as well as overall satisfaction with care, to show that the specific complications of prostate cancer treatment are more common than previously reported. There was no difference between the quality of life experience of patients receiving surgery versus radiation, although those undergoing both modalities were more likely to suffer more negative quality of life outcomes than with only one modality. These and other studies [69–73] emphasize the significant role for HRQOL studies in men with prostate cancer.

In an innovative study of patient utilities, Singer and colleagues [74] demonstrated that many men would select treatment with a lower survival rate in order to maintain sexual function. This observation emphasizes the importance of including patient values when considering various treatment options.

In men with localized prostate cancer, other studies examining HRQOL using psychometrically valid general and disease-specific HRQOL instruments are presently under way at numerous sites in the United States and throughout the world.

Health-related quality of life in patients with bladder cancer

HRQOL research in patients treated for bladder cancer has been more limited. Bjerre and colleagues [75] assessed HRQOL with a structured interview in men undergoing cystectomy followed by either ileal conduit or orthotopic urethral Kock bladder substitution. They showed that urine leakage caused much less distress in those undergoing bladder substitution, while body image was surprisingly similar in both groups. Global satisfaction with life was high and similar in both groups. In a similar study that used established instruments — the Beck Depression Inventory and the Profile of Mood States (POMS) — Boyd and colleagues [76] showed that self image was worse among patients with ileal conduits, compared to those with continent cutaneous Kock reservoirs. No differences were seen in the mental and emotional health indices, and levels of satisfaction were similar in both groups, partly owing to the decreased expectations among those undergoing conduit diversions. Mansson and colleagues [77] used an unvalidated, self-administered HRQOL instrument in patients undergoing cystectomy to compare those reconstructed by continent cutaneous ileocecal diversion with those undergoing simple conduit diversion. Patients in both groups suffered equivalent declines in HRQOL related to sexual problems, disturbed partner relationships, and emotional dysfunction. Participation in sports, leisure activities, and travel was significantly better in those undergoing continent diversions. Other evaluations of quality of life with a urinary stoma have confirmed that body image and sexual function are disturbed [78] and that patients are embarrassed even by continent stomas [79], but that overall HRQOL does not seem to be affected [80]. Such findings underscore the importance of using both generic and disease-specific instruments when assessing HRQOL. Follow-up care with interval cystoscopy and intravesical chemotherapy has also been shown to impact negatively on patients' sexual HRQOL, although data are mixed [81,82].

Lynch and colleagues [83] compared HRQOL in complete responders to radiotherapy for muscle-invasive bladder carcinoma by administering the Nottingham Health Profile to patients and an age- and sex-matched control group without urinary tract disease. They found no differences between groups on all scales of the NHP, suggesting that those who respond to radiotherapy maintain good HRQOL.

Health-related quality of life in patients with testicular cancer

HRQOL research in patients treated for testis cancer has been more limited. Gritz et al. [84] compared the outlooks of patients and their wives several years after the couple had gone through testicular cancer treatment. Patients reported higher levels of anxiety over sexual performance as compared to their wives, who reported high levels of satisfaction. Long-term psychosocial adjustment was good. Rieker et al. [85,86] showed that men previously treated for testis cancer expressed distress with performance and infertility, though not with libido. Those with ejaculatory dysfunction noted more strained intimate relationships and more psychological problems. Compared to healthy controls, testis cancer patients as a group did not reveal any more difficulty with relationships, employment, divorce, or overall mental outlook. In another study, Douchez et al. [87] compared 109 long-term survivors of nonseminomatous testicular cancer with a group of health controls, using an unvalidated HRQOL questionnaire, and found more anxiety, insomnia, irritability, and depression in the patient group. Fossa et al. [88] also used an unvalidated instrument to compare long-term survivors with healthy controls. Although anxiety and depression were significantly more common in the patient group, these patients expressed much more general satisfaction with life. Interestingly, when the same group reported results from the Hopkin symptom checklist, a published anxiety/depression instrument, they found no group differences between patients and healthy controls [89]. In a comparison of long-term survivors cured by chemotherapy versus those cured by radiotherapy, Stuart et al. [90] used another unvalidated instrument to demonstrate more anxiety and depression in the radiotherapy group. The chemotherapy group reported that the illness had had a more positive impact on their relationship with family and friends. While these studies are interesting, their methodologies have been appropriately criticized when they did not use established, validated instruments to measure HRQOL [91]. Conversely, Bloom et al. [92] used a new, well-validated instrument and a series of established, validated scales to compare HRQOL in testicular cancer patients with that in men with Hodgkin's disease. Men with testicular cancer showed more specific HRQOL disruptions in areas such as sexual enjoyment and health habits, while men with Hodgkin's showed more general HRQOL disruptions in areas such as fatigue and work impairment. Both groups had similar levels of erectile dysfunction. More comprehensive studies of HRQOL in men with testis cancer have not been undertaken.

Health-related quality of life in patients with other genitourinary malignancies

Published HRQOL research in patients with renal [93], penile [94], and other urological cancers has been almost nonexistent. Further work is needed in these areas.

Directions for future research in health-related quality of life

Specific research questions begin with the need for basic descriptive analysis of quality of life in patients treated for urological cancers. Depiction of the fundamental elements in quality of life for these individuals requires study of their health perceptions and how their daily activities are impacted by both their general health and their cancer. Physical and emotional well-being form the cornerstone of this approach, but research must also extend to issues such as eating and sleeping habits, anxiety and fatigue, depression, rapport with physician, interactions with spouse or partner, social interactions, and specific pelvic functions, such as sexual, urinary, and bowel. Characterization of all domains must address not only the actual functions, but also the relative importance of these issues to patients and how bothered they are by any dysfunction that is present.

Beyond the descriptive analysis, HRQOL outcomes must be compared in patients undergoing different modes of therapy. General and disease-specific

HRQOL must be measured to facilitate comparison with patients treated for diabetes, heart disease, arthritis, and other common chronic conditions. Quality of life outcomes must also be controlled for variations in comorbidity or in sociodemographic variables such as age, race, education, income, insurance status, geographic region, and access to health care. In this context, HRQOL may be linked with many factors other than the traditional medical ones. Research initiatives must rely on established HRQOL instruments with proven records of statistical reliability and validity administered by objective third parties. Quality of life can have many different definitions and interpretations, but its measurement must adhere to the strict scientific application of psychometric science.

With better information on quality of life, as well as clinical outcomes, we will develop a richer database that is more useful to patients. We will be better able to evaluate new treatment modalities, educate our patients, and counsel them individually on what to do and expect when treated for urological malignancies.

References

1. Patrick DL, Erickson P (1993). Assessing health-related quality of life for clinical decision-making. In Walker SR, Rosser RM (eds), Quality of Life Assessment: Key Issues in the 1990s. Kluwer Academic Publishers: Dordrecht, p. 19.
2. World Health Organization (1948). Constitution of the World Health Organization, Basic Documents. World Health Organization: Geneva, ••.
3. Fayers PM, Jones DR (1983). Measuring and analyzing quality of life in cancer clinical trials: a review. Stat Med 2:429–446.
4. Sadura A, Pater J, Osoba D, Levine M, Palmer M, Bennett K (1992). Quality of life assessment: patient compliance with questionnaire completion. J Natl Cancer Inst 84:1023–1026.
5. Litwin MS (1994). Measuring health-related quality of life in men with prostate cancer. J Urol 152:1882–1887.
6. Patrick DL, Deyo RA (1989). Generic and disease-specific measures in assessing health status and quality of life. Med Care 27:S217–S232.
7. Zwinderman AH (1990). The measurement of change of quality of life in clinical trials. Stat Med 9:931–942.
8. Olschewski M, Schumacher M (1990). Statistical analysis of quality of life data in cancer clinical trials. Stat Med 9:749–763.
9. Gelber RD, Gelman RS, Goldhirsch A (1989). A quality-of-life-oriented endpoint for comparing therapies. Biometrics 45:781–795.
10. Karnovsky DA, Buchenal JH (1949). The clinical evaluation of chemotherapeutic agents in cancer. In Macleod CM (ed), Evaluation of Chemotherapeutic Agents. Columbia University Press: New York.
11. Mor V, Laliberte L, Morris JN (1984). The Karnofsky Performance Status Scale. An examination of its reliability in a research setting. Cancer 53:2002–2007.
12. Osoba D (1991). Measuring the effect of cancer on quality of life. In Osoba D (ed), Effect of Cancer on Quality of Life. CRC Press: Boca Raton, p. 31.
13. Tulsky DA (1990). An introduction to test theory. Oncology 4:43–48.
14. Cronbach LJ (1951). Coefficient alpha and the internal structure of tests. Psychometrika 16:297–334.
15. Messick S (1988). The once and future issues of validity: assessing the meaning and conse-

quences of measurement. In Wainer H, Braun HI (eds), Test Validity. Lawrence Erlbaum Associates: Hillside, NJ.
16. Tannock IF (1990). Management of breast and prostate cancer: how does quality of life enter the equation? Oncology 4:149–156.
17. Moinpour CM, Feigl P, Metch B, Hayden KA, Meyskens FL, Crowley J (1989). Quality of life endpoints in clinical trials: review and recommendations. J Natl Cancer Inst 81:485–495.
18. Moinpour CM (1990). Quality of life assessment in Southwest Oncology Group trials. Oncology 4:79–89.
19. Tarlov AR, Ware JE, Greenfield S, Nelson EC, Perrin E, Zubkoff M (1989). Medical outcomes study: an application of methods for evaluating the results of medical care. JAMA 262:907–913.
20. Ware JE, Sherbourne CD, Davies AR (1992). Developing and testing the MOS 20-item short-form health survey: a general population application. In Stewart AL, Ware JE (eds), Measuring Functioning and Well-Being: The Medical Outcomes Study Approach. Duke University Press: Durham, NC.
21. Stewart AL, Hays RD, Ware JE (1988). The MOS short-form general health survey: reliability and validity in a patient population. Med Care 26:724–735.
22. Ware JE, Sherbourne CD (1992). The MOS 36-item short-form health survey (SF-36): I. Conceptual framework and item selection. Med Care 30:473–483.
23. McHorney CA, Ware JE, Rogers W, Raczek AE, Lu JF (1992). The validity and relative precision of MOS short- and long-form health status scales and Dartmouth COOP charts in discriminating among adults with medical and psychiatric conditions: results from the medical outcomes study. Med Care 30(Suppl):MS253–265.
24. Hays RD, Hayashi T (1990). Beyond internal consistency reliability: rationale and user's guide for multitrait scaling analysis program on the microcomputer. Behav Res Methods Instruments Computers 22:167–175.
25. McDowell I, Ewell C (1987). Measuring Health: A Guide to Rating Scales and Questionnaires. Oxford University Press: New York.
26. Kaplan RM, Anderson JP (1988). A general health policy model: update and applications. Health Serv Res 23:203–235.
27. Kaplan RM, Bush JW (1982). Health-related quality of life measurement for evaluation research and policy analysis. Health Psychol 1:61–80.
28. Hays RM, Shapiro MF (1992). An overview of generic health-related quality of life measures for HIV research. Quality of Life Res 1:91–98.
29. Kaplan RM, Bush JW, Berry CC (1976). Health status: types of validity and the index of well-being. Health Serv Res 11:478–507.
30. Bergner M, Bobbitt RA, Carter WB, Gilson BS (1981). The sickness impact profile: development and final revision of a health status measure. Med Care 19:787–805.
31. Bergner M, Bobbitt RA, Pollard WE, Martin DP, Gilson BS (1976). The sickness impact profile: validation of a health status measure. Med Care 14:57–67.
32. Deyo RA, Inui TS, Leininger JD, Overman SS (1983). Measuring functional outcomes in chronic disease: a comparison of traditional scales and a self-administered health status questionnaire in patients with rheumatoid arthritis. Med Care 21:180–192.
33. Moinpour CM, Feigl P, Metch B, Kayden KA, Meyskens FL, Crowley J (1989). Quality of life end points in cancer clinical trials: review and recommendations. J Natl Cancer Inst 81:485–495.
34. Martini CJM, McDowell I (1978). Socio-medical measurements of health in primary care. Report submitted to Social Sciences Research Council, London, England, December.
35. Hunt SM, McEwen J, McKenna SP (1985). Measuring health status: a new tool for clinicians and epidemiologists. J Royal Coll Gen Pract 35:185–188.
36. McDowell IW, Martini CJM, Waugh W (1978). A method for self-assessment of disability before and after hip replacement operations. Br Med J 2:57–58.
37. Martini CJ, McDowell I (1976). Health status: patient and physician judgements. Health Serv Res 11:508–515.

38. Stewart AL, Greenfield S, Hays RD (1989). Functional status and well-being of patients with chronic conditions. JAMA 262:907–913.
39. Ganz PA, Schag CAC, Lee JJ, Sim MS (1992). The CARES: a generic measure of health-related quality of life for patients with cancer. Quality of Life Res 1:19–29.
40. Schag CAC, Heinrich RL (1990). Development of a comprehensive quality of life measurement tool: CARES. Oncology 4:135–138.
41. Schag CAC, Heinrich RL (1988). Cancer Rehabilitation Evaluation System (CARES) Manual. Cares Consultants: Los Angeles.
42. Schag CAC, Heinrich RL, Ganz PA (1989). The Cancer Rehabilitation Evaluation System (CARES): the short form (CARES-SF). Proc Amer Soc Clin Oncol 8:316.
43. Cella DF, Tulsky DS (1990). Measuring quality of life today. Oncology 4:29–38.
44. Tulsky DS, Cella DF, Bonomi A, Lee-Riordan D, Silberman M (1990). Development and validation of new quality of life measures for patients with cancer. Proc Soc Behav Med 11:45–46.
45. Cella DF, Cherin EA (1988). Quality of life during and after cancer treatment. Compr Ther 14:69–75.
46. Cella DF, Orofiamma B, Holland JC, Silberfarb PM, Tross S, Feldstein M, Orav EJ, Perry M, Maurer LH, Comis R, Green M (1987). Relationship of psychological distress, extent of disease, and performance status in patients with lung cancer. Cancer 60:239–245
47. Tchekmedyian NS, Cella DF (1991). Quality of Life in Current Oncology Practice and Research. Dominus: Williston Park, NY.
48. Schipper H, Clinch J, McMurray A, Levitt M (1984). Measuring quality of life in cancer patients: the Functional Living Index–Cancer: development and validation. J Clin Oncol 2:472–483.
49. Finkelstein DM, Cassileth BR, Bonomic PD, Ruckdeschel JC, Ezdinli EZ, Wolter JM (1988). A pilot study of the Functional Living Index–Cancer (FLIC) scale for the assessment of quality of life for metastatic lung cancer patients. Am J Clin Oncol 11:630–633.
50. Waterhouse J, Metcalfe MC (1986). Development of the sexual adjustment questionnaire. Oncol Nurs Forum 13:53–59.
51. Cassileth BR, Soloway MS, Vogelzang NJ, Schellhammer PS, Seifmon EJ, Hait HI, Kennealey GT (1989). Patients' choice of treatment in stage D prostate cancer. Urology 33(Suppl):57–62.
52. Cassileth BR, Soloway MS, Vogelzang NJ, Chou JM, Schelhammer PD, Seidmon EJ, Kennealey GT, Zoladex Prostata Cancer Study Group (1992). Quality of life and psychosocial status in stage D prostate cancer. Qual Life Res 1:323–329.
53. Herr HH, Kornblith AB, Ofman U (1993). A comparison of the quality of life of patients with metastatic prostate cancer who received or did not receive hormonal therapy. Cancer Suppl 71:1143–1150.
54. Tannock IF, Gospodarowicz M, Panzarella T, Stewart L, Rider W (1989). Treatment of metastatic prostate cancer with low-dose prednisone: evaluation of pain and quality of life as pragmatic indices of response. J Clin Oncol 7:1–7.
55. Melzack R (1975). The McGill Pain Questionnaire: major properties and scoring methods. Pain 1:277–299.
56. Ganz PA, Schag CAC, Lee JJ, Sim MS (1992). The CARES: a generic measure of health-related quality of life for patients with cancer. Quality of Life Res 1:19–29.
57. Kornblith AB, Herr HW, Ofman US, Scher HI, Holland JC (1994). Quality of life of patients with prostate cancer and their spouses. Cancer 73:2791–2802.
58. Calais da Silva F (1993). Quality of life in prostatic carcinoma. Eur Urol 24(Suppl):113–117.
59. Pedersen KV, Carlsson P, Rahmquist M, Varenhorst E (1993). Quality of life after radical retropubic prostatectomy for carcinoma of the prostate. Eur Urol 24:7–11.
60. Litwin MS, Hays RD, Fink A, Ganz PA, Leake B, Leach GE, Brook RH (1995). Quality of life outcomes in men treated for localized prostate cancer. JAMA 273:129–135.
61. Litwin MS, Fink A, Hays RD, Ganz PA, Brook RH, Duan N, Rosenthal JT, deKernion JB (1993). Quality of life in men with prostate cancer: a pilot study. J Urol 149:494A.

62. Rieker P, Clark J, Kalish L, Coleman N, Talcott J, Weeks J, Kantoff P (1993). Health-related quality of life following treatment for early stage prostate cancer. Proc Am Soc Clin Oncol 12:452A.
63. Herr HW (1994). Quality of life of incontinent men after prostatectomy. J Urol 151:652–654.
64. Pedersen KV, Carlsson P, Rahmquist M, Varenhorst E (1993). Quality of life after radical retropubic prostatectomy for carcinoma of the prostate. Eur Urol 24:7–11.
65. Leandri P, Rossignol G, Gautier JR, Ramon J (1992). Radical retropubic prostatectomy: morbidity and quality of life. Experience with 620 consecutive cases. J Urol 147:883–887.
66. Fowler FJ, Barry MJ, Lu-Yao G, Roman A, Wasson J, Wennberg JE (1993). Patient-reported complications and follow-up treatment after radical prostatectomy. Urology 42:622–629.
67. Fowler FJ, Barry MJ, Lu-Yao G, Wasson J, Roman A, Wennberg J (1995). Effect of radical prostatectomy for prostate cancer on patient quality of life: results from a Medicare survey. Urology 45:1007–1015.
68. Gburek B, Harmon B, Chodak GW (1992). Quality of life assessment in patients with prostate cancer treated by radical prostatectomy, radiation therapy, or a combination. J Urol 147:466A.
69. Fossa S, Kaasa S, Calais da Silva F, Suciu S, Hengeveld M (1992). Quality of life in prostate cancer patients. Prostate 4(Suppl):145–148.
70. Calais da Silva F, Reis E, Costa T, Denis L, Quality of Life Committee of the EORTC Genitourinary Group (1993). Quality of life in patients with prostatic cancer: a feasibility study. Cancer Suppl 71:1138–1142.
71. Sharp JW (1993). Expanding the definition of quality of life for prostate cancer. Cancer Suppl 71:1078–1082.
72. Aaronson NK, Calais da Silva F (1987). Prospects for the future: quality of life evaluation in prostatic cancer protocols. Prog Clin Biol Res 243B:501–512.
73. Friedland JL, Pow-Sang J, Johnson DJ, Byrnes J (1995). Quality-of-life issues associated with the treatment of prostate cancer. Cancer Contr 12:42–46.
74. Singer PA, Tasch ES, Stocking C, Rubin S, Siegler M, Weichselbaum R (1991). Sex or survival: tradeoffs between quality and quantity of life. J Clin Oncol 9:328–334.
75. Bjerre BD, Johansen C, Steven K (1995). Health-related quality of life after cystectomy: bladder substitution compared with ileal conduit diversion. A questionnaire survey. Br J Urol 75:200–205.
76. Boyd SD, Feinberg SM, Skinner DG, Lieskovsky G, Baron D, Richardson J (1987). Quality of life survey of urinary diversion patients: comparison of ileal conduits versus continent Kock ileal reservoirs. J Urol 138:1386–1389.
77. Mansson A, Johnson G, Mansson W (1988). Quality of life after cystectomy. Br J Urol 62:240–245.
78. Schover LR, Von Eschenbach AC (1985). Sexual function and female radical cystectomy: a case series. J Urol 134:465–468.
79. Oishi K, Arai Y, Hashimura T, Takeuchi H, Yoshida O, Okada Y (1993). Quality of life in patients with continent urinary reservoir. Hinyokika Kiyo Acta Urol Jpn 39:7–14.
80. Fossa SD, Reitan JB, Ous S, Kaalhus O (1987). Life with an ileal conduit in cystectomized bladder cancer patients: expectation and experience. Scand J Urol Nephrol 21:97–101.
81. Schover LR, Evans RB, Von Eschenbach AC, Smith DB, Gonzalez J (1986). Sexual rehabilitation and male radical cystectomy. J Urol 136:1015–1017.
82. Schover LR (1987). Sexuality and fertility in urologic cancer patients. Cancer 60(Suppl):553–558.
83. Lynch WJ, Jenkins BJ, Fowler CG, Hope-Stone HF, Blandy JP (1992). The quality of life after radical radiotherapy for bladder cancer. Br J Urol 70:519–521.
84. Gritz ER, Wellisch DK, Wang HJ, Siau J, Landsverk JA, Cosgrove MD (1989). Long-term effects of testicular cancer on sexual functioning in married couples. Cancer 64:1560–1567.
85. Rieker PP, Fitzgerald EM, Kalish LA, Richie JP, Lederman GS, Edbril SD, Garnick MB (1989). Psychosocial factors, curative therapies, and behavioral outcomes. A comparison of testis cancer survivors and a control group of health men. Cancer 64:2399–2407.

86. Rieker PP, Edbril SD, Garnick MB (1985). Curative testis cancer therapy: psychosocial sequelae. J Clin Oncol 3:1117–1126.
87. Douchez J, Droz JP, Desclaux B, Allain Y, Fargeot P, Caty A, Charrot P (1993). Quality of life in long-term survivors of nonseminomatous germ cell testicular tumors. J Urol 149:498–501.
88. Fossa SD, Aass N, Ous S, Waehre H (1991). Long-term morbidity and quality of life in testicular cancer patients. Scand J Urol Nephrol Suppl 138:241–246.
89. Kaasa S, Aass N, Mastekaasa A, Lund E, Fossa SD (1991). Psychosocial well-being in testicular cancer patients. Eur J Cancer 27:1091–1095.
90. Staurt NSA, Grundy R, Woodroffe CM, Cullen MH (1990). Quality of life after treatment for testicular cancer — the patient's view. Eur J Cancer 26:291–294.
91. Maguire P (1992). Psychosocial well-being in testicular cancer patients. Eur J Cancer 28A:722.
92. Bloom JR, Fobair P, Gritz E, Wellisch D, Spiegel D, Varghese A, Hoppe R (1993). Psychosocial outcomes of cancer: a comparative analysis of Hodgkin's disease and testicular cancer. J Clin Oncol 11:979–988.
93. Osband ME, Lavin PT, Babayan RK, Graham S, Lamm DL, Parker B, Sawczuk I, Ross S, Krane RJ (1990). Effect of autolymphocyte therapy on survival and quality of life in patients with metastatic renal-cell carcinoma. Lancet 335:994–998.
94. Witkin MH, Kaplan HS (1983). Sex therapy and penectomy. J Sex Marit Ther 8:209–221.

Index